Complications in Vascular and Endovascular Surgery

How to avoid them and how to get out of trouble

Edited by Jonothan J Earnshaw & Michael G Wyatt

A Joint Vascular Research Group book

tfm Publishing Limited, Castle Hill Barns, Harley, Nr Shrewsbury, SY5 6LX, UK.

Tel: +44 (0)1952 510061; Fax: +44 (0)1952 510192

E-mail: nikki@tfmpublishing.com; Web site: www.tfmpublishing.com

Design & Typesetting: Nikki Bramhill BSc Hons Dip Law

First Edition: © 2012

ISBN: 978 1 903378 80 9

Printed by Gutenberg Press Ltd., Gudja Road, Tarxien, PLA 19, Malta.

Tel: +356 21897037; Fax: +356 21800069.

Contents

Contents

Contributors

Marc A. Bailey MB ChB BSc MRCS(Eng) Academic Clinical Fellow in Vascular Surgery, The Leeds Vascular Institute, The General Infirmary at Leeds, Leeds, UK

Daryll Baker PhD FRCS Consultant Vascular Surgeon, Royal Free Hospital, London, UK

Jonathan D. Beard ChM MEd FRCS Consultant Vascular Surgeon, Sheffield Vascular Institute and Honorary Professor of Surgical Education, University of Sheffield, Sheffield, UK

Bruce Campbell MS FRCP FRCS Consultant Vascular Surgeon, Royal Devon and Exeter Hospital and Professor, Peninsula Medical School, Exeter, UK

Roderick T. A. Chalmers MD FRCS(Ed) Consultant Vascular Surgeon, Edinburgh Vascular Surgical Service, Royal Infirmary of Edinburgh, Edinburgh, UK

Rachel E. Clough MB BS BSc MRCS NIHR BRC Clinical Training Fellow, Department of Vascular Surgery, NIHR Comprehensive Biomedical Research Centre of Guy's and St Thomas' NHS Foundation Trust and King's College London, and King's Health Partners, London, UK

Jason Constantinou MD MRCS Specialist Registrar in Vascular Surgery, Multidisciplinary Endovascular Team, University College London and University College London Hospital, London, UK

Alun H. Davies MA DM FRCS FHEA FEBVS FACPh Professor of Vascular Surgery, Academic Department of Vascular Surgery, Imperial College London, London, UK

Duncan Drury MD FRCS Specialist Registrar in Vascular Surgery, Sheffield Vascular Institute, Sheffield, UK

Jonothan J. Earnshaw DM FRCS Consultant Vascular Surgeon, Gloucestershire Royal Hospital, Gloucester, UK

Robert K. Fisher FRCS MD Consultant Vascular & Endovascular Surgeon, Department of Vascular Surgery, Royal Liverpool University Hospital, Liverpool, UK

Jonathan Ghosh FRCS MD Endovascular Fellow, Department of Vascular Surgery, Royal Liverpool University Hospital, Liverpool, UK

Manj Gohel MD FRCS Specialist Registrar in Vascular Surgery & Honorary Lecturer, St Mary's Hospital, Imperial College London, London, UK

Michael J. Gough ChM FRCS Professor of Vascular Surgery, The Leeds Vascular Institute, The General Infirmary at Leeds, Leeds, UK

Perbinder Grewal MBBS MRCS (Ed) FRCS (Gen Surg) Senior Vascular Fellow, Royal Free Hospital, London, UK

George Hamilton MD FRCS FRCS (Glas) Professor of Vascular Surgery, Royal Free Hospital, London, UK

Peter L. Harris MD FRCS Head of Multidisciplinary Endovascular Team, Multidisciplinary Endovascular Team, University College London and University College London Hospital, London, UK

Teik K. Ho FRCS Specialist Registrar in Vascular Surgery, Royal Free Hospital, London, UK

Peter Holt PhD FRCS Clinical Lecturer in Vascular Surgery, St George's NHS Trust, London, UK

Russell W. Jamieson MChir MRCS(Ed) Specialist Registrar in Vascular Surgery, Edinburgh Vascular Surgical Service, Royal Infirmary of Edinburgh, Edinburgh, UK

Michael Jenkins BSc MS FRCS FEBVS Consultant Vascular Surgeon & Honorary Senior Lecturer, St Mary's Hospital, Imperial College London, London, UK

Rakesh Kapur MBBS MS FRCS (Glasg) FRCS (Gen Surg) PCME (Postgrad Cert in Med Edu) Specialist Registrar in Vascular Surgery, Department of Vascular and Endovascular Surgery, Nottingham University Hospital, Nottingham, UK

Peter M. Lamont MD FRCS Consultant Vascular Surgeon, Bristol Royal Infirmary, Bristol, UK

Sumaira Macdonald MBChB (Comm.) FRCR FRCP PhD Consultant Interventional Radiologist, Freeman Hospital, Newcastle upon Tyne, UK

Shane MacSweeney MA MB BChir MChir FRCSEng Consultant Vascular Surgeon, Department of Vascular and Endovascular Surgery, Nottingham University Hospital, Nottingham, UK

James McCaslin MBBS MRCS MD Specialist Registrar in Vascular Surgery, Freeman Hospital, Newcastle upon Tyne, UK

Garrett McGann FRCR Consultant Radiologist, Cheltenham General Hospital, Cheltenham, UK

Felicity Jane Meyer MA FRCS Consultant Vascular Surgeon and Honorary Senior Lecturer, Norfolk and Norwich University Hospital, University of East Anglia, Norwich, UK

David C. Mitchell MA MS FRCS Consultant Vascular and Transplant Surgeon, Southmead Hospital, Bristol, UK

Robert Morgan MRCP FRCR Consultant Vascular and Interventional Radiologist, Radiology Department, St George's NHS Trust, London, UK

A. Ross Naylor MD FRCS Professor of Vascular Surgery, Leicester Royal Infirmary, Leicester, UK

Ian Nordon MD FRCS Specialist Registrar in Vascular Surgery, Department of Vascular Surgery, Southampton General Hospital, Southampton, UK

Simon Parvin MD FRCS Consultant Vascular Surgeon, Royal Bournemouth Hospital, Bournemouth, UK

David Ratliff MD FRCP FRCS (Eng & Ed) Consultant Vascular Surgeon, Northampton General Hospital, Northampton, UK

Cliff Shearman MS FRCS Professor of Vascular Surgery, Department of Vascular Surgery, Southampton General Hospital, Southampton, UK

Sidhartha Sinha MA MRCS Clinical Research Fellow in Vascular Surgery, St George's NHS Trust, London, UK

Frank C. T. Smith BSc MD FRCS FRCSEd Reader & Honorary Consultant Vascular Surgeon, University of Bristol & Bristol Royal Infirmary, Bristol, UK

Kaji Sritharan MD FRCS Specialist Registrar in Vascular Surgery, Academic Department of Vascular Surgery, Imperial College London, London, UK

Peter R. Taylor MA MChir FRCS Professor of Vascular Surgery, Department of Vascular Surgery, NIHR Comprehensive Biomedical Research Centre of Guy's and St Thomas' NHS Foundation Trust and King's College London, and King's Health Partners, London, UK

John F. Thompson MS FRCSEd FRCS Consultant Surgeon, Exeter Vascular Service, Peninsula College of Medicine and Dentistry, Exeter, UK

Alex Torrie MRCS Orthopaedic Specialist Registrar, Gloucestershire Royal Hospital, Gloucester, UK

Alex B. Watson MSc FRCS Specialist Registrar in Vascular Surgery, Bristol Royal Infirmary, Bristol, UK

Catherine Western BSc MBBS MRCS Specialist Registrar in Vascular Surgery, Southwest Peninsula Deanery, Peninsula Medical School, Royal Cornwall Hospitals Trust, Truro, Cornwall, UK

Mark Whyman MB BS FRCS MS Consultant Surgeon, Cheltenham General Hospital, Cheltenham, UK

David Williams MD FRCS Endovascular Fellow, Sheffield Vascular Institute, Sheffield, UK

Robin Windhaber MD FRCS Specialist Registrar in Vascular Surgery, Royal Bournemouth Hospital, Bournemouth, UK

Peng Foo Wong MB ChB MD FRCS (Gen Surg) Specialist Registrar in Vascular Surgery, Freeman Hospital, Newcastle upon Tyne, UK

Kenneth R. Woodburn MD FRCSG(Gen) Consultant Vascular and Endovascular Surgeon, Cornwall Vascular Unit, Honorary Clinical Lecturer, Peninsula Medical School, Royal Cornwall Hospitals Trust, Truro, Cornwall, UK

Michael G. Wyatt MSc MD FRCS Consultant Vascular Surgeon and Honorary Reader, Freeman Hospital, Newcastle upon Tyne, UK

Foreword

No surgeon, however experienced or confident, wants to pin their reputation on being recognised as an expert in complications. The following paraphrases common sentiments:

"None of us, of course, ever has any complication with whatever operation we perform... And if we do have complications, they occur much less frequently anyway than those of others, and are never serious... And if they are serious, of course, they are not life-threatening... And if they are life-threatening, we never had a patient die from them... And if a patient does die from a complication, it is always the resident who is at fault."
David Ligtenstein

This volume acknowledges the fact that complications can and do occur in vascular and endovascular surgery. Some of the procedures we use as vascular specialists are at the forefront of medical technological development. Others are well established with a sound evidence base. All, however, have some degree of inherent risk and our cohort of patients often has significant comorbidities. Some complications are specifically associated with particular disease processes. The advent of good audit practice and clinical databases provides insight into potential problems, but the experienced clinician anticipates the unexpected and develops an armamentarium of technical tips and tricks to deal with complications they encounter.

This book brings together the collective experience of members of the Joint Vascular Research Group in dealing with, and managing a wide variety of complications that occasionally bedevil the practice of vascular surgery. We hope that this will enable the reader to avoid some of the trials and errors that the authors have encountered.

The JVRG wishes to acknowledge the tireless work of the editors of this volume, Jonothan Earnshaw and Michael Wyatt, in bringing together this collection of experiences. Our thanks are also due to Ms Nikki Bramhill, our publisher at tfm, for her expert overview and long-term patience!

The contributors to this book have been challenged by their encounters with the problems described therein, but in dealing with these problems, have built up a combined repository of experience, and, occasionally, wisdom. They have enjoyed the fellowship of the JVRG and the collaboration required to bring the fruits of their labours to us, the readers.

"*Good surgeons operate well... Great surgeons know how to manage their complications.*"

If this book helps you to avoid a single major complication or to deal successfully with a tricky vascular problem, then it will have achieved its goal. We hope you enjoy reading it!

Frank C. T. Smith BSc MD FRCS FRCSEd
Chair, Joint Vascular Research Group
Reader & Honorary Consultant Vascular Surgeon
University of Bristol & Bristol Royal Infirmary, Bristol, UK

Introduction

Complications in Vascular and Endovascular Surgery – how to avoid them and how to get out of trouble is the third in a highly successful series of publications from the Joint Vascular Research Group, which includes *The Evidence for Vascular Surgery* and *Rare Vascular Disorders – A practical guide for the vascular specialist*. The present title has been inspired by the rapid development in the treatment of patients with vascular disease, which embraces the new endovascular techniques and changes to medical management that are revolutionising our treatment of these patients.

Each chapter is written to present up-to-date evidence-based information on the prevention and treatment of vascular and endovascular complications. Each author has been chosen to provide a particular expertise and experience to the presentation of their subject. There is a particular emphasis on the tips and tricks of how to get out of trouble, and we hope this will help you in your practice of vascular and endovascular surgery.

The editors are both past Chairmen of the Joint Vascular Research Group and present and past Secretaries of The Vascular Society of Great Britain and Ireland. We are very aware that vascular surgery continues to develop rapidly and that we all need to be kept updated on not only the new treatments available, but also on their risks and the management of their associated complications. We hope you enjoy this book and that it will help you manage the often complex complications associated with intervention on patients with vascular disease.

Jonothan J. Earnshaw DM FRCS
Consultant Vascular Surgeon
Gloucestershire Royal Hospital, Gloucester, UK
Michael G. Wyatt MSc MD FRCS
Consultant Vascular Surgeon and Honorary Reader
Freeman Hospital, Newcastle upon Tyne, UK

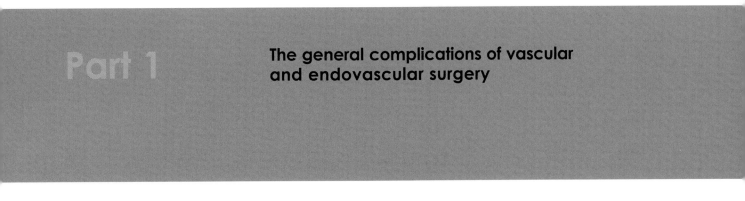

Part 1

The general complications of vascular and endovascular surgery

Chapter 1   How do complications influence outcome?

Sidhartha Sinha MA MRCS, Clinical Research Fellow in Vascular Surgery
Peter Holt PhD FRCS, Clinical Lecturer in Vascular Surgery
St George's NHS Trust, London, UK

Introduction

Vascular surgical procedures carry an intrinsic risk, since they are performed on patients with multiple, often severe comorbidities [1]. It is unrealistic to expect no postoperative complications in this cohort of patients therefore, and the way in which adverse events are handled is important in determining final peri-operative and longer-term outcomes. As high quality is central to any modern surgical service, an understanding of the reporting and interpretation of outcomes data, and the impact of peri-procedural complications on outcomes is important for the vascular specialist. The ways in which the detection and management of complications can lead to quality improvements in vascular surgery are paramount.

The quality agenda and outcomes assessment

The most recent report on health care delivery in the National Health Service in the UK places critical importance on the achievement of high quality [2]. In defining quality, the report identifies three key domains (Figure 1) and builds on an existing model of clinical governance to propose the necessary means to achieve high quality health care. It is noteworthy that, in contrast to previous iterations, the most recent

changes propose to drive up quality standards predominantly by improvements in (and the transparent publication of) clinical outcomes [3, 4].

Which outcomes to measure in vascular surgery?

Understanding how complications influence outcomes requires a knowledge of which current metrics are informative. In general, outcome measures are visible and quantifiable endpoints of clinical pathways that are commonly employed in the assessment of quality, underpinning quality improvement frameworks and informing the commissioning of health care services. An increasing number of quality metrics are being proposed to assess surgical care. Critically, when each is reported, it should be placed into context such that the reported outcome is valid for the specific condition or procedure assessed.

Mortality

Postoperative mortality rates are objective and easily measurable. Despite some conceptual and methodological difficulties associated with their use, they are the most commonly employed outcomes

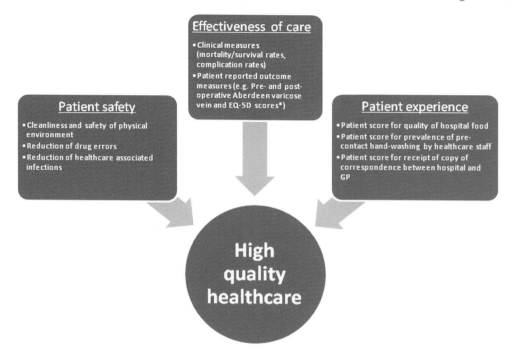

Figure 1. Darzi model of the domains of high quality health care – with specific examples. * European Quality of Life 5-dimension questionnaire.

measure in studies assessing health care quality and remain the most valid proxy [5-7]. Postoperative mortality can be reported at differing intervals; commonly used variations are in-hospital, 30-day and 1-year mortality rates. Increasingly, longer-term mortality rates are reported in the literature. Although in-hospital mortality is reliably quantified, it may be confounded by institutional, political and financial factors favouring more rapid discharge [8]. One-year mortality is also susceptible to confounding by factors unrelated to the structure and process of care delivered, such as the extent/nature of underlying disease and social circumstances. It may, however, be a more meaningful outcome statistic from the patient's point of view [8, 9].

Morbidity

Although postoperative morbidity refers to untoward or adverse events after surgery, traditionally this has been interpreted from a clinical viewpoint. Thus postoperative morbidity has become synonymous with postoperative complications, including deep venous thrombosis and surgical site infection [10]. A more holistic appraisal of the concept envisages a model where several other inter-related

metrics could be interpreted as components of morbidity: reintervention (return to theatre) rate, length of stay, readmission rate and discharge destination (Figure 2) [5].

Complication rates

There is increasing interest in the use of postoperative complication rates as an index of quality. Concerns remain over the lack of standardisation in defining and recording complications; however, postoperative complication rates in modern surgical practice tend to be sufficiently frequent to yield stable statistical estimates when used as outcome measures [8]. Furthermore, it has been demonstrated that postoperative complications are significantly related to other outcome measures such as mortality and hospital length of stay [11, 12].

Readmission rates

Emergency readmission has been defined as a quality metric by the UK Department of Health for a number of surgical procedures, including abdominal aortic aneurysm (AAA) repair [5]. This is based on the

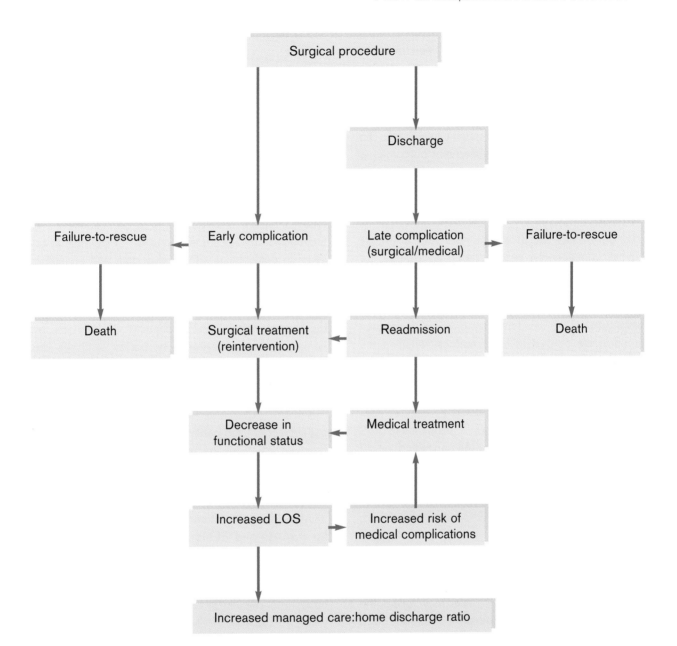

Figure 2. Inter-relationship between components of postoperative mortality and morbidity. LOS = length of stay.

assumption that unplanned readmission reflects a deficiency in the quality of care during the index admission. Retrospective studies from both North America and the UK have shown that patients requiring either medical or surgical readmission at 30 days, or even up to 1 year after open or endovascular aneurysm repair (EVAR) had higher mortality than patients not requiring readmission [5, 13]. Yet readmission rates vary considerably between surgical specialties and are highly influenced by case-mix, being much more common in the elderly and those with chronic medical conditions [14]. Within vascular surgery, most readmissions are related to medical comorbidities. Context is therefore crucial when publishing outcomes, allowing the reason for readmission (surgical, medical or social) to be understood and appropriately reimbursed.

Reintervention rates

Surgical reintervention rates have been used as secondary outcome measures in clinical studies including the EVAR trials [15, 16]. They have been proposed as surrogate quality markers in AAA repair, as the need for reintervention may reflect technical failure during surgery and poor patient selection [5]. The impact of reintervention on subsequent outcomes is discussed later.

Length of stay

Length of stay (LOS) is a current political priority and has consequently been adopted as a metric for outcomes assessment. It is suggested that a reduced LOS improves the cost-effectiveness of care and may be a surrogate marker for peri-operative complications [5, 8, 11]. This can only be true when placed in the context of other metrics including the use of managed care facilities for patient discharge, the emergency readmission rate and mortality.

LOS is also significantly affected by clinical, non-clinical and demographic factors [17]. Variations in LOS may actually reflect variations in the capacity of social services, or in the effectiveness of liaison between hospital and community care, rather than measuring quality directly [5, 17].

Discharge destination

Patients who have peri-operative complications have an increased LOS and a lower probability of being discharged home [11, 13]. This may reflect the seriousness of the complication suffered and subsequent decrease in functional status requiring discharge to a managed care facility [18]. With specific reference to vascular surgery, a retrospective study on open AAA repair and EVAR found that after adjusting for LOS and complication rate, variables that predicted likelihood of discharge to a rehabilitation facility rather than home were: type of procedure (open repair), age and comorbidity [19]. Similarly, a retrospective study using UK administrative data found that EVAR was associated with a lower rate of discharge to managed care instead of home than open AAA repair [5].

Patient satisfaction

Patient-reported outcome measures (PROMs) are standardised, validated questionnaires completed by patients to measure their perceptions of their own health and health care experiences [20]. They are gaining popularity in a number of fields, especially in the management of chronic disease. In vascular surgery, PROMs have been adopted as quality indicators for varicose vein surgery using pre- and postoperative scores on the disease-specific Aberdeen Varicose Vein Questionnaire and the generic European Quality of Life 5-dimension (EQ-5D) questionnaire [21]. PROMs may be taken in conjunction with survival data and economic assessment of services to provide information on the incremental cost-effectiveness ratio (ICER) and quality-adjusted life-years (QALYs), which are key indicators for the planning and purchasing of services by commissioners and regulatory bodies such as the National Institute for Health and Clinical Excellence (NICE) [22].

Patient experience measures (PEMs) refer to patient scores for generic aspects of the care they received, such as the quality of food, availability of assistance with eating when required, cleanliness of environment and hand-washing practice of staff [23].

As with other outcomes measures, response rates for PROMs and PEMs are significantly affected by demographics such as race/ethnicity, language, level of education and socioeconomic status, and thus require advanced case-mix adjustment to yield meaningful results for comparisons [20, 24]. The way in which PROMs and PEMs will influence future health service configuration remains unclear.

Can outcomes be improved by reducing complications?

The rate of postoperative complications influences the incidence of other outcome measures and so may be considered a useful marker of quality. A focus on reducing the rate of postoperative complications is predicated on the assumption that this will lead to reductions in postoperative mortality, reintervention rate, length of stay, readmission rate and discharge

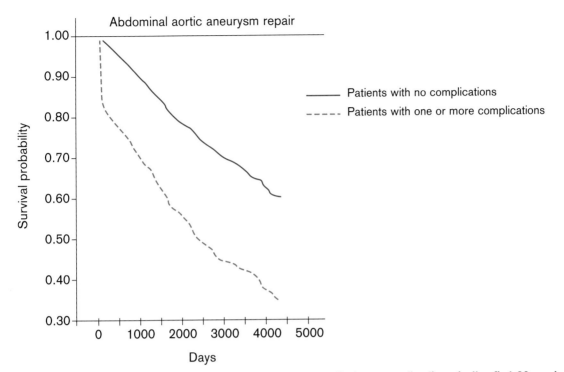

Figure 3. Patient survival curves after AAA repair in those suffering complications in the first 30 postoperative days versus those who did not. *Reproduced with permission from Khuri SF, et al* [12].

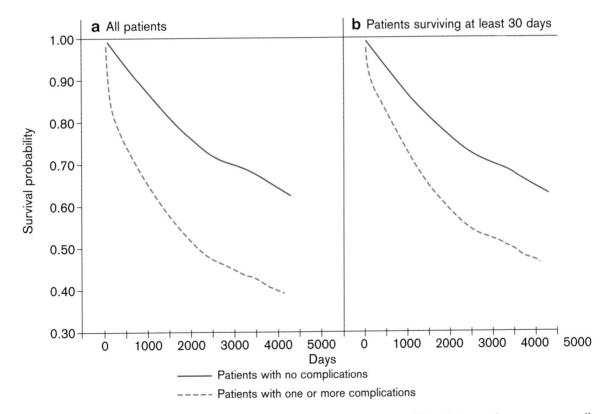

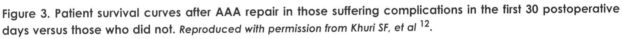

Figure 4. a) Survival curves of all patients who sustained a complication within 30 days of surgery versus those who did not. b) Survival curves of all patients surviving more than 30 days after surgery and who sustained a complication within 30 days of surgery versus those who did not. *Reproduced with permission from Khuri SF, et al* [12].

destination – and therefore represents a global improvement in quality and patient experience. Indeed in the USA, the Centers for Medicare and Medicaid Services (CMS) now deny reimbursement to hospitals for certain preventable postoperative adverse events, including urinary tract infection, pressure ulcers and surgical site infection [25].

Whilst improving outcomes by reducing complication rates seems intuitive, it is noteworthy that, the relationship between peri-procedural complications and outcomes is complex and can show attenuation with proper risk adjustment [26]. Patients who have a complication fare worse both early and in the longer term, as shown for AAA repair (Figure 3) [12]. Patients with any complication in the peri-operative period fare worse in the long run, even after excluding those who do not survive the first 30 days after surgery (Figure 4) [12]. This is true for a number of specific complications of AAA repair, lower limb arterial bypass and carotid endarterectomy (CEA) [12].

The relationship between postoperative mortality and complications

In attempting to explain why certain hospitals had improved outcomes for high-risk procedures, one retrospective study from North America found a lower incidence of complication rates in high-volume hospitals for three complex procedures (pancreatic resection, oesophagectomy and AAA repair). It was proposed that this explained volume-related differences in mortality rates [27]. However, whilst it is not surprising that a hospital with high postoperative mortality rates would also have high postoperative complication rates, research suggests that the rate of complications may be a function of underlying patient characteristics rather than hospital characteristics, whereas mortality rates reflect both of these [28].

There is mounting evidence that postoperative complication rates may not be related to caseload. Risk-adjusted retrospective studies on open AAA repair and CEA using UK administrative data failed to

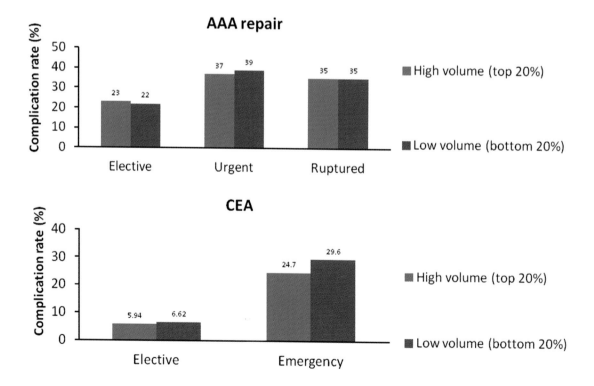

Figure 5. Complication rates according to volume for AAA repair and CEA (differences not significant). *Adapted from Holt PJE, et al* [29, 30].

demonstrate any difference in peri-operative complication rates underlying significant volume-outcome relationships for these two procedures (Figure 5) [29, 30]. Two risk-adjusted retrospective studies from North America, one specifically examining AAA repair, and using routine data, found much larger differences in complication-related mortality rates than in the incidence of complications, when comparing hospitals with the highest and lowest procedural mortality rates (Figure 6) [25, 31].

Failure-to-rescue (FTR)

The above findings focused interest on complication-related mortality rates as a more robust measure of health care quality than either isolated mortality or complication rates. Termed failure-to-rescue (FTR), the concept of this finding is that FTR is more reflective of a hospital's structure and processes of care, than of patient factors or disease severity. Thus, a patient in a hospital with better overall outcomes who develops a postoperative complication will be identified promptly, appropriate resuscitative and corrective measures will be instituted more quickly and death from that complication will be prevented [32]. FTR correlates well with overall mortality rates, and requires less risk adjustment than overall complication rates, as it is less dependent on patient factors, and is likely to increase in use as an outcome measure [32, 33].

Although specific evidence for FTR in vascular surgical procedures is lacking, a recent study attempted to identify the structural characteristics associated with lower FTR rates after pancreatectomy [34]. Characteristics associated with lower FTR rates included teaching hospital status, larger overall hospital size, increased nurse-to-patient ratios and the provision of modern technology. Each of these systemic factors could apply similarly to optimal vascular surgery.

Improvements in outcomes are likely to be maximized by focusing both on reducing the actual rate of postoperative complications, and also preventing FTR events. This might potentially be achieved through delivering specialist care in vascular institutes with 24/7 vascular specialist cover.

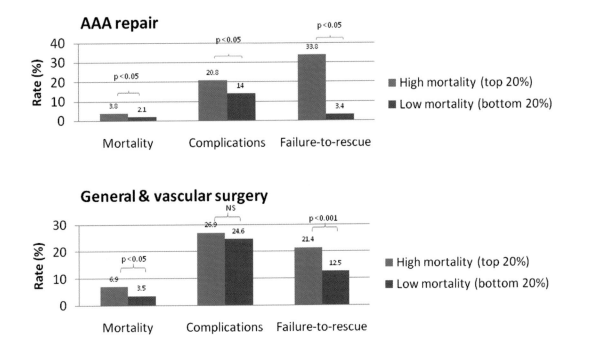

Figure 6. Overall mortality rate, complications rate and complication-related mortality (failure-to-rescue) rate according to top and bottom mortality quintiles. *Adapted from Ghaferi AA, et al* [25, 31].

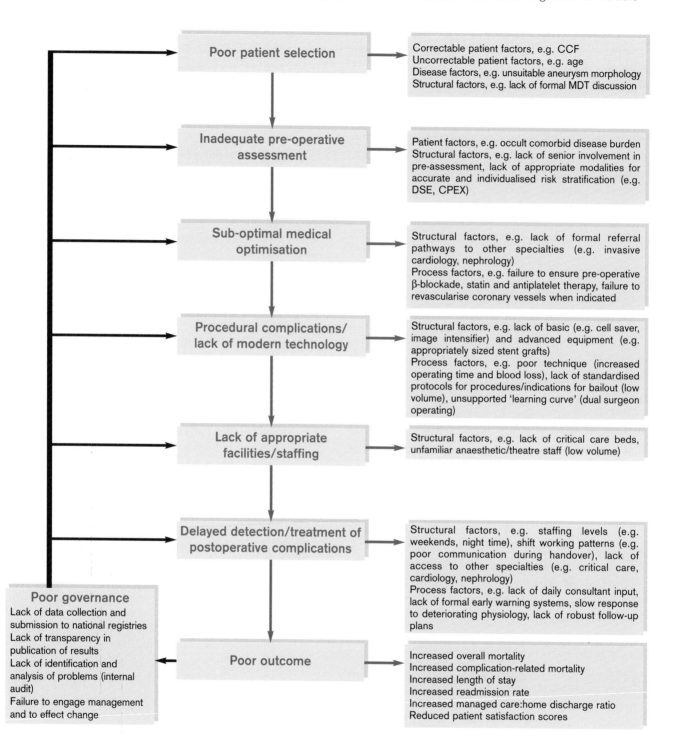

Figure 7. The complications pathway with specific reference to vascular surgery. CCF = congestive cardiac failure; MDT = multidisciplinary team; DSE = dobutamine stress echocardiography; CPEX = cardiopulmonary exercise testing.

The complications pathway

When considering health care quality in the dimensions of structure, process and outcome, it is possible to construct an optimal pathway of surgical care (Figure 7). There are several obvious steps along the pathway where deficiencies in structures and processes of care could increase the likelihood of postoperative complications (or FTR events).

Patient selection

Outcomes are often determined by decisions made long before a surgical procedure. Inappropriate patient selection is a major risk factor for subsequent postoperative complications. Some patient factors are fixed and not amenable to optimisation – such as advanced age – but confer significant risk of postoperative complications, increased LOS and death [35]. Correctable factors in this patient group reside within their co-existing comorbidities, which may be numerous and occult [36].

Risk stratification

The aim of pre-operative assessment is to stratify patients according to risk, allowing appropriate allocation of postoperative care resources and to identify and optimise medical comorbidities [37]. Traditional reliance on scoring systems (e.g. P-POSSUM) and clinical risk indices (e.g. the revised cardiac risk index) is poorly supported by high quality evidence and there is increasing interest in the use of modern assessment methods to stratify risk [38, 39]. Dobutamine stress echocardiography (DSE) can identify patients at greatest risk of postoperative cardiac events, and who may benefit from pre-operative coronary revascularisation [39-41]. Cardiopulmonary exercise testing (CPEX) is an objective measure of cardiorespiratory reserve that may also identify surgical patients at increased risk of postoperative complications, although further evidence is needed to define its precise role [11]. Involvement of a specialist vascular anaesthetist in the pre-assessment process for major vascular surgery can improve risk stratification, medical optimisation (and patient satisfaction), although the effect on outcome has yet to be proven [37].

Medical optimisation

The significant and frequently occult comorbid disease burden of vascular surgical patients presents considerable scope for pre-operative optimisation. Accurate identification of occult disease may require the involvement of experienced clinicians, whilst optimal risk factor modification requires co-located specialist medical services such as cardiology and nephrology [36, 37, 42]. Appropriate pre-operative medical therapy including antiplatelet agents and statins in all patients, and β-blockers in selected patients, has been shown to reduce the incidence of postoperative complications in vascular surgery patients [1].

Access to technology

Availability of, and experience with, modern technology provides minimally invasive treatment options for surgical pathologies that can reduce the incidence of postoperative complications including acute kidney injury, respiratory failure and infection [1]. In tandem with minimally invasive techniques, other technological adjuncts can further reduce complication rates. For example, the routine availability of CT angiography has been shown to increase the detection of significant endoleak following EVAR, facilitating on-table correction and preventing early return to theatre; the latter has an 8% mortality rate within 30 days of the original procedure [43].

Procedural complications

Intra-operative difficulties may be associated with structural factors such as lack of consignment endovascular stock, limiting bailout options, and process factors such as poor surgical technique, manifesting as increased operating time or blood loss. An association between operating time and postoperative complications has been demonstrated for AAA repair, leg bypass and CEA [44-46]. Some of the

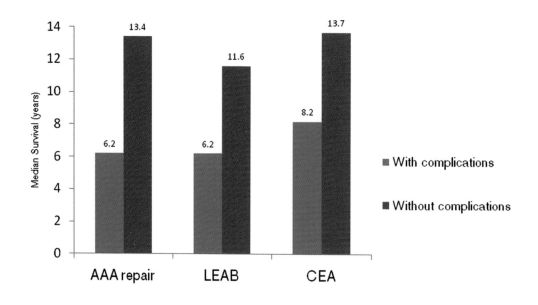

Figure 8. Median survival of patients undergoing vascular surgical procedures with or without any postoperative complication (all differences significant at p <0.001). LEAB = lower extremity arterial bypass. *Adapted from Khuri SF, et al* [12].

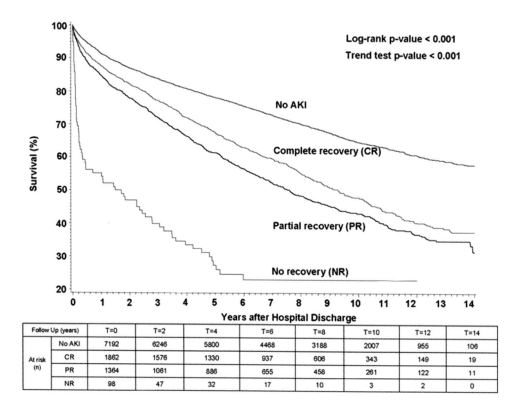

Follow Up (years)		T=0	T=2	T=4	T=6	T=8	T=10	T=12	T=14
At risk (n)	No AKI	7192	6246	5800	4468	3188	2007	955	106
	CR	1862	1576	1330	937	606	343	149	19
	PR	1364	1061	886	655	458	261	122	11
	NR	98	47	32	17	10	3	2	0

Figure 9. Survival curves of patients with and without an episode of acute kidney injury during hospitalisation, stratified by degree of recovery. *Reproduced with permission from Bihorac A, et al* [18].

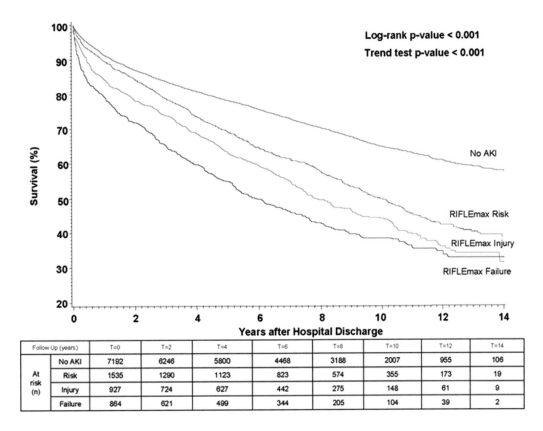

Figure 10. Survival curves of patients with and without acute kidney injury, stratified by RIFLE classification. *Reproduced with permission from Bihorac A, et al* [18].

benefits in outcome that follow surgical specialization at both hospital and surgeon level may be the result of improvements in this area [47, 48].

Facilities and staffing

Structural factors such as the standard care bed:augmented care bed ratio and the specialization of all staff involved in peri-operative care of the vascular surgical patient will affect the rate of postoperative complications [42]. This includes the availability of a dedicated vascular ward with nursing and junior medical staff experienced in the management of patients following vascular surgical procedures. On site 24-hour cover from vascular and interventional specialists is likely to drive improvements in outcome, and is a requirement of a modern vascular service.

Specific postoperative complications

Postoperative complications reduce both short- and long-term survival after AAA repair, leg bypass and CEA (Figure 8) [12]. The effects of individual complications are discussed further below.

Acute kidney injury

Postoperative acute kidney injury (AKI) is associated with increased peri-procedural and longer-term mortality, even when there is complete recovery of renal function (Figure 9) [18]. Mortality is associated with both the severity of AKI and the degree of recovery (Figures 9 and 10). Therefore, it is important to ensure renal protection during vascular surgical procedures, especially in patients with pre-existing chronic renal dysfunction [49].

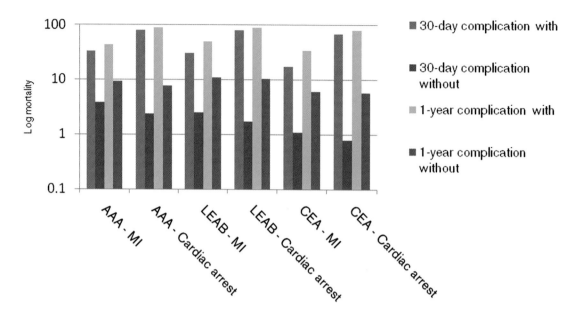

Figure 11. Mortality rates for myocardial infarction (MI) and cardiac arrest by procedure (AAA, LEAB, CEA) and by time from procedure (30 days and 1 year). For each complication, the development of the specific complication was associated with a significant increase in 30-day and 1-year mortality. Five-year outcomes were similarly affected (not shown here). Mortality rate is shown on a log scale. *Adapted from Khuri SF, et al* [12].

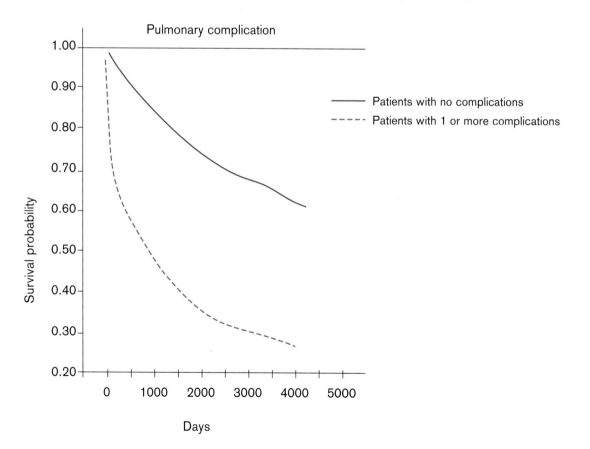

Figure 12. Survival curves of all patients who sustained one or more pulmonary complications (pneumonia, prolonged intubation and failure to wean) in the first 30 postoperative days versus those who did not. *Reproduced with permission from Khuri SF, et al* [12].

Cardiac complications

Postoperative myocardial infarction (and cardiac arrest) both confer significant reductions in short, medium and long-term survival after AAA repair, leg bypass and CEA (Figure 11) [12]. This underscores the importance of medical optimisation of cardiovascular risk factors before surgery and the need to identify patients who might benefit from coronary revascularisation.

Pulmonary complications

Pneumonia and prolonged intubation are also associated with significant reductions in postoperative survival (Figure 12) [12]. With specific reference to vascular surgery, this relationship persists at 30 days, 1 year and 5 years after AAA repair, leg bypass and CEA. This illustrates the importance of good surgical technique and evidence-based intensive care management protocols and preventative ward-based measures such as effective chest physiotherapy [12].

Wound complications

Wound complications including both superficial and deep infection are associated with reductions in postoperative survival, although the relationship is weaker for vascular surgical procedures in comparison to cardiopulmonary complications (Figure 13) [12].

Detection of postoperative complications

Central to the concept of FTR is the early detection and treatment of postoperative complications [32]. Detection of complications is likely to be affected by structural factors, such as ward staffing levels and staff working patterns, and processes of care, such as the use of formal early warning systems to identify patients with deteriorating physiology. Optimal management of postoperative complications and prevention of FTR events requires associated specialist services such as 24/7 on-site interventional

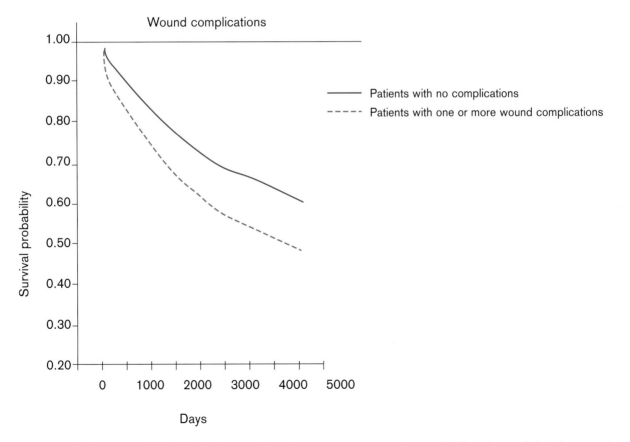

Figure 13. Survival curves of all patients who sustained one or more wound complications (superficial, deep and wound dehiscence) in the first 30 postoperative days versus those who did not. *Reproduced with permission from Khuri SF, et al* [12].

radiology, coronary revascularisation, renal replacement therapy and the provision of appropriate critical care facilities [42].

Clinical governance

Good governance practices such as complete and accurate data collection, internal audit, transparent publication of results, and benchmarking against defined quality standards perpetuate good performance. In the context of AAA repair, it has been shown that lack of formal mortality and morbidity review of critical care at least monthly was associated with an increased hospital LOS [50]. Similarly, in the setting of colorectal surgery it has been shown that non-submitters to the national audit process have a higher peri-operative mortality rate than clinicians from hospitals that submit data routinely [51]. This makes a strong argument for the submission of both surgeon-specific and hospital-level data to national audits and their subjection to peer review.

Reporting of surgical outcomes data

All surgeons have an obligation towards accurate and complete data collection and audit. This must include surgical turndown rates to assess risk-averse behaviour and to place outcomes into context. Current reporting standards of surgical outcomes are undermined by data inaccuracies due to over-simplistic identification of cases from administrative data and weak statistical analyses which fail to identify outliers [52]. Gauging improvement against national Quality Improvement Frameworks requires transparent reporting of outcomes and may necessitate service remodelling.

How to minimise complications

A number of structural and process measures that might lead to reductions in peri-operative mortality and morbidity have been discussed above. The aim is to manage patients within a system that allows full and accurate pre-operative assessment and risk stratification, performance of surgery in a safe environment using modern surgical (and endovascular) techniques, bailout options and postoperative nursing on appropriately staffed and equipped intensive care units and wards. Finally, vascular units should scrutinise, publish and understand their results, investigating how quality assurance and improvement measures might be implemented. In the case of arterial surgery in the UK, this should include contributing data to the National Vascular Database.

Not every hospital can deliver all of these standards and this might contribute to FTR events and peri-operative mortality. For many complex surgical procedures, a clear association between hospital volume and outcome has been demonstrated [53]. Within vascular surgery, significant volume-outcome relationships have been proven for open AAA repair, EVAR, CEA and lower limb bypass [29, 30, 54-57]. Wide variations in outcome have also been demonstrated across England for major leg amputations [58]. The strength and reproducibility of this volume-outcome relationship is driving service remodelling by informing the commissioning process [59, 60]. The relationship appears to exist for individual surgeons and whole units. One way to reduce the FTR rate appears to be to centralize major arterial surgery into specialist units.

Conclusions

Poor outcomes such as postoperative mortality, complication and FTR rates are the result of systematic failures in the care pathway. Complications and FTR events contribute to short-term and long-term mortality. These failures may be minimised by concentrating services in fewer, more specialized centres with an appropriate clinical governance framework. Meticulous pre-operative work-up, surgical planning including risk stratification, active postoperative surveillance and timely reintervention reduces mortality from postoperative complications. Improving surgical outcomes by focusing on reducing postoperative complications is likely to be most effective if process changes occur that reduce FTR rates.

Key points

- Assessment of quality of health care delivery is increasingly important.
- Assessment of quality in surgery has traditionally relied on outcome measures such as postoperative mortality and complication rates.
- Outcome measures are imperfect surrogates for quality of care, particularly when associated structures and processes of care are not considered.
- Vascular patients are a high-risk group undergoing high-risk surgery and thus complications are inevitable.
- The rate of postoperative complications can be minimised by careful pre-operative assessment, risk stratification, medical optimisation, surgical planning and postoperative surveillance.
- Postoperative death resulting from complications (failure-to-rescue) more closely reflects underlying structures and processes of care and thus may be a more valid marker of quality.
- Improvement in quality is more likely if efforts are made to improve FTR rates as well as to reduce the incidence of postoperative complications.

References

1. Garrioch MA, Pichel AC. Reducing the risk of vascular surgery. *Curr Anaesth Crit Care* 2008; 19: 128-37.
2. Darzi A. High quality care for all: NHS next stage review final report. London: Department of Health, 2008.
3. Darzi A. Quality and the NHS next stage review. *Lancet* 2008; 371(9624): 1563-4.
4. Lansley A. Equity and excellence: liberating the NHS. London: Department of Health, 2010.
5. Holt PJE, Poloniecki JD, Hofman D, et al. Re-interventions, readmissions and discharge destination: modern metrics for the assessment of the quality of care. *Eur J Vasc Endovasc Surg* 2010; 39: 49-54.
6. Rubin HR, Pronovost P, Diette GB. The advantages and disadvantages of process-based measures of health care quality. *Int J Qual Health Care* 2001; 13: 469-74.
7. Iezzoni LI. The risks of risk adjustment. *JAMA* 1997; 278: 1600-7.
8. Daley J, Henderson WG, Khuri SF. Risk-adjusted surgical outcomes. *Ann Rev Med* 2001; 52: 275-87.
9. Edwards MB, Taylor KM. Is 30-day mortality an adequate outcome statistic for patients considering heart valve replacement? *Ann Thorac Surg* 2003; 76: 482-5.
10. Grocott MPW. Improving outcomes after surgery. *BMJ* 2010; 340(7737): 62.
11. Snowden CP, Prentis JM, Anderson HL, et al. Submaximal cardiopulmonary exercise testing predicts complications and hospital length of stay in patients undergoing major elective surgery. *Ann Surg* 2010; 251: 535-41.
12. Khuri SF, Henderson WG, DePalma RG, et al. Determinants of long-term survival after major surgery and the adverse effect of postoperative complications. *Ann Surg* 2005; 242: 326-43.
13. Gioia LC, Filion KB, Haider S, et al. Hospital readmissions following abdominal aortic aneurysm repair. *Ann Vasc Surg* 2005; 19: 35-41.
14. Leng GC, Walsh D, Fowkes FGR, Swainson CP. Is the emergency readmission rate a valid outcome indicator? *Qual Health Care* 1999; 8: 234-8.
15. EVAR Trial Participants. Endovascular aneurysm repair versus open repair in patients with abdominal aortic aneurysm (EVAR trial 1): randomised controlled trial. *Lancet* 2005; 365(9478): 2179-86.
16. EVAR Trial Participants. Endovascular aneurysm repair and outcome in patients unfit for open repair of abdominal aortic aneurysm (EVAR trial 2): randomised controlled trial. *Lancet* 2005; 365(9478): 2187-92.
17. Brasel KJ, Lim HJ, Nirula R, Weigelt JA. Length of stay: an appropriate quality measure? *Arch Surg* 2007; 142: 461-6.
18. Bihorac A, Yavas S, Subbiah S, et al. Long-term risk of mortality and acute kidney injury during hospitalization after major surgery. *Ann Surg* 2009; 249: 851-8.
19. Bosch JL, Beinfeld MT, Halpern EF, et al. Endovascular versus open surgical elective repair of infrarenal abdominal aortic aneurysm: predictors of patient discharge destination. *Radiology* 2001; 220: 576-80.
20. Dawson J, Doll H, Fitzpatrick R, et al. The routine use of patient reported outcome measures in healthcare settings. *BMJ* 2010; 340: c186.
21. Department of Health. Guidance on the routine collection of Patient Reported Outcome Measures (PROMS). London: Department of Health, 2008.
22. Phillips C, Thompson G. What is a QALY? London: Hayward Medical Communications, 2009.
23. The NHS Information Centre. Indicators for quality improvement. London: The NHS Information Centre, 2009.
24. Johnson ML, Rodriguez HP, Solorio MR. Case-mix adjustment and the comparison of community health center performance on patient experience measures. *Health Serv Res* 2010; 45: 670-90.
25. Ghaferi AA, Birkmeyer JD, Dimick JB. Variation in hospital mortality associated with inpatient surgery. *New Engl J Med* 2009; 361: 1368-75.

26. Silber JH, Rosenbaum PR. A spurious correlation between hospital mortality and complication rates: the importance of severity adjustment. *Med Care* 1997; 35(10 Suppl): OS77-92.

27. Dimick JB, Pronovost PJ, Cowan JA, Jr., *et al*. Variation in postoperative complication rates after high-risk surgery in the United States. *Surgery* 2003; 134: 534-40.

28. Silber JH, Williams SV, Krakauer H, Schwartz JS. Hospital and patient characteristics associated with death after surgery - a study of adverse occurrence and failure to rescue. *Med Care* 1992; 30: 615-29.

29. Holt PJE, Poloniecki JD, Loftus IM, *et al*. Epidemiological study of the relationship between volume and outcome after abdominal aortic aneurysm surgery in the UK from 2000 to 2005. *Br J Surg* 2007; 94: 441-8.

30. Holt PJE, Poloniecki JD, Loftus IM, Thompson MM. The relationship between hospital case volume and outcome from carotid endarterectomy in England from 2000 to 2005. *Eur J Vasc Endovasc Surg* 2007; 34: 646-54.

31. Ghaferi AA, Birkmeyer JD, Dimick JB. Complications, failure to rescue, and mortality with major inpatient surgery in medicare patients. *Ann Surg* 2009; 250: 1029-34.

32. Silber JH, Romano PS, Rosen AK, *et al*. Failure-to-rescue: comparing definitions to measure quality of care. *Med Care* 2007; 45: 918-25.

33. Silber JH, Rosenbaum PR, Williams SV, *et al*. The relationship between choice of outcome measure and hospital rank in general surgical procedures: implications for quality assessment. *Int J Quality Health Care* 1997; 9: 193-200.

34. Ghaferi AA, Osborne NH, Birkmeyer JD, Dimick JB. Hospital characteristics associated with failure to rescue from complications after pancreatectomy. *J Am Coll Surg* 2010; 211: 325-30.

35. Polanczyk CA, Marcantonio E, Goldman L, *et al*. Impact of age on perioperative complications and length of stay in patients undergoing noncardiac surgery. *Ann Int Med* 2001; 134: 637-43.

36. Dawson J, Vig S, Choke E, *et al*. Medical optimisation can reduce morbidity and mortality associated with elective aortic aneurysm repair. *Eur J Vasc Endovasc Surg* 2007; 33: 100-4.

37. Cantlay KL, Baker S, Parry A, Danjoux G. The impact of a consultant anaesthetist led pre-operative assessment clinic on patients undergoing major vascular surgery. *Anaesthesia* 2006; 61: 234-9.

38. Pearse RM, Rhodes A, Grounds RM. Clinical review: how to optimize management of high-risk surgical patients. *Crit Care* 2004; 8: 503-7.

39. Atkinson D, Carter A. Pre-operative assessment for aortic surgery. *Curr Anaesth Crit Care* 2008; 19: 115-27.

40. McFalls EO, Ward HB, Moritz TE, *et al*. Coronary-artery revascularization before elective major vascular surgery. *New Engl J Med* 2004; 351: 2795-804.

41. Poldermans D, Schouten O, Vidakovic R, *et al*. A clinical randomized trial to evaluate the safety of a noninvasive approach in high-risk patients undergoing major vascular surgery: the DECREASE-V Pilot Study. *J Am Coll Cardiol* 2007; 49: 1763-9.

42. Healthcare for London. Cardiovascular services - case for change. London: NHS Commissioning Support for London, 2010.

43. Biasi L, Ali T, Hinchliffe R, Morgan R, *et al*. Intraoperative DynaCT detection and immediate correction of a type 1a endoleak following endovascular repair of abdominal aortic aneurysm. *Cardiovasc Intervent Radiol* 2009; 32: 535-8.

44. Diehl JT, Cali RF, Hertzer NR, Beven EG. Complications of abdominal aortic reconstruction - an analysis of perioperative risk factors in 557 patients. *Ann Surg* 1983; 197: 49-56.

45. Edwards WH, Martin RS, Jenkins JM, Mulherin JL. Primary graft infections. *J Vasc Surg* 1987; 6: 235-9.

46. Allen BT, Anderson CB, Rubin BG, *et al*. The influence of anesthetic technique on perioperative complications after carotid endarterectomy. *J Vasc Surg* 1994; 19: 834-43.

47. Young EL, Holt PJE, Poloniecki JD, *et al*. Meta-analysis and systematic review of the relationship between surgeon annual caseload and mortality for elective open abdominal aortic aneurysm repairs. *J Vasc Surg* 2007; 46: 1287-94.

48. Hall BL, Hsiao EY, Majercik S, *et al*. The impact of surgeon specialization on patient mortality: examination of a continuous Herfindahl-Hirschman index. *Ann Surg* 2009; 249: 708-16.

49. Park B, Mavanur A, Drezner AD, *et al*. Clinical impact of chronic renal insufficiency on endovascular aneurysm repair. *Vasc Endovasc Surg* 2007; 40: 437-45.

50. Pronovost PJ, Jenckes MW, Dorman T, *et al*. Organizational characteristics of intensive care units related to outcomes of abdominal aortic surgery. *JAMA* 1999; 281: 1310-7.

51. Almoudaris AM, Burns EM, Bottle A, *et al*. A colorectal perspective on voluntary submission of outcome data to clinical registries. *Br J Surg* 2010; 98: 132-9.

52. Holt PJ, Poloniecki JD, Thompson MM. Interpret surgical outcome data with care. *BMJ* 2008; 337: a1401.

53. Birkmeyer JD, Siewers AE, Finlayson EVA, *et al*. Hospital volume and surgical mortality in the United States. *New Engl J Med* 2002; 346: 1128-37.

54. Holt PJE, Poloniecki JD, Khalid U, *et al*. Effect of endovascular aneurysm repair on the volume-outcome relationship in aneurysm repair. *Circulation: Cardiovasc Qual Outcomes* 2009; 2: 624-32.

55. Awopetu AI, Moxey P, Hinchliffe RJ, *et al*. Systematic review and meta-analysis of the relationship between hospital volume and outcome for lower limb arterial surgery. *Br J Surg* 2010; 97: 797-803.

56. Holt PJE, Poloniecki JD, Gerrard D, *et al*. Meta-analysis and systematic review of the relationship between volume and outcome in abdominal aortic aneurysm surgery. *Br J Surg* 2007; 94: 395-403.

57. Holt PJE, Poloniecki JD, Loftus IM, Thompson MM. Meta-analysis and systematic review of the relationship between hospital volume and outcome following carotid endarterectomy. *Eur J Vasc Endovasc Surg* 2007; 33: 645-51.

58. Moxey PW, Hofman D, Hinchliffe RJ, *et al*. Epidemiological study of lower limb amputation in England between 2003 and 2008. *Br J Surg* 2010; 97: 1348-53.

59. Holt PJE, Poloniecki JD, Hinchliffe RJ, *et al*. Model for the reconfiguration of specialized vascular services. *Br J Surg* 2008; 95: 1469-74.

60. Birkmeyer JD, Finlayson EVA, Birkmeyer CM. Volume standards for high-risk surgical procedures: potential benefits of the Leapfrog initiative. *Surgery* 2001; 130: 415-22.

Chapter 2

Complications related to cardiorespiratory comorbidity

Teik K. Ho FRCS, Specialist Registrar in Vascular Surgery
Daryll Baker PhD FRCS, Consultant Vascular Surgeon
Royal Free Hospital, London, UK

Introduction

Vascular disease tends to affect the older age group, with the associated risk factors of diabetes, hypertension, hypercholesterolaemia and a history of cigarette smoking. They, therefore, have an increased incidence of underlying cardiorespiratory comorbidities, which are likely to be exacerbated by surgical intervention. Following elective vascular surgery, cardiac and respiratory causes of death contribute up to 40% and 35% of mortality, respectively [1].

To reduce cardiorespiratory complications it is necessary to:

◆ pre-operatively identify patients at risk of cardiorespiratory complications;
◆ take measures to reduce identified risks;
◆ identify early and treat postoperative cardio-respiratory complications.

Pre-operative assessment of cardiorespiratory comorbidities

Pre-operative assessment identifies patients at risk of cardiorespiratory peri-operative complications and therefore:

◆ provides the opportunity to optimise medical condition;
◆ allows the risk of adverse events to be discussed with the patient, and hence enables informed consent;
◆ enables the planning of anticipated critical care resource.

Targeted pre-operative assessment of the cardiac and respiratory systems involves obtaining a thorough medical history, performing a physical examination, and arranging appropriate investigations. According to the NICE guidelines [2], the only initial investigations necessary for patients aged 60 years or older in all American Society of Anaesthesiologists (ASA) grades (Table 1) are a set of routine blood tests (full blood count and renal function) and an ECG. NICE recommends that ASA grade 2 and 3 patients with cardiorespiratory morbidities should also be considered for arterial blood gas analysis and undergo respiratory function tests.

From the history, physical examination, and initial investigations, further pre-operative investigations are undertaken based on a structured assessment of the individual's cardiorespiratory risk and fitness for surgery. Examples of structured assessments are discussed below.

Table 1. ASA grades.

ASA grade	Definitions
1	Normal healthy patient without any clinically important comorbidity or clinically significant past medical history
2	A patient with mild systemic disease
3	A patient with severe systemic disease
4	A patient with severe systemic disease that is a constant threat to life

ASA grades are a simple scale describing fitness to undergo general anaesthesia. These grades often relate to functional capacity – that is comorbidity that does not (ASA grade 2) or that does (ASA grade 3) limit a patient's activity.

Table 2. Physical activities and associated METs (metabolic equivalents).

Physical activity	MET
Light	*<3*
Watching television	1.0
Playing musical instrument	2.0
Walking, 1.7 mph, level ground, strolling	2.3
Walking, 2.5 mph	2.9
Moderately vigorous	*3 to 6*
Calisthenics, home exercise, light or moderate effort	3.5
Walking briskly (1 mile every 20 min)	3.5
Climbing stairs	4.0
Bicycling, <10 mph, leisurely	4.0
Slow swimming	4.5
Stationary bicycling	5.5
Vigorous	*>6*
Aerobic calisthenics	8.0
Jogging (1 mile every 12 min)	8.0
Running 6 mph (10 min mile)	10.0

The highest possible MET the patient can reportedly undertake is determined on direct questioning using the table above. The lower the maximum MET achievable, the greater the risk of cardiovascular complications.

Metabolic equivalents (METs)

Objective functional cardiorespiratory capacity is measured in metabolic equivalents (METs). One MET equals the basal metabolic rate, which is equivalent to 3.5ml oxygen/kg/minute. From direct questioning the highest possible MET the patient can achieve is determined (Table 2). The inability to climb two flights of stairs or run a short distance (<4 METs) indicates poor functional capacity and is associated with an increased incidence of postoperative cardiac events [3].

General cardiorespiratory risk assessment according to ASA grade

NICE has outlined features according to the patient's ASA grade which places them into a moderate or high surgical risk group (Table 3) [2].

Specific cardiac risk assessment

The Lee cardiac risk index [4] was developed to predict major cardiac complications in non-cardiac surgery patients and assigns 1 point to each of the following contributing factors: high-risk surgery, ischaemic heart disease, heart failure,

Table 3. Characterisation of 'mild' and 'severe' comorbidity, corresponding to ASA grades 2 and 3, for cardiovascular and respiratory comorbidities. *Adapted from "CG 3 Pre-operative tests: the use of routine pre-operative tests for elective surgery". London: NICE. Available from www.nice.org.uk.*

	ASA grade 2: Mild systemic disease	ASA grade 3: Severe systemic disease
Cardiovascular disease		
Current angina	Occasional use of GTN spray (2-3 times per month). Does not include patients with unstable angina who would be ASA 3	Regular use of GTN spray (2-3 times per week) or unstable angina
Exercise tolerance	Not limiting activity	Limiting activity
Hypertension	Well controlled using a single anti-hypertensive medication.	Not well controlled, requiring multiple antihypertensive medications.
Diabetes	Well controlled, no obvious diabetic complications	Not well controlled, diabetic complications (e.g. claudication, impaired renal function)
Previous coronary revascularisation	Not directly relevant – depends on current signs and symptoms	Not directly relevant – depends on current signs and symptoms
Respiratory disease		
COAD/COPD	Productive cough; wheeze well controlled by inhalers; occasional episodes of acute chest infection	Breathlessness on minimal exertion (for example, stair climbing, carrying shopping); distressingly wheezy much of the time; several episodes per year of acute chest infection
Asthma	Well controlled by medications/inhalers; life-style; not limiting life-style	Poorly controlled; limiting on high dose of inhaler/oral steroids; frequent hospital admission on account of asthma exacerbation

COAD = chronic obstructive airways disease; COPD = chronic obstructive pulmonary disease; GTN = glyceryl trinitrate

cerebrovascular disease, renal impairment with plasma creatinine more than 177µmol/L, and diabetes mellitus requiring insulin. The incidence of major cardiac complications is estimated at 0.4, 0.9, 7, and 11% in patients with an index of 0 (low risk), 1, 2 (intermediate risk), and 3 or more points (high risk), respectively. Patients who have undergone cardiac bypass surgery in the previous 5 years or percutaneous coronary intervention from 6 months to 5 years, and who have no clinical evidence of ischaemia, generally have a low risk of cardiac complications from surgery. They may proceed without further testing, particularly if they are functionally very active and asymptomatic [5]. Ongoing cardiac conditions, for which the patient should undergo evaluation and treatment before vascular surgery, are unstable coronary syndromes, decompensated heart failure, significant arrhythmias, and severe valvular disease [5].

Specific pulmonary risk assessment

Pulmonary complications are as common as cardiac complications following vascular surgery [6]. The most significant of these are atelectasis, pneumonia, respiratory failure, and exacerbations of underlying chronic lung disease. All patients need to be clinically assessed for significant risk factors for postoperative pulmonary complications; i.e. chronic obstructive pulmonary disease, age older than 60 years, ASA class of II or greater, functionally dependent, and congestive heart failure [7]. A structured method involves the use of the postoperative pneumonia risk index [8] (Table 4). A major limitation of this index is the absence of arterial blood gas and spirometry values. Arterial blood gas analysis may be useful in patients with poor lung function and may reveal underlying respiratory failure.

From the history, physical examination, initial investigations and structured assessment of the individual's cardiorespiratory risk, a clear indication of their fitness for surgery should have been obtained. Additional pre-operative investigations to further define cardiorespiratory risk are only valid when they are likely to change the management plan for the patient and lead to a specific intervention.

Specific cardiac investigations

Transthoracic echocardiography

A high ejection fraction is associated with a low peri-operative cardiac risk, but a normal ejection fraction cannot exclude severe coronary artery disease. However, transthoracic echocardiography does play an important role in evaluating the severity of stenotic and regurgitant valvular lesions.

Table 4. Postoperative pneumonia index. *Arozullah AM, et al* [8].

Pre-operative risk factor	Point value
Type of surgery	
Abdominal aortic aneurysm repair	15
Thoracic	14
Upper abdominal	10
Neck	8
Neurosurgery	8
Vascular	3
Age	
>80 y	17
70-79 y	13
60-69 y	9
50-59 y	4
Functional status	
Totally dependent	10
Partially dependent	6
Weight loss >10% in past 6 months	7
History of COPD	5
General anaesthesia	4
Sensory impairment	4
History of cerebrovascular accident	4
Blood urea nitrogen level	
<2.86mmol/L (<8mg/dL)	4
7.85-10.7mmol/L (22-30mg/dL)	2
>10.7mmol/L (>30mg/dL)	3
Transfusion >4 units	3
Emergency surgery	3
Steroid use for chronic condition	3
Current smoker within 1 year	3
Alcohol intake >2 drinks/d in past 2 weeks	2
COPD = chronic obstructive pulmonary disease	

Exercise tolerance test

A meta-analysis of the reported studies using treadmill testing in vascular surgery patients shows a rather low sensitivity of 74%, and a specificity of 69%; these figures are comparable with daily clinical practice [9]. The positive predictive value (PPV) was as low at 10%, but the negative predictive value (NPV) was very high at 98%. The conclusion is that the exercise tolerance test has not yet been proven to be reliable.

Stress echocardiography

The heart can be stressed by exercise or pharmacologically. Since patients often have a limited exercise ability, pharmacological agents are more commonly used and have been proven to be safe and sensitive with a good NPV [10]. Dobutamine is a beta-receptor agonist which increases both heart rate and contractility and is the most common pharmacological agent used to stress the heart. In conjunction with echocardiography, stress-induced regional wall motion abnormalities and, therefore, myocardial ischaemia, may be determined. The mean sensitivity and specificity of a dobutamine stress test is 81% and 80%, whereas the PPV and NPV were 77% and 85%, respectively [10]. Nevertheless, this test is operator-dependent and should be avoided in patients with a history of ventricular tachyarrhythmia.

Myocardial perfusion imaging

Two agents, thallium 201 and technetium-99 sestamibi, are widely used for myocardial perfusion scanning. Images are usually obtained by single-photon emission computed tomography (SPECT) (Figure 1) [11]. Comparison of the myocardial distribution of the radiopharmacological agent after stress by exercise or pharmacologic agent, and at rest, provides information on myocardial viability, inducible perfusion abnormalities, and, when ECG gated imaging is used, global and regional myocardial function. The test can discriminate between regions of inducible ischaemia at risk for future myocardial infarction and areas that have already been irreversibly damaged by prior myocardial infarction. The mean sensitivity and specificity are 86% and 59%; the mean PPV and NPVs are 69% and 80% [10]. In contrast to dobutamine stress echocardiography, a positive result of myocardial perfusion imaging has a significantly lower prognostic value [12]. In addition, myocardial perfusion imaging exposes the patient to radiation.

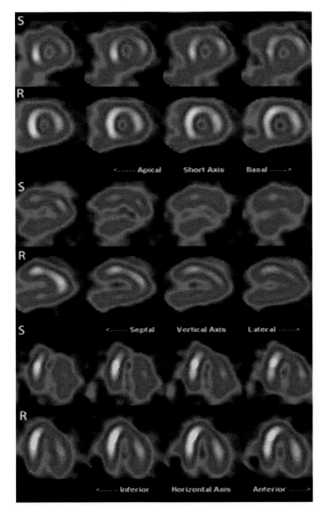
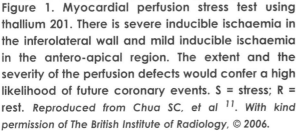

Figure 1. Myocardial perfusion stress test using thallium 201. There is severe inducible ischaemia in the inferolateral wall and mild inducible ischaemia in the antero-apical region. The extent and the severity of the perfusion defects would confer a high likelihood of future coronary events. S = stress; R = rest. *Reproduced from Chua SC, et al [11]. With kind permission of The British Institute of Radiology, © 2006.*

Cardiac computed tomography (CT) angiography

CT can be used to detect coronary calcium, which reflects coronary atherosclerosis (Figures 2 and 3) [13]. A meta-analysis using ischaemic heart disease detected by conventional coronary angiography as a reference, demonstrated a sensitivity and a specificity of 82% and 91% on a vessel basis (eight studies, 2726 vessels); on a patient basis (21 studies, 1570 patients), the sensitivity and specificity were 96% and 74% [14]. However, data in the setting of pre-operative risk stratification are lacking and, in addition, there are concerns of the risk of radiation.

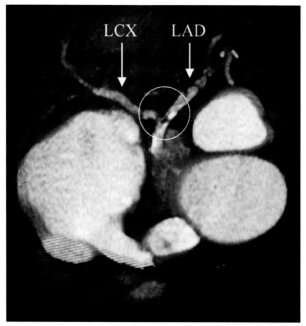

Figure 2. Volume-rendered CT angiogram shows a high-grade proximal left anterior descending coronary artery (LAD) lesion with a moderate- to low-grade stenosis of the proximal left circumflex artery (LCX) (lesion site circled). *Reproduced from Hoffmann MHK, et al [13]. Reprinted with permission from the American Journal of Roentgenology.*

Coronary angiography

There is a lack of evidence derived from randomised clinical trials on the usefulness of routine coronary angiography in patients scheduled for non-cardiac surgery. Coronary angiography is indicated for:

♦   patients with suspected or proven coronary artery disease (Figure 4);

♦   patients considered high risk from non-invasive testing, e.g. stress echocardiography, myocardial perfusion imaging, etc; angina pectoris unresponsive to medical therapy;

♦   patients with unstable angina pectoris;

♦   high-risk patients with a positive non-diagnostic or equivocal non-invasive test undergoing a high-risk procedure [5].

Coronary angiography should not be performed routinely in all vascular patients. In patients with known ischaemic heart disease, indications for pre-operative coronary angiography and revascularisation are similar to angiography indications in the non-surgical setting [5, 15].

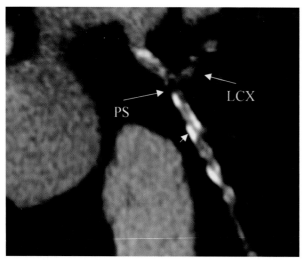

Figure 3. Corresponding curved planar reformation. The figure demonstrates fibrous plaque stenosis (PS), wall calcifications (short arrow) of the proximal LAD, and sectioned branch of the LCX. *Reproduced from Hoffmann MHK, et al [13]. Reprinted with permission from the American Journal of Roentgenology.*

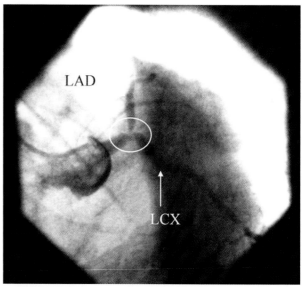

Figure 4. Corresponding conventional coronary catheterisation radiograph. This shows bifurcational stenosis (circle) in a spider view (left anterior oblique view caudally tilted). *Reproduced from Hoffmann MHK, et al [13]. Reprinted with permission from the American Journal of Roentgenology.*

Cardiopulmonary exercise testing (CPET)

CPET is a non-invasive test which provides objective assessment of both cardiac and pulmonary functions. The patient is exercised preferably on a bicycle ergometer, or a treadmill as an alternative, during which he/she breathes through a mouthpiece which is a minaturised pressure differential pneumotachygraph. The most commonly used data from this test are O_2 consumption at peak exercise (VO_{2peak}) (Figure 5) and at anaerobic threshold (VO_{2AT}), defined as the point when metabolic demands exceed oxygen delivery, and anaerobic metabolism begins to occur (Figure 6). The thresholds for classifying patients as low risk are

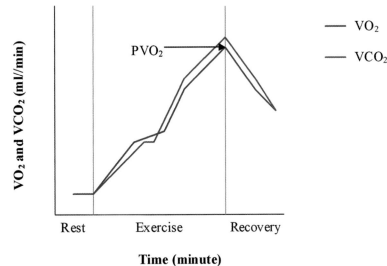

Figure 5. Determination of peak oxygen consumption. Progressive increase in VO_2 is noted in the initial first few minutes of exercise, reaching a peak (PVO_2) before commencement of the recovery period.

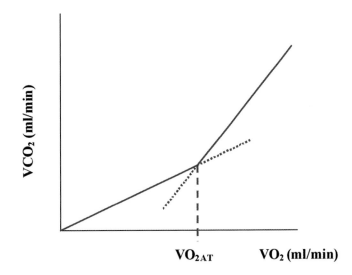

Figure 6. Determination of the anaerobic threshold. Anaerobic threshold (VO_{2AT}), defined as the point when metabolic demands exceed oxygen delivery, and anaerobic metabolism begins to occur, is represented in the graph by the point at which the slope of VCO_2 increases relative to VO_2 changes.

usually taken as VO_{2peak} >15mL/kg/min and VO_{2AT} >11mL/kg/min. These thresholds roughly equate to 4 METs [16]. Non-cardiac and non-respiratory factors such as skeletal muscle function and physical training can underestimate aerobic metabolic activity. A further consideration must be that CPET testing is not available in all centres. The role of CPET in pre-operative risk assessment is not yet conclusive and it should not yet be considered to be a substitute for stress testing in routine clinical practice [15].

Specific pulmonary investigations

Spirometry

Spirometry is one of the most common lung function tests and is used to measure the severity, type (restrictive/obstructive) and reversibility of respiratory disease. A forced expiratory volume in 1 second (FEV_1) of <70% predicted or a FEV_1/FVC (forced vital capacity) ratio of <65% indicates a high risk of peri-operative complications. There is a lack of evidence for the use of spirometry as a pre-operative assessment test in predicting risk effectively for individual patients. It is reserved mainly for patients who are thought to have undiagnosed chronic obstructive pulmonary disease [7].

Chest X-ray

Chest X-ray (CXR) is not routinely indicated except in the likelihood of admission to an intensive care unit or for patients with suspected malignancy or tuberculosis [17]. They may also be requested for dyspnoeic patients, those with known cardiac disease and the very elderly. Many patients with cardio-respiratory disease who have a recent CXR available do not need a repeat [17].

Serum albumin

A low serum albumin level (<35g/L) is a powerful marker of increased risk for postoperative pulmonary complications. It should be measured in all patients who are clinically suspected of having hypoalbuminaemia and measurement should be considered in patients with one or more risk factors for peri-operative pulmonary complications [7]. A guideline from the American College of Physicians reported postoperative pulmonary complication rates according to serum albumin level by using a threshold of 36g/L to define low levels. It found that the postoperative pulmonary complication rates for patients with low and normal serum albumin levels were 27.6% and 7% [7].

Cardiorespiratory risk reduction strategies

Cardiac risk reduction

Pharmacological

Beta-blocker medication

The rationale for using beta-blocker medications peri-operatively is to decrease myocardial oxygen consumption by decreasing myocardial contractility and heart rate. The evidence suggests that peri-operative beta-blocker therapy effectively reduces cardiovascular morbidity and mortality among patients with clinical risk factors undergoing major vascular surgery [18]. Meta-analyses gave consistent results showing a significant reduction in peri-operative myocardial ischaemia, myocardial infarction, and cardiac mortality in patients receiving beta-blockers [19, 20]. However, there were concerns on hypotension and bradycardia resulting in stroke and death, as highlighted in the Peri-Operative Ischemic Evaluation (POISE) trial [21]. Vascular surgery patients treated with beta-blockers should be monitored carefully during the peri-operative period to avoid adverse consequences of overtreatment. A recent review of data by Bauer *et al* indicated that initiation of treatment should begin at the first patient encounter in high-risk patients and selected intermediate-risk patients [22]. Bauer *et al* [22] also recommended the use of beta-1 selective agents with a longer half-life and suggested a 2.5-5mg fixed dose of bisoprolol in intermediate-risk patients as it is likely to achieve long-term effects. By contrast, upward dosage titration is indicated in patients at high risk for myocardial ischaemia in order to achieve a desired heart rate. For these patients, bisoprolol should be started 30 days before vascular surgery and a higher systolic blood pressure threshold of 120mmHg is appropriate to lower the dose or stop upward titration when trying to achieve a therapeutic heart rate of around 70 beats/minute [22]. Current data do not support the peri-operative use of these agents among patients at low cardiac risk [18].

Statin medications

3-Hydroxy-3-methylglutaryl co-enzyme A (3-HMG-CoA) reductase inhibitors, more commonly known as statins, have a lipid-lowering effect as well as pleiotropic effects of inducing atherosclerotic plaque stabilization, thus, preventing plaque rupture and subsequent myocardial infarction. There is strong evidence from randomised controlled trials and large retrospective studies that statins have beneficial effects in reducing cardiovascular events after vascular surgery [23, 24]. The use of statins has been widely accepted by vascular surgeons for secondary prevention and cardiac risk reduction. Statins with a long half-life, or extended-release formulations such as atorvastatin and fluvastatin, are recommended [15, 22], and treatment should be commenced as early as possible, preferably 30 days before their procedure. In addition, these patients should be maintained on statins for life, providing no adverse effects are noted (muscle weakness, hepatic dysfunction etc.).

Antiplatelet therapy

Antiplatelet therapy is widely prescribed to vascular patients with concomitant coronary artery disease and as best medical treatment of peripheral vascular disease. In a review by Bauer *et al*, antiplatelet therapy has been shown to reduce the risk of cardiovascular events in patients with coronary artery disease. Low-dose aspirin is just as effective as high-dose aspirin therapy in decreasing the combined endpoint of vascular death, myocardial infarction and stroke [25, 26]. However, specific evidence of benefit for the use of aspirin in the peri-operative setting is limited [15]. The concern is that peri-operative bleeding may be associated with the use of antiplatelet therapy and it should, therefore, only be discontinued if the risk of bleeding outweighs the cardiac benefits [15]. For patients receiving antiplatelet therapy, i.e. aspirin, clopidogrel, or both, with excessive or life-threatening peri-operative bleeding, transfusion of platelets and/or administration of other prohaemostatic agents is recommended [15].

Alpha-2 agonist medication

Alpha-2 agonists are centrally-acting sympatholytic vasodilators which are occasionally used to treat hypertension. There is some evidence that alpha-2 agonist therapy can reduce cardiovascular events in vascular surgery [27]. Fluid retention and oedema are problems associated with chronic therapy and sudden discontinuation of alpha-2 agonists can lead to rebound hypertension due to excessive sympathetic activity.

Calcium channel blocker medication

The favourable effect of calcium channel blockers on the balance between myocardial oxygen supply and demand makes them theoretically suitable for risk reduction strategies. However, it is necessary to distinguish between dihydropyridines that do not act directly on heart rate and diltiazem or verapamil that lower the heart rate. Calcium channel blockers significantly reduce ischaemia and supraventricular tachycardia and are associated with a trend toward reduced rates of death and myocardial infarction [28]. Although heart rate-reducing calcium channel blockers are not indicated in patients with heart failure and systolic dysfunction, in patients who have contra-indications to beta-blockers, the continuation or the introduction of heart rate-reducing calcium channel blockers may be considered [15].

Pre-operative coronary revascularisation

Coronary angiography and revascularisation before non-cardiac surgery [5] is indicated for patients with stable angina who have:

◆ significant left main coronary artery stenosis;
◆ three-vessel disease (survival benefit is greater when left ventricular ejection fraction <0.50);
◆ two-vessel disease with a significant proximal left anterior descending stenosis and either an ejection fraction <0.50 or a demonstrable ischaemia on non-invasive evaluation.

Coronary revascularisation is also recommended in patients with unstable angina or non-ST-segment elevation myocardial infarction, or with acute ST-elevation myocardial infarction. It is not routinely indicated in patients with stable coronary artery disease [5]. Several randomised trials have shown that pre-operative coronary artery revascularisation before elective major vascular surgery does not alter the long-term outcome in patients with stable coronary artery disease. Furthermore, pre-operative percutaneous coronary intervention does not reduce the risk of death, myocardial infarction, or other major cardiovascular events when added to optimal medical therapy [29].

A coronary stent is used in most percutaneous revascularisation procedures. In this case, further delay in non-cardiac surgery may be beneficial. Elective non-cardiac surgery is not recommended within 4-6 weeks of bare-metal coronary stent implantation, within 12 months of drug-eluting coronary stent implantation, or in patients who need to discontinue thienopyridine therapy (e.g. clopidrogel, ticlopidine) or aspirin and thienopyridine therapy peri-operatively [5]. Discontinuing antiplatelet therapy may cause acute stent thrombosis with very high morbidity and mortality.

Pulmonary risk reduction

Pre-operative smoking cessation

Periods of at least 4 weeks of smoking cessation decrease the incidence of postoperative respiratory complications [30].

Lung expansion modalities

Lung expansion modalities include incentive spirometry, chest physical therapy, including deep breathing exercises, cough, postural drainage, percussion and vibration, suctioning and ambulation, intermittent positive-pressure breathing, and continuous positive-airway pressure. The available evidence suggests that for patients undergoing abdominal surgery, any type of lung expansion intervention is better than no prophylactic intervention; however, no one modality is superior [7]. Incentive spirometry may be the least labour-intensive. However, nasal continuous positive-airway pressure may be especially beneficial in patients who are unable to perform incentive spirometry or deep breathing exercises [7].

Analgesic techniques

Postoperative epidural pain management seems superior to other routes of opioid analgesia delivery in preventing postoperative pulmonary complications [7]. Nevertheless, the frequent use of heparin in vascular surgery contributes to the risk of epidural haemorrhage and may influence decisions against this method of analgesia.

Surgical techniques

Evidence is lacking comparing pulmonary complications in different types of vascular operations; however, as vascular surgery becomes ever increasingly less invasive and the procedures can be undertaken without the need for long general anaesthetics, it is likely that this will reduce respiratory complications.

Nutritional support, pulmonary artery catheterisation, and nasogastric tube decompression

There is no strong evidence to suggest a significant role of nutritional support, pulmonary artery catheterisation and routine use of nasogastric tube decompression in reducing pulmonary complications in vascular surgery.

Early identification and treatment of postoperative cardiorespiratory complications

Vascular surgical patients require close monitoring which mandates that they be triaged to the appropriate postoperative care environment to enable early identification and treatment of complications. This is frequently influenced by a patient's comorbidity and peri-operative haemodynamic stability.

Cardiac complications

Myocardial infarction is the most common cause of morbidity and mortality following major vascular surgery. The majority of MIs in postoperative vascular patients are asymptomatic. A high index of suspicion is required for diagnosis, based on clinical examination and ECG findings. An increase in postoperative cardiac troponin I is consistent with a cardiac event and is associated with increased mortality. Such postoperative cardiac events can be categorised into non-ST elevated myocardial infarction and ST elevated myocardial infarction. Most postoperative vascular patients are diagnosed with non-ST elevated myocardial infarction, manifesting as ST-segment depression on the ECG.

Generally, the initial treatment of non-ST elevated myocardial infarction includes medical stabilization and risk stratification, whereas, ST elevated myocardial infarction requires acute reperfusion therapy with fibrinolytic agents or percutaneous coronary intervention. Fibrinolytic therapy is not currently recommended in non-ST elevated myocardial infarction and in fact may be detrimental. The treatment options for postoperative MI are limited by the risk of surgical site bleeding in the early postoperative period.

Respiratory complications

Postoperative respiratory complications include atelectasis, bronchopneumonia, bronchospasm and respiratory failure. The factors contributing to postoperative respiratory complications are related to the patient's prior health status and the effects of surgery and anaesthesia.

Early postoperative respiratory complications are suspected on clinical findings, arterial blood gas analysis, sputum specimens for microscopy, culture and sensitivity, chest X-ray and ECG. Active treatment is encouraged, with a combination of antibiotics, chest physiotherapy, and mechanical ventilatory support as indicated. When acute postoperative respiratory failure develops, non-invasive continuous positive airway pressure is the recommended first-line treatment in order to avoid re-intubation. Invasive mechanical ventilation may be required if respiratory failure progresses and/or there is evidence of acute lung injury.

Conclusions

Not all patients undergoing vascular surgery need extensive pre-operative investigations. Clinical risk factors alone may identify intermediate- or low-risk patients and they should be simply optimised with medical therapy. The decision to recommend further testing for the individual patient has to take into consideration the estimated probabilities of effectiveness versus risk. High-risk patients, as defined by the Lee index [4], should be considered for stress testing with the intention to identify patients at increased risk for myocardial ischaemia induced by the stress response of vascular surgery. Similarly, risks factors for pulmonary complications can be identified clinically and by using the postoperative pneumonia index and low serum albumin as predictors for pulmonary complications. The information can be used to intensify medical therapy and possibly modify the operative approach to avoid high-risk surgery in favour of less invasive procedures.

Key points

Pre-operative assessment
- Clinical history, examination, basic laboratory tests and data stratification identify those at risk of cardiopulmonary morbidity during vascular surgical intervention:
  - the inability to climb two flights of stairs or run a short distance (<4 METs) indicates poor functional capacity and is associated with increased postoperative cardiac events;
  - the Lee cardiac risk index is the best currently available cardiac risk prediction index in non-cardiac surgery;
  - a low serum albumin level (<35g/L) is a powerful marker of increased risk for postoperative pulmonary complications.
- Investigations to further define cardiorespiratory risk are only valid if likely to change the planned management and lead to a specific intervention.

Pre-operative intervention
- Statins with a long half-life or extended-release formulations are recommended.
- Antiplatelets should only be discontinued if the risk of bleeding outweighs the cardiac benefits.
- Elective vascular surgery is not recommended within 4-6 weeks of bare-metal coronary stent implantation or within 12 months of drug-eluting coronary stent implantation.
- Patients should stop smoking 6 weeks before surgery.
- Lung expansion modalities and analgesic techniques reduce postoperative pulmonary complications.

References

1. McFalls EO, Ward HB, Santilli S, *et al*. The influence of perioperative myocardial infarction on long-term prognosis following elective vascular surgery. *Chest* 1998; 113: 681-6.

2. Guideline Development Group. Pre-operative tests - the use of routine pre-operative tests for elective surgery. National Institute for Clinical Excellence (NICE) Guidelines, 2003.

3. Reilly DF, McNeely MJ, Doerner D, *et al*. Self-reported exercise tolerance and the risk of serious perioperative complications. *Arch Intern Med* 1999; 159(18): 2185-92.

4. Lee TH, Marcantonio ER, Mangione CM, *et al*. Derivation and prospective validation of a simple index for prediction of cardiac risk of major noncardiac surgery. *Circulation* 1999; 100(10): 1043-9.

5. Fleisher LA, Beckman JA, Brown KA, *et al*. ACC/AHA 2007 Guidelines on Perioperative Cardiovascular Evaluation and Care for Noncardiac Surgery: Executive Summary: A Report of the American College of Cardiology/American Heart Association Task Force on Practice Guidelines (Writing Committee to Revise the 2002 Guidelines on Perioperative Cardiovascular Evaluation for Noncardiac Surgery) Developed in Collaboration With the American Society of Echocardiography, American Society of Nuclear Cardiology, Heart Rhythm Society, Society of Cardiovascular Anesthesiologists, Society for Cardiovascular Angiography and Interventions, Society for Vascular Medicine and Biology, and Society for Vascular Surgery. *J Am Coll Cardiol* 2007; 50(17): 1707-32.

6. Fleischmann KE, Goldman L, Young B, *et al*. Association between cardiac and noncardiac complications in patients undergoing noncardiac surgery: outcomes and effects on length of stay. *Am J Med* 2003; 115: 515-20.

7. Qaseem A, Snow V, Fitterman N, *et al*. Risk assessment for and strategies to reduce perioperative pulmonary complications for patients undergoing noncardiothoracic surgery: a guideline from the American College of Physicians. *Ann Intern Med* 2006; 144: 575-80.

8. Arozullah AM, Khuri SF, Henderson WG, *et al*. Development and validation of a multifactorial risk index for predicting postoperative pneumonia after major noncardiac surgery. *Ann Intern Med* 2001; 135(10): 847-57.

9. Kertai MD, Boersma E, Bax JJ, *et al*. A meta-analysis comparing the prognostic accuracy of six diagnostic tests for predicting perioperative cardiac risk in patients undergoing major vascular surgery. *Heart* 2003; 89(11): 1327-34.

10. Bax JJ, Poldermans D, Elhendy A, *et al*. Sensitivity, specificity, and predictive accuracies of various noninvasive techniques for detecting hibernating myocardium. *Curr Probl Cardiol* 2001; 26: 147-86.

11. Chua SC, Ganatra RH, Green DJ, Groves AM. Nuclear cardiology: myocardial perfusion imaging with SPECT and PET. *Imaging* 2006; 18: 166-77.

12. Kertai MD, Boersma E, Sicari R, *et al*. Which stress test is superior for perioperative cardiac risk stratification in patients undergoing major vascular surgery? *Eur J Vasc Endovasc Surg* 2002; 24: 222-9.

13. Hoffmann MHK, Shi H, Schmid FT, *et al*. Noninvasive coronary imaging with MDCT in comparison to invasive conventional coronary angiography: a fast-developing technology. *AJR* 2004; 182: 601-8.

14. Hamon M, Biondi-Zoccai GG, Malagutti P, *et al*. Diagnostic performance of multislice spiral computed tomography of coronary arteries as compared with conventional invasive coronary angiography: a meta-analysis. *J Am Coll Cardiol* 2006; 48: 1896-910.

15. Poldermans D, Bax JJ, Boersma E, *et al*. Guidelines for pre-operative cardiac risk assessment and perioperative cardiac management in non-cardiac surgery: the Task Force for Preoperative Cardiac Risk Assessment and Perioperative Cardiac Management in Non-cardiac Surgery of the European Society of Cardiology (ESC) and European Society of Anaesthesiology (ESA). *Eur Heart J* 2009; 30(22): 2769-812.

16. Reilly CS. Can we accurately assess an individual's perioperative risk? *Br J Anaesth* 2008; 101: 747-9.

17. The Royal College of Radiologists. Making the Best Use of a Department of Clinical Radiology. Guidelines for Doctors, 4th ed. London: The Royal College of Radiologists, 1998.

18. Brooke BS. Perioperative beta-blockers for vascular surgery patients. *J Vasc Surg* 2010; 51: 515-9.

19. Bangalore S, Wetterslev J, Pranesh S, *et al*. Perioperative beta blockers in patients having non-cardiac surgery: a meta-analysis. *Lancet* 2008; 372(9654): 1962-76.

20. Wiesbauer F, Schlager O, Domanovits H, *et al*. Perioperative beta-blockers for preventing surgery-related mortality and morbidity: a systematic review and meta-analysis. *Anesth Analg* 2007; 104: 27-41.

21. Devereaux PJ, Yang H, Yusuf S, *et al*. Effects of extended-release metoprolol succinate in patients undergoing non-cardiac surgery (POISE trial): a randomised controlled trial. *Lancet* 2008; 371(9627): 1839-47.

22. Bauer SM, Cayne NS, Veith FJ. New developments in the preoperative evaluation and perioperative management of coronary artery disease in patients undergoing vascular surgery. *J Vasc Surg* 2010; 51: 242-51.

23. O'Neil-Callahan K, Katsimaglis G, Tepper MR, *et al*. Statins decrease perioperative cardiac complications in patients undergoing noncardiac vascular surgery: the Statins for Risk Reduction in Surgery (StaRRS) study. *J Am Coll Cardiol* 2005; 45: 336-42.

24. Schouten O, Boersma E, Hoeks SE, *et al*. Fluvastatin and perioperative events in patients undergoing vascular surgery. *N Engl J Med* 2009; 361(10): 980-9.

25. Sillesen H. What does 'best medical therapy' really mean? *Eur J Vasc Endovasc Surg* 2008; 35: 139-44.

26. Taylor DW, Barnett HJ, Haynes RB, *et al*. Low-dose and high-dose acetylsalicylic acid for patients undergoing carotid endarterectomy: a randomised controlled trial. ASA and Carotid Endarterectomy (ACE) Trial Collaborators. *Lancet* 1999; 353(9171): 2179-84.

27. Wijeysundera DN, Naik JS, Beattie WS. Alpha-2 adrenergic agonists to prevent perioperative cardiovascular complications: a meta-analysis. *Am J Med* 2003; 114: 742-52.

28. Wijeysundera DN, Beattie WS. Calcium channel blockers for reducing cardiac morbidity after noncardiac surgery: a meta-analysis. *Anesth Analg* 2003; 97: 634-41.

29. Boden WE, O'Rourke RA, Teo KK, *et al*. Optimal medical therapy with or without PCI for stable coronary disease. *N Engl J Med* 2007; 356(15): 1503-16.

30. Mills E, Eyawo O, Lockhart I, *et al*. Smoking cessation reduces postoperative complications: a systematic review and meta-analysis. *Am J Med* 2011; 124: 144-54.

Chapter 3

Prevention and management of renal complications in vascular surgery

Perbinder Grewal MBBS MRCS (Ed) FRCS (Gen Surg), Senior Vascular Fellow
George Hamilton MD FRCS FRCS (Glas), Professor of Vascular Surgery
Royal Free Hospital, London, UK

Introduction

Acute kidney injury (AKI) is a spectrum of renal impairment ranging from early injury to advanced kidney failure. Clinically, AKI results in a rapid reduction in renal function commencing with oliguria, anuria and/or biochemical abnormalities. This is often accompanied by significant morbidity and mortality [1]. A recent clarification of the definition and classification of AKI has been proposed (Kidney Diseases: Improving Global Outcomes [2], Table 1).

AKI secondary to vascular surgery can be multifactorial and depends on the type of surgery performed and/or the type of contrast injected (Table 2).

The incidence of renal failure after abdominal aortic aneurysm (AAA) surgery is 2-7%, and after thoraco-abdominal aneurysm surgery as high as 15-50%. This is predominantly the result of renal hypoperfusion and ischaemia. Renal failure complicating aortic surgery is associated with mortality rates from 50-90% [3].

Table 1. Staging of acute kidney injury.

Stage	Serum creatinine (SCr) criteria	Urine output criteria
1	SCr increase ≥26µmol/L or SCr increase ≥1.5- to 2-fold from baseline	<0.5ml/kg/hour for >6 consecutive hours
2	SCr increase ≥2 to 3-fold from baseline	<0.5ml/kg/hour for >12 hours
3	SCr increase ≥3-fold from baseline or SCr increase 354µmol/L or Commenced on renal replacement therapy (RRT) irrespective of stage	<0.3ml/kg/hour for >24 hours or anuria for 12 hours

Table 2. Causes of AKI in vascular and endovascular surgery.

Patient-related	Procedure-related
Comorbidity	Long clamp time in open AAA surgery
Nephrotoxic medication (NSAIDs, ACE inhibitor)	Contrast media used (non-ionic versus ionic)
Previous kidney disease	Hypotension
Hypovolaemia	Hypothermia
Poor nutritional status	Sepsis

NSAIDs = non-steroidal anti-inflammatory drugs; ACE = angiotensin-converting enzyme

Chronic kidney disease

Prior chronic kidney disease is a major risk factor in developing AKI. Chronic kidney disease is defined as a glomerular filtration rate (GFR) less than 60ml/minute/1.73m^2 for 3 or more months. The National Kidney Foundation: Kidney Disease Outcome Quality Initiative proposed a definition and staging for chronic kidney disease to allow stratification for risk (Table 3) [4].

Serum creatinine is a poor biomarker for kidney function [5]. It takes several hours for creatinine to rise after a reduction in renal function. The GFR is considered to be the most accurate measure of the filtering capacity of the kidneys. A low GFR is a good indicator of poor renal function. Estimated GFR (eGFR) provides a more accurate and convenient measure of kidney function than serum creatinine alone, but it is important to understand that this measurement is only an estimate and does have limitations.

The Modification of Diet in Renal Disease (MDRD) multicentre trial developed an equation to predict GFR from serum creatinine levels [6]. The GFR was

Table 3. Staging of acute kidney injury.

Stage	Description	GFR (ml/min/1.73m^2)
1	Normal GFR with other evidence of chronic kidney damage	>90
2	Mild impairment with other evidence of chronic kidney damage	60-89
3	Moderate impairment	30-59
4	Severe impairment	15-29
5	Established renal failure (ERF) on dialysis	<15

measured using ^{125}I-iothalamate renal clearance and creatinine clearance was calculated from a 24-hour urine collection and plasma creatinine. Stepwise logistic regression analysis determined the variables that best predicted GFR. This was expressed as an equation, which was later adjusted to the reference isotope-dilution mass spectrometry method [7].

Equation:

MDRD eGFR = 175 x [Plasma Creatinine (μmol/L) x 0.0011312] $^{-1.154}$
x [age (years)]$^{-0.203}$
x [0.742 if female] x [1.212 if black]

The MDRD equation has been validated in diabetic, renal transplant and African-American patients with renal disease. It has not been validated in children under 18 years old, pregnancy, patients over 70 years of age and in ethnic groups other than African-Americans. It has also not been validated in obese and slim individuals. The MDRD formula performs poorly in people with a low plasma creatinine [8].

Contrast-induced acute kidney injury

Contrast-induced AKI, formerly known as contrast-induced nephropathy, occurs 48-72 hours after the intravascular administration of iodinated contrast media and usually recovers over 5 days. It is associated with an increased duration of hospital stay, and short- and long-term morbidity and mortality [9]. Contrast agents used in vascular and endovascular imaging and surgery are either iodine-based (iodinated) or gadolinium-based.

Iodinated contrast agents

The incidence of contrast-induced AKI correlates with the volume of iodinated contrast given, the type of contrast, the osmolality (Table 4) and viscosity of the contrast agent.

These agents are water-soluble derivatives of tri-iodinated benzoic acid and can be monomeric (contain one benzene ring) or dimeric (two benzene rings). Once in solution these agents can be sub-divided into ionic (forms charged moieties) or non-ionic (forms neutral moieties). These classes possess different properties. For example, non-ionic monomers have higher osmolality and lower viscosity than non-ionic dimers (Table 4).

The viscosity of contrast agents depends on the iodine concentration within the solution. Viscosity increases exponentially as a function of concentration and as such increases during renal excretion as part of the concentration process in the renal tubules.

Table 4. Osmolality of iodinated contrast agents compared to plasma.	
	Osmolality (mOsm/kg)
Plasma	275-299
Iso-osmolar (non-ionic) – iodixanol (Visipaque™), iopamidol (Ultravist®), iohexol (Omnipaque™), iopromide (Isovue®)	400-750
Low osmolar (ionic) – ioxaglate (Hexabrix®)	600-850
High osmolar (ionic) – iothalamate (Conray®), diatrizoate (Hypaque®)	1500-1800

Pathophysiology

There are two possible mechanisms whereby contrast media cause acute kidney injury, which have complementary effects:

- contrast is directly toxic to the renal tubule cell, causing mitochondrial dysfunction, generation of reactive oxygen species and apoptosis [10-11];
- contrast is hyperosmolar compared to plasma causing rapid shifts of water from renal cells into the vasculature resulting in vasodilation to compensate for the increased volume. There is a compensatory release of vasoconstrictors which reduces medullary blood flow, specifically to the loop of Henle [12], resulting in natriuresis, increased oxygen demand, release of nitric oxide and prostaglandins. Overall, this results in intense renal vasoconstriction (possibly via adenosine and endothelin) resulting in reduced blood flow, reduced GFR and medullary ischaemia.

Risk factors (Table 5)

The recognition of high-risk groups is a very important part of the strategy to prevent contrast-induced AKI. Chronic kidney disease is a major risk factor: a baseline serum creatinine of 177-256μmol/L and >256μmol/L is associated with a seven-fold and 12-fold risk of contrast-induced AKI, respectively [13]. Diabetes mellitus is associated with a five-fold risk. The hyperosmolarity of the contrast is also clinically important in patients with heart failure and appropriate measures must be taken.

Strategies to prevent contrast-induced AKI

The main priority is to identify patients at high risk and assess whether the imaging modality is absolutely necessary or whether an alternative is available, e.g. MR angiography with gadolinium, or an alternative such as carbon dioxide (Figure 1).

Table 5. Risk factors for contrast-induced AKI.

Patient-related	Procedure-related
Chronic kidney disease	Volume of contrast
Diabetes mellitus	Osmolality of contrast
Hypovolaemia	Viscosity of contrast
Chronic heart failure	
Hypertension	
Age	
Myocardial infarction	
Left ventricular ejection fraction <40%	

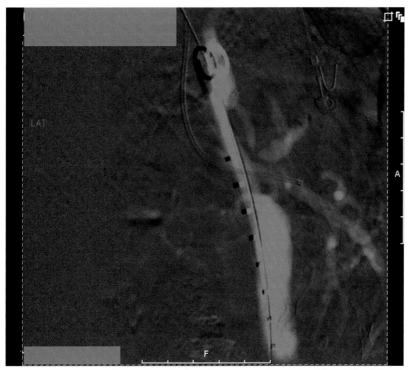

Figure 1. CO_2 angiography during fenestrated EVAR. This patient had stage IV renal impairment pre-operatively. Total contrast load was 30ml Visipaque™, and his renal function was unchanged after the procedure.

If there is no alternative then strategies need to be used to reduce the risk. Potentially nephrotoxic medication should be withheld. Non-steroidal anti-inflammatory agents inhibit prostaglandins in the kidney, increasing the risk of vasoconstriction associated with iodinated contrast [14]. These drugs should be stopped 10-14 days before, and for 3-5 days after the procedure.

Metformin is a biguanide that reduces blood sugar levels. Its precise mechanism of action in unknown but its predecessor, phenformin, was withdrawn from clinical practice in 1978 for a strong causal association with lactic acidosis [15]. Metformin-associated metabolic acidosis is a serious side effect and may be associated with a mortality of 50% [16]. Metformin is not nephrotoxic but is exclusively excreted by the kidneys, thus it may accumulate in renal impairment, and there is a theoretical risk of lactic acidosis after contrast administration.

The Royal College of Radiologists recommends stopping metformin for 48 hours after the procedure if the serum creatinine is greater than normal, or the eGFR is less than 60, after discussion with the referring physician [17].

Contrast-related strategies

If there is no alternative to iodinated contrast, then the dose must be minimised and given in a single episode. No further contrast should be administered until full recovery of renal function, and the serum creatinine should be checked 48-72 hours after the procedure.

A meta-analysis from 1993 suggested nephrotoxicity was reduced with low osmolar compared to high osmolar contrast agents [18]. This was confirmed in a prospective randomised trial 2 years later, where iohexol, a low osmolar agent, was compared to diatrizoate, a high osmolar agent [19]. A recent meta-analysis involving 16 trials and 2463 patients showed an increased risk of contrast-induced AKI with ioxaglate and iohexol comparing low and iso-osmolar agents [20]. Based on this, the American

College of Cardiology/American Heart Association Guidelines advocate the use of iso-osmolar or low-osmolar contrast other than iohexol and ioxaglate in patients with chronic kidney disease who need angiography [21].

Overall, it is safer to use non-ionic contrast agents than ionic agents. Unfortunately, non-ionic agents are more expensive and tend to be reserved for patients with renal impairment and contrast hypersensitivity.

Pharmacological strategies (Figure 2)

Hydration with intravenous fluids

Increasing the intravascular volume with intravenous fluids reduces vasoconstriction caused by iodinated contrast agents by inhibiting vasopressin secretion, inhibiting the renin-angiotensin axis, and increasing prostaglandins [22]. This reduces the concentration and viscosity of the contrast, thereby reducing the direct toxic effects on the renal tubule cells.

Intravenous saline undoubtedly works in the reduction of AKI; 0.9% normal saline 1mg/kg/hour

for 12 hours pre- and post-procedure is superior to 0.45% saline [23].

Sodium bicarbonate

Sodium bicarbonate is an anti-oxidant and scavenges reactive free radicals, which play an important role in AKI [24]. An isotonic bicarbonate infusion of 3ml/kg/hour for 1 hour before the procedure and 1ml/kg/hour for 6 hours afterwards is better than saline alone [25]. There have, however, also been many negative trials and a large RCT (Evaluation of Sodium Bicarbonate to Reduce the Incidence of Contrast-Induced Chronic Kidney Injury in Patients with Kidney Disease [BOSS]) is underway, with results expected in late 2011 [26].

N-acetylcysteine (NAC)

NAC scavenges oxygen free radicals, reduces the depletion of glutathione and stimulates the production of vasodilator mediators, such as nitric oxide. Administration of NAC has been shown to protect the renal tubule from apoptosis in animal models [27]. A benefit has been shown for NAC given intravenously in cardiac imaging, but not in patients undergoing angiography for peripheral vascular disease [28]. Since two meta-analyses have now shown no advantage

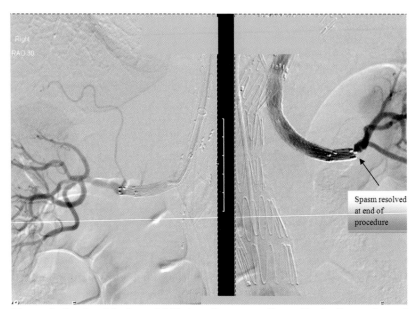

Figure 2. Contrast-induced AKI despite precautions. Illustrations of renal artery stenting during branched EVAR for a 7cm thoraco-abdominal aneurysm. This patient developed stage I AKI due to contrast load (250ml Omnipaque™) despite prehydration, N-acetylcysteine and intravenous sodium bicarbonate.

with the use of NAC for prevention of AKI [29-30], many clinicians have stopped using NAC unless further evidence becomes available.

Atrial natriuretic peptide (ANP)

ANP is secreted by cardiac myocytes and increases GFR and renal medullary blood flow [31]. It has been shown to improve renal function in AKI [32]. A recent single-centre, randomised trial, in 254 patients with chronic kidney disease undergoing coronary angiography, suggested that intravenous ANP and normal saline slightly reduced the rise in serum creatinine compared to normal saline alone [33]. It did not reduce rates of subsequent dialysis or heart failure. Further large controlled studies are needed to define any potential benefits from ANP administration.

Statins

Statins have anti-oxidant and anti-inflammatory properties and also positively affect endothelial function. Two studies by the same group showed improved creatinine levels, reduced length of stay, reduced rates of acute renal failure and reduced rates of dialysis with the use of statins [34-35]. Unfortunately, two other controlled trials reported no benefit in the prevention of acute kidney injury with statins [36-37]. They do, however, reduce long-term morbidity and mortality from cardiac adverse events after vascular procedures [38]. They also improve cardiovascular outcomes in diabetic patients undergoing angiography [39]. Thus, overall, statins should be recommended in these patients, particularly if they have other cardiovascular risk factors.

Prostaglandin/prostacyclin analogues

Vasodilation modulated via PGI2 and PGE2 receptors attenuated the severe vasoconstriction associated with iodinated contrast in an animal model [40]. A recent randomised study that included 208 patients with chronic kidney disease undergoing coronary angiography showed a reduction in rates of contrast-induced AKI with iloprost (8%) compared with placebo (25%) [41].

Fenoldopam

Fenoldopam is a selective dopamine A1-receptor agonist, which reduces vascular resistance and increases renal blood flow to the cortex and medulla [42]. Several small studies have been performed, with subsequent meta-analysis, showing a reduced need for renal replacement therapy and reduced mortality in AKI [43]. It remains unproven whether the reduced vascular resistance in the renal bed produced by this agent is clinically relevant.

Contrast allergy

Contrast anaphylaxis can cause acute bronchospasm, hypotension and urticaria and can be life-threatening. It can occur without previous exposure to contrast. Many patients with a supposed contrast allergy are not allergic but have had a reaction to the contrast, e.g. flushing, pain, nausea and vomiting. Caution is, however, needed when this history is present.

Recommendations to prevent contrast reactions are:

- use the smallest amount of contrast necessary;
- where there is a genuine possibility of an allergy, the procedure should be covered with intravenous hydrocortisone and loratadine (a non-sedating antihistamine);
- use non-ionic, low-osmolality agents as these are associated with fewer adverse reactions;
- consider alternative agents (gadolinium, carbon dioxide);
- if anaphylaxis occurs then adrenaline should be given as an intramuscular injection 500μg, i.e. 0.5ml of 1mg/ml (1 in 1000), repeated every 5 minutes, if necessary.

Nephrogenic systemic fibrosis (NSF) due to gadolinium

Adverse events with gadolinium are uncommon (0.46%) [44]. However, gadolinium administration in patients with severe renal impairment occasionally causes NSF [45] (200 known cases) with mortality reported at 28% [46]. More recently, studies have shown that macrocyclic chelates of gadolinium-based contrast agents have reduced risk of NSF [47]. Macrocyclic chelates of gadolinium are caged in the cavity of the ligand as opposed to linear (open-chain) chelates. Macrocyclic chelates are more stable thermodynamically and kinetically.

GFR:	>60 CKD 1/2	45-59 CKD3A	30-44 CKD 3B	15-29 CKD 4	Dialysis CKD 5
Table 6. Indicat...					
Iodinated	Safe	Small risk	High risk	High risk	Safe
Gadolinium	Safe	Low/medium risk	Low/medium risk	Low risk only	Contra-indicated

Table 6. Indications for iodinated versus gadolinium contrast agents.

In 2010, the Medicines & Healthcare products Regulatory Agency (MHRA) produced guidelines on the use of gadolinium-based agents for patients with chronic kidney disease, based on the European Committee for Medicinal Products for Human Use (CHMP) guidance [48]. They classified gadolinium agents into high, medium and low risk for NSF. Their recommendations are:

- patients with severe renal impairment, a GFR <30, should only receive low-risk or medium-risk agents, with no repeat contrast within 7 days;
  - low-risk agents (macrocyclic compounds): gadobutrol (Gadovist®), gadoteridol (ProHance®), gadoteric acid (Dotarem®);
  - medium-risk agents (linear chelates): gadobenic acid (MultiHance®), gadoxetic acid (Primovist®), gadofosveset (Vasovist®);
- patients with moderate renal impairment can receive the high-risk gadolinium-based contrast agents only if absolutely necessary in a single, lowest dose:
  - high-risk agents: gadodiamide (Omniscan™), gadoversetamide (OptiMARK™), gadopentetic acid (Magnevist®).

Adherence to these guidelines is recommended, but the blanket ban on the use of gadolinium in acute or chronic kidney disease is no longer justified. In patients allergic to iodinated agents, gadolinium-based agents are a useful alternative (Table 6).

Renal failure after aortic surgery

The risk of AKI after endovascular surgery is largely related to the exposure to contrast agents, as described above. Open aortic surgery is associated with additional haemodynamic disturbances, which can result in AKI (Table 7). These other factors are the reason that the development of AKI after open aneurysm repair is less clearly related to pre-operative serum creatinine levels [49].

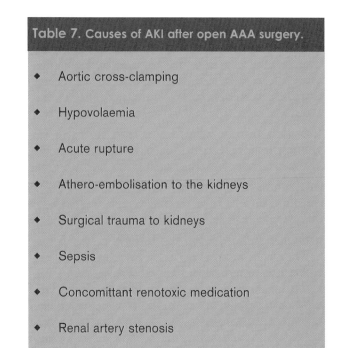

Table 7. Causes of AKI after open AAA surgery.

- Aortic cross-clamping
- Hypovolaemia
- Acute rupture
- Athero-embolisation to the kidneys
- Surgical trauma to kidneys
- Sepsis
- Concomittant renotoxic medication
- Renal artery stenosis

Aortic cross-clamping

Aortic cross-clamping produces profound changes in renal haemodynamics, which can lead to renal impairment. It is important that the anaesthetist maintains adequate renal perfusion both during and after AAA repair to prevent AKI [50]. It is also important to keep the aortic clamp time as short as possible, and to mobilise the aorta gently to prevent embolisation into the renal vessels. For reasons of turbulence and haemodynamics it is advisable to clamp the aorta below the renal arteries first, and then clamp the iliac arteries second [51].

The position of the clamp in relation to the renal arteries is fundamental. Suprarenal cross-clamping causes renal ischaemia which is associated with increased morbidity and mortality; the need for suprarenal clamping probably also reflects the more advanced stage of arteriosclerosis in these patients.

Indications for renal replacement therapy (Table 8)

Patients identified at risk of AKI should have a full assessment of renal function, with advice from a nephrologist before any procedure, where possible. Haemofiltration, as temporary renal replacement therapy, is a major advance deliverable in intensive care units without the need for dialysis facilities. Haemodialysis will be needed in some cases when prolonged renal failure develops, or in patients previously on dialysis. Such patients are best treated in a centre with nephrology and dialysis support.

Renal replacement therapy is indicated early in the therapy of AKI, and also in critically ill patients [52-53]. Early haemofiltration reduces morbidity and mortality in patients with AKI.

Conclusions

Acute kidney injury associated with vascular and endovascular surgery is a major complication, that increases morbidity and mortality. Early recognition and prevention is the key. Multidisciplinary teamworking with nephrologists, radiologists, and anaesthetists, where necessary, produces optimal outcomes. Patients with chronic kidney disease must be pre-assessed and preventative strategies employed. AKI is preventable in the majority of patients undergoing angiography or vascular surgery, and can be avoided with appropriate protocols (Figure 3).

Table 8. Indications for renal replacement therapy.	
Biochemical	**Clinical**
Refractory hyperkalaemia	Urine output <0.3ml/kg for 24 hours or anuria for 12 hours
Serum urea >27mmol/L	AKI with multiple organ failure
Refractory metabolic acidosis	Refractory volume overload
Refractory hyponatraemia	End organ involvement – pericarditis, encephalopathy, neuropathy, myopathy, uraemic bleeding
Refractory hypernatraemia	To increase intravascular space for blood products and parenteral nutrition
Refractory hypercalcaemia	Severe hypo- or hyperthermia

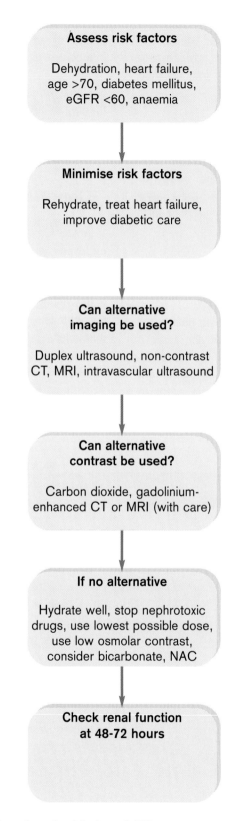

Figure 3. Strategy for the prevention of contrast-induced AKI.

Key points

♦ Risk assessment should be performed early to identify patients at risk of AKI.

♦ Prevention: intravenous fluids should be initiated early if risk has been identified; sodium bicarbonate can be added to saline if appropriate; N-acetylcysteine can be given orally.

♦ Investigation: serum creatinine should be measured at baseline and at 48-72 hours; eGFR should be calculated at baseline and at every creatinine measurement.

♦ Management: early nephrology input should be used where indicated for joint care.

♦ Management: initiation of renal replacement therapy should occur as soon as possible if there is no recovery of renal function.

♦ Renal replacement: haemofiltration is appropriate for some cases but haemodialyis will be needed for high-risk patients.

♦ Renal replacement: early haemofiltration reduces mortality and morbidity in AKI.

References

1. Mehta RL, Kellum JA, Shah SV, *et al*. Acute Kidney Injury Network: report of an initiative to improve outcomes in acute kidney injury. *Critical Care* 2007; 11: R31. http://ccforum.com/content/11/2/R31.

2. Kidney Disease: Improving Global Outcomes (KDIGO). http://www.kdigo.org/.

3. Bertolissi M. Prevention of acute renal failure in major vascular surgery. *Minerva Anesthesiol* 1999; 65: 867-77.

4. K/DOQI Clinical Practice Guidelines for Chronic Kidney Disease: Evaluation, Classification, and Stratification. Kidney Disease Outcome Quality Initiative. *Am J Kidney Dis* 2002; 39: S1-246.

5. Rashid ST, Salman M, Agarwal S, Hamilton G. Occult renal impairment is common in patients with peripheral vascular disease and normal serum creatinine. *Eur J Vasc Endovasc Surg* 2006; 32: 294-9.

6. Levey AS, Bosch JP, Lewis JB, *et al*. A more accurate method to estimate glomerular filtration rate from serum creatinine: a new prediction equation. Modification of Diet in Renal Disease Study Group. *Ann Intern Med* 1999; 130: 461-70.

7. Levey AS, Coresh J, Greene T, *et al*. Using standardized serum creatinine values in the Modification of Diet in Renal Disease study equation for estimating glomerular filtration rate. *Ann Intern Med* 2006; 145: 247-54.

8. Lin J, Knight EL, Hogan ML, Singh AK. A comparison of prediction equations for estimating glomerular filtration rate in adults without kidney disease. *J Am Soc Nephrol* 2003; 14: 2573-80.

9. Levy EM, Viscoli CM, Horwitz RI. The effect of acute renal failure on mortality: a cohort analysis. *JAMA* 1996; 275: 1489-94.

10. Romano G, Briguori C, Quintavalle C, *et al*. Contrast agents and renal cell apoptosis. *Eur Heart J* 2008; 29: 2569-76.

11. Bakris G, Lass N, Gaber AO, *et al*. Radiocontrast medium-induced declines in renal function: a role for oxygen free radicals. *Am J Physiol* 1990; 258: F115-20.

12. Persson BP, Hansell P, Liss P. Pathophysiology of contrast medium-induced nephropathy. *Kidney Int* 2005; 68: 14-22.

13. Goldenberg I, Matetzky S. Nephropathy induced by contrast media: pathogenesis, risk factors and preventive strategies. *CMAJ* 2005; 172: 1461-71.

14. Ruiz J, Lowenthal T. NSAIDs and nephrotoxicity in the elderly. *Geriatr Nephrol Urol* 1997; 7: 51-7.

15. Dembo AJ, Marliss EB, Halperin ML. Insulin therapy in phenformin-associated lactic acidosis; a case report, biochemical considerations and review of the literature. *Diabetes* 1975; 24: 28e35.

16. Monson JP. Metformin and lactic acidosis. *Prescriber Journal* 1993; 33: 170-3.

17. Metformin: updated guidance for use in diabetics with renal impairment. London: The Royal College of Radiologists www.RCR.ac.uk 2009.

18. Barrett BJ, Carlisle EJ. Meta-analysis of the relative nephrotoxicity of high- and low-osmolality iodinated contrast media. *Radiology* 1993; 188: 171-8.

19. Rudnick MR, Goldfarb S, Wexler L, *et al*. Nephrotoxicity of ionic and non-ionic contrast media in 1196 patients: a randomized trial. The Iohexol Cooperative Study. *Kidney Int* 1995; 47: 254-61.

20. Reed M, Meier P, Tamhane UU, *et al*. The relative renal safety of iodixanol compared with low-osmolar contrast media: a meta-analysis of randomized controlled trials. *J Am Coll Cardiol* 2009; 2: 645-54.

21. Kushner FG, Hand M, Smith SC Jr, *et al*. 2009 focused updates: ACC/AHA Guidelines for the Management of Patients with ST-elevation Myocardial Infarction (updating the 2004 guideline and 2007 focused update) and ACC/AHA/SCAI Guidelines on Percutaneous Coronary Intervention (updating the 2005 guideline and 2007 focused update). A report of the American College of Cardiology Foundation/American Heart Association Task Force on Practice Guidelines. *J Am Coll Cardiol* 2009; 54: 2205-41.

22. Weisbord SD, Palevsky PM. Prevention of contrast-induced nephropathy with volume expansion. *Clin J Am Soc Nephrol* 2008; 3: 273-80.

23. Mueller C, Buerkle G, Buettner HJ, *et al.* Prevention of contrast media associated nephropathy: randomised comparison of 2 hydration regimens in 1620 patients undergoing coronary angioplasty. *Arch Intern Med* 2002; 162: 329-36.

24. Halliwell B, Gutteridge JMC. Role of free radicals and catalytic metal ions in human diseases: an overview. *Methods Enzymol* 1990; 186: 1-85.

25. Merten GJ, Burgess WP, Gray LV, *et al.* Prevention of contrast-induced nephropathy with sodium bicarbonate: a randomized controlled trial. *JAMA* 2004; 291: 2328-34.

26. Evaluation of Sodium Bicarbonate to Reduce the Incidence of Contrast Induced Chronic Kidney Injury in Patients With Kidney Disease (BOSS). http://clinicaltrials.gov/ct2/show/NCT00930436.

27. Meyer M, LeWinter MM, Bell SP, *et al.* N-acetylcysteine-enhanced contrast provides cardiorenal protection. *J Am Coll Cardiol Cardiovasc Interv* 2009; 2: 215-21.

28. Rashid ST, Salman M, Myint F, *et al.* Prevention of contrast-induced nephropathy in vascular patients undergoing angiography: a randomized controlled trial of intravenous N-acetylcysteine. *J Vasc Surg* 2004; 40: 1136-41.

29. Kshirsagar AV, Poole C, Mottl A, *et al.* N-acetylcysteine for the prevention of radio contrast-induced nephropathy: a meta-analysis of prospective controlled trials. *J Am Soc Nephrol* 2004; 15: 761-9.

30. Nallamothu BK, Shojania KG, Saint S, *et al.* Is N-acetylsysteine effective in preventing contrast-related nephropathy? A meta-analysis. *Am J Med* 2004; 117: 938-47.

31. Huang CL, Lewicki J, Johnson LK, Cogan MG. Renal mechanism of action of rat atrial natriuretic factor. *J Clin Invest* 1985; 75: 769-73.

32. Rahman SN, Kim GE, Mathew AS, *et al.* Effects of atrial natriuretic peptide in clinical acute renal failure. *Kidney Int* 1994; 45: 1731-8.

33. Morikawa S, Sone T, Tsuboi H, *et al.* Renal protective effects and the prevention of contrast-induced nephropathy by atrial natriuretic peptide. *J Am Coll Cardiol* 2009; 53: 1040-6.

34. Attallah N, Yassine L, Musial J, *et al.* The potential role of statins in contrast nephropathy. *Clin Nephrol* 2004; 62: 273-8.

35. Khanal S, Attallah N, Smith DE, *et al.* Statin therapy reduces contrast-induced nephropathy: an analysis of contemporary percutaneous interventions. *Am J Med* 2005; 118: 843-9.

36. Jo SH, Koo BK, Park JS, *et al.* Prevention of radiocontrast medium-induced nephropathy using short-term high-dose simvastatin in patients with renal insufficiency undergoing coronary angiography (PROMISS) trial: a randomized controlled study. *Am Heart J* 2008; 155: 499 e1-499; e8.

37. Toso A, Maioli M, Leoncini M, *et al.* Usefulness of atorvastatin (80mg) in prevention of contrast-induced nephropathy in patients with chronic renal disease. *Am J Cardiol* 105: 288-92.

38. Sadowitz B, Maier KG, Gahtan V. Basic science review: statin therapy-Part I: the pleiotropic effects of statins in cardiovascular disease. *Vasc Endovasc Surg* 2010; 44: 241-51.

39. Athyros VG, Mitsiou EK, Tziomalos K, *et al.* Impact of managing atherogenicdyslipidemia on cardiovascular outcome across different stages of diabetic nephropathy. *Expert Opin Pharmacother* 2010; 11: 723-30.

40. Agmon Y, Peleg H, Greenfeld Z, *et al.* Nitric oxide and prostanoids protect the renal outer medulla from radiocontrast toxicity in the rat. *J Clin Invest* 1994; 94: 1069-75.

41. Spargias K, Adreanides E, Demerouti E, *et al.* Iloprost prevents contrast-induced nephropathy in patients with renal dysfunction undergoing coronary angiography or intervention. *Circulation* 2009; 120: 1793-9.

42. Mathur VS, Swan SK, Lambrecht LJ, *et al.* The effects of fenoldopam, a selective dopamine receptor agonist, on systemic and renal haemodynamics in normotensive subjects. *Crit Care Med* 1999; 29: 1832-7.

43. Landoni G, Biondi-Zoccai GGL, Tumlin JA, *et al.* Beneficial impact of fenoldopam in critically ill patients with or at risk for acute renal failure: a meta-analysis of randomised clinical trials. *Am J Kidney Dis* 2007; 49: 56-68.

44. Li A, Wong C, Wong M, *et al.* Acute adverse reactions to magnetic resonance contrast media - gadolinium chelates. *Br J Radiol* 2006; 79: 368-71.

45. Cowper S, Robin H, Steinberg S, *et al.* Scleromyxoedema-like cutaneous diseases in renal dialysis patients. *Lancet* 2000; 356: 1000-1

46. Mendoza F, Artlett C, Sandorfi N, *et al.* Description of 12 cases of nephrogenicfibrosingdermopathy and review of the literature. *Semin Arthritis Rheum* 2006; 35: 238-49.

47. Mendichovszky IA, Marks SD, Simcock CM, *et al.* Gadolinium and nephrogenic systemic fibrosis: time to tighten practice. *Pediatr Radiol* 2008; 38: 489-96.

48. MHRA. Gadolinium-containing contrast agents: new advice to minimise the risk of nephrogenic systemic fibrosis. Drug Safety Update, Jan 2010. http://www.mhra.gov.uk/Safety information/DrugSafetyUpdate/CON087741.

49. Kim GS, Ahn HJ, Kim WH, *et al.* Risk factors for postoperative complications after open infrarenal abdominal aortic aneurysm repair in Koreans. *Yonsei Med J* 2011; 52: 339-46.

50. Gamulin Z, Forster A, Morel D, *et al.* Effects of infrarenal aortic cross-clamping on renal haemodynamics in humans. *Anesthesiology* 1984; 61: 394-9.

51. Thompson MM, Nasim A, Sayers RD, *et al.* Oxygen free radical and cytokine generation during endovascular and conventional aneurysm repair. *Eur J Vasc Endovasc Surg* 1996; 12: 70-5.

52. Seabra VF, Balk EM, Liangos O, *et al.* Timing of renal replacement therapy initiation in acute renal failure: a meta-analysis. *Am J Kidney Dis* 2008; 52: 272-84.

53. Bagshaw SM, Uchino S, Bellomo R, *et al.* Beginning and ending supportive therapy for the kidney I: timing of renal replacement therapy and clinical outcomes in critically ill patients with severe acute kidney injury. *J Crit Care* 2009; 24: 129-40.

Chapter 4

Complications related to diabetes in vascular patients

Bruce Campbell MS FRCP FRCS, Consultant Vascular Surgeon
Royal Devon and Exeter Hospital and Professor, Peninsula Medical School, Exeter, UK

Introduction

As a result of its worldwide increase in incidence and prevalence, diabetes mellitus is a leading risk factor in the pathogenesis of atherosclerotic occlusive disease.

The occlusive lesions of diabetics resemble generic atheromatous disease, but diabetic vascular disease has some distinctive features – in particular, medial arterial calcification and a tendency to affect distal arteries. Diabetics present special challenges and are prone to a wide range of complications after both endovascular and open surgical interventions [1-2]. Nowhere are these challenges and complications more evident than in the lower extremity. Infra-inguinal diabetic vascular disease is now the primary cause for non-traumatic major and minor amputation in all western countries and most emerging nations [3]. The care of the diabetic foot and prevention of amputation in diabetics have therefore become major health care and political issues both in the United Kingdom and internationally (see Chapter 21), so this aspect of vascular practice is under a bright spotlight [4].

A notable feature of diabetic patients with lower extremity arterial disease is that they may remain asymptomatic until foot problems develop – either because of ischaemia and/or as a result of trauma in the insensate, neuropathic foot. Lacking the protective effect of pain, any damaged area or ulcer may go unnoticed and unattended until it becomes infected; sometimes the patient's first complaint may be that of foot odour noticed by a family member. Doctors attending the patient may overlook the presence of ischaemia because the patient often has an excellent popliteal pulse and weak foot pulses may be identified. This insidious presentation of ischaemia resembles diabetic coronary artery disease that may not herald its presence with angina pectoris but instead lead to silent myocardial infarction. Comorbidities such as coronary disease and renal dysfunction pose general risks for diabetics having procedures on their peripheral arteries [5]. The risks are particularly high for insulin-dependent diabetics.

Control of diabetes and other medical problems

Diabetics presenting with infected feet and those requiring major surgery have specific risks of failure to control their diabetes (resulting in hypoglycaemia or ketoacidosis), cardiac complications, and renal failure [5, 6]. Good control of diabetes with oral medication and/or insulin is fundamental and requires a basis of written protocols agreed with diabetologists and with anaesthetists. There should be a very low threshold for involving the medical diabetes team in any decisions about control of diabetes for patients under vascular care; close liaison between vascular surgeons and diabetologists is important for managing both inpatients and outpatients. Similar comments apply to collaboration with other specialties in the management of the variety of medical problems that diabetics may suffer – in particular with cardiologists and renal physicians. Optimising the medical state of diabetics before they undergo surgical interventions is a very important aspect of avoiding complications.

Delay in referral is an important reason for the poor outcome of many diabetics presenting with infected and/or ischaemic feet. It is worth emphasizing the need to keep up educational pressure on family doctors and on all physicians involved in admitting emergencies, to be sure that diabetics with infected feet are referred for vascular surgical advice without delay. Delayed referral can result in the need to deal with extensive sepsis, involving greater loss of tissue, more likelihood of major amputation, and an increased risk of general complications. Early referral for possible surgery must be combined with continued attention to the medical control of diabetes and appropriate antibiotic treatment.

Diagnosis and assessment

Clinical and Doppler assessment of the lower limb arteries

Clinical examination is the most important assessment. Focus on special investigations can distract from the most important features which should determine management. Incorrect clinical assessment can lead to poor management decisions and subsequent complications. In assessing the arterial supply to the foot, a good popliteal pulse indicates distal disease. This may argue against a decision for early endovascular intervention in a patient whose infected foot looks potentially well enough perfused to heal after local surgical intervention. Intervention on the arteries can be done later if healing is delayed after local surgery on an infected foot.

Assessment of the level of arterial perfusion to the foot is vital, but uncritical use of Doppler systolic pressures is dangerous in diabetics: measurements are often spurious due to arterial calcification [7]. When the arteries are incompressible, the problem is obvious. It is when pressures are recorded which are in a credible range that they can be misinterpreted, because readings may be falsely high. Listening to the Doppler sounds with an experienced ear is much more reliable than depending on ankle pressure measurements in diabetics. Some advocate the use of toe pressures and these may be useful, but after brief experience I have not adopted their use.

It is important to listen routinely to the peroneal artery in diabetics during hand-held Doppler assessment, specifically when the posterior tibial and dorsalis pedis signals are absent or poor. The peroneal may be the best, and sometimes the only, patent artery at ankle level in patients with diabetes [8].

Arterial imaging, renal dysfunction and metformin

Imaging of calcified arteries in diabetics with multilevel disease and poor flow can be difficult and there are risks of failing to demonstrate patent vessels properly [9]. In addition, contrast-induced acute kidney injury (see Chapter 3) (a rise in serum creatinine 24-72 hours following the use of radiological contrast, which can occasionally progress to renal failure) is a risk in diabetics, many of whom have renal function which is already compromised. Metformin increases this risk and the fact that a diabetic is taking metformin must always be flagged up on any vascular radiology request. Although the evidence only supports a risk of worsening renal function in patients with pre-existing renal impairment, it is usual practice to stop metformin for the duration of contrast arteriography: 24-48 hours before and afterwards [10]. Other measures which are regularly taken to minimise the risk of contrast-induced acute kidney injury are:

◆   keeping the patient well hydrated (saline infusion);
◆   using iso-osmolar contrast such as Visipaque™ (GE Healthcare, Chalfont St Giles, HP8 4SP, UK) [11];

- diluting the contrast 50:50 with saline;
- in high-risk cases, considering the use of N-acetylcysteine, although the evidence for its effectiveness is limited (see Chapter 3).

Revascularisation procedures on the lower limbs in diabetes

Endovascular procedures

Endovascular treatment has become the treatment of first choice for revascularisation in diabetics with threatened legs, but careful planning, involving both surgeons and radiologists is important [2, 12]. As for surgery, the fact that many diabetics present late, with advanced infection and ischaemia, can make limb salvage a challenge.

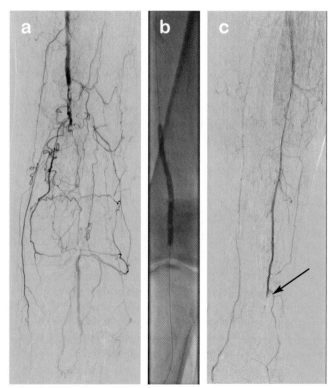

Figure 1. a) Angiogram of a diabetic patient with occlusion of the popliteal artery with patent anterior and posterior tibial arteries distally. b) Following technically successful angioplasty. c) Imaging showed embolism of a fragment of atheroma to the distal peroneal artery which could not be removed.

Distal angioplasty

The main challenge is the need to deal with distal occlusive disease in tibial and foot arteries which are small in calibre, calcified, and frequently affected by long occlusions and/or multiple stenoses. The capacity to achieve successful revascularisation has been greatly improved in recent years by the development of fine guide wires and angioplasty balloons which are both narrow in calibre and long in length (for example 1.5mm diameter and 25cm long). The ability to reopen a diseased foot arch, by passage of wires and balloons down one tibial artery, through the arch, and up another has opened new horizons in the revascularisation of the diabetic foot, in a similar way to the introduction of bypasses to distal arteries in the 1980s. Adventurous endovascular procedures like these carry a risk of failure or even making the situation worse, and they should be reserved for diabetics who would otherwise be facing limb loss. These are not procedures for anyone other than highly experienced endovascular specialists.

A number of local complications can occur when performing endovascular procedures on the difficult calcified arteries of diabetics, including distal embolisation, dissection and arterial perforation or rupture.

Distal embolisation (Figure 1)

This becomes apparent when the main tibial artery has been recanalised, but there is then an occlusion distally – usually due to dislodgement of a piece of atheromatous material. Use of thrombolysis will not be successful for material of this kind and aspiration thrombectomy is required. This is best done using a catheter that is not tapered, and that has as wide a lumen as the vessel will allow, and that is flat (not oblique) across its tip.

Extraction of atheromatous debris can be awkward. Continuous aspiration is needed to keep the fragment applied to the end of the catheter and it is withdrawn into a sheath, usually placed in the femoral artery. Getting embolic fragments out of the sheath, without 'losing' them back down into the artery can be achieved by removing the valve from the proximal end of the sheath, while quickly flicking out the distal end of the catheter, with its attached debris. Any debris which might otherwise be left inside the sheath is eluted with a jet of backbleed, which is then controlled. This process can be repeated if more atheromatous debris needs to be extracted.

Dissection (Figure 2)

This can often be dealt with by further dilatation using a long balloon and prolonged inflation (for example, 3-5 minutes). The angiographic appearance thereafter is less important than observing rapid flow. If flow into the dissection channel persists, or if flow remains poor, then use of a stent may resolve the problem.

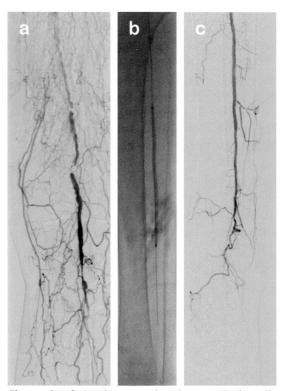

Figure 3. a) Angiogram showing occlusive disease extending from the popliteal artery well down the anterior tibial artery in a diabetic with critical ischaemia. b) During attempted subintimal angioplasty, contrast extravasation indicates perforation of the anterior tibial artery. c) The procedure was continued, gaining re-entry to the arterial lumen. After balloon inflation a good result was seen, with no residual extravasation.

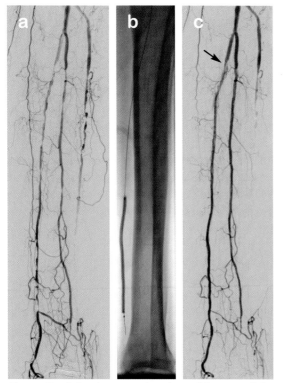

Figure 2. a) Angiogram showing widespread stenotic disease of the tibial arteries and an ischaemic foot with infection. b) Following balloon angioplasty of both arteries there was a dissection of the posterior tibial. c) Further balloon inflation produced good flow, but the appearance of residual dissection is seen in the proximal part of the posterior tibial artery.

Arterial perforation or rupture (Figure 3)

Perforation may become obvious because the guide wire is seen to have advanced away from the line of the artery; this seldom has any adverse effect if the vessel is occluded (as usually it is). Perforation or rupture which allows escape of contrast usually seals spontaneously, but it may result in the need to terminate the procedure. If a perforation occurs which allows continued escape of contrast then the defect can be coil embolised.

Subintimal angioplasty

Extensive arterial calcification in diabetics often means that subintimal angioplasty is not possible: specifically, it may prove impossible to break back into the lumen. If a guide wire is advanced much beyond the distal extent of the occlusion, then dissection with worsening of blood flow is a risk. The introduction of 're-entry' devices for achieving subintimal angioplasty in larger arteries holds out the prospect of similar technology for smaller calibre arteries in due course.

Surgical revascularisation procedures

In common with endovascular intervention, most of the problems relate to distal occlusive disease and to arterial calcification. Good planning, avoidance of technical errors and continual attention to antisepsis are fundamental, especially in diabetics with their propensity to poor healing and infection.

Infection

Diabetics have a generally increased risk of infection, and wound infection rates after vascular surgery are higher in diabetics than in other patients [13, 14]. When operating on the arteries of an ischaemic and infected extremity in a diabetic, my own practice includes:

◆ avoiding prosthetic bypass grafts whenever possible (Figure 4);

◆ taking great care to exclude the operative wounds from any infected tissue by planning cleaning, draping and the sequence of any combined surgery for revascularisation and debridement;

◆ using appropriate systemic antibiotic prophylaxis – both for the organisms known to be present and for prophylaxis against current 'hospital-acquired' organisms (because these patients have often been in hospital for some time before operation);

◆ placing a gentamicin-collagen sponge adjacent to synthetic graft (or patch) material in any wound.

Choice of bypass graft

When revascularisation is needed in the presence of infection in a diabetic foot, then autogenous vein is preferable to any synthetic infra-inguinal graft, not only because of the risk of infection is likely to be lower, but because of its greater likelihood of long-term patency.

Choice of distal artery

To maximise the chance of both immediate and prolonged graft patency, the best distal vessel – with continuity into the foot – should be chosen. That may mean the peroneal artery, or sometimes the posterior tibial distal to the ankle, or the dorsalis pedis [15]. I

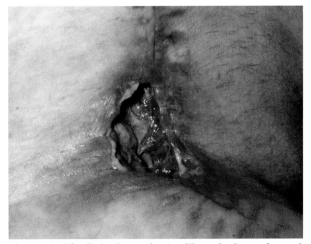

Figure 4. This diabetic patient, with an ischaemic and infected foot had no vein suitable for a bypass. A PTFE femoropopliteal bypass graft was inserted, which restored flow to the foot. However, infection occurred in the groin wound, exposing the PTFE graft. The infection could not be resolved: the graft was removed and transtibial amputation performed.

would only use vein to anastomose to the very distal arteries. Use of the popliteal artery for the origin of the vein graft, when possible, means the need for a shorter graft than if it is taken from groin level.

Tunnelling vein grafts

Tunnelling always poses a risk of twisting a vein graft: care should be taken with the orientation as the graft is pulled through the tunneller. Flushing it with heparinised saline when it is in position, and performing the proximal anastomosis first, to observe and check distal blood flow before suturing the distal anastomosis, are methods for minimising the risk of a twist. Some surgeons mark the vein with blue dye before tunnelling it, but twists of 360° can occur despite this precaution.

Operating on calcified arteries

This is a particular problem in diabetics [16]. Application of vascular clamps can break the calcified atheroma and lead to occlusion or dissection. Cushioned clamps (Fogarty cushion clamps for larger arteries – carefully applied with only two or three 'clicks' to just stop flow – or disposable cushioned spring clamps for distal arteries) are generally preferable to clamps with metallic jaws. Occluding the arteries by traction on slings around them is another option.

If arteries contain a circumferential layer of calcium, all the above may be ineffective in controlling blood flow and intraluminal occlusion may be safer than risking plaque fracture by external control. Some surgeons use commercial vessel occluders, placed in the lumen of distal vessels or specially produced gel which can subsequently be eluted by saline infusion. An alternative is a Number 6 (or Number 4) umbilical catheter, introduced into the distal vessel (with the additional purpose of flushing it with heparinised saline) as an occluder, with a little tension around it from a sling if necessary. Performing all but the last few sutures with the catheter in the distal artery provides haemostasis and also guarantees patency of the outflow from the anastomosis.

If it proves impossible to pass a calcium-cutting needle through the atheroma in any part of the arteriotomy, one or two sutures can be passed between the outer layer of the arterial wall and the calcified atheromatous layer. Atheroma so calcified will not separate or dissect, particularly if there is a suture through all layers of the arterial wall on each side of the affected area.

Keeping high-risk grafts patent

Evidence on the best pharmacological means of enhancing the patency of high-risk grafts to distal arteries remains sparse [17]. All patients should be on an antithrombotic agent (at the time of surgery). In addition, I have used dextran 40 in the early postoperative period because there is some evidence that this enhances the early patency of high-risk distal bypasses (but note that there have been recent problems obtaining dextran 40 in the UK in recent times) [18]. In the longer term I have a low threshold for combined antplatelet therapy (aspirin with clopidogrel) or for antiplatelet and anticoagulant therapy for high-risk distal bypasses. The choice between aspirin and clopidogrel versus warfarin and an antithrombotic is based more on personal preference than on any good evidence: one or other combination is worth considering to reduce the

chance of occlusion of any high-risk distal bypass in the long term.

Patent graft with a persistently non-healing foot

This is a most disappointing situation [19, 20]. A distal bypass graft (or angioplasty) restores blood flow into the foot and continues to work well, but the foot shows no sign of healing and major amputation is required (Figure 5). Whether restoration of blood flow beyond the ankle will result in well-vascularised pink tissues, or persistence of tissue with a grey/brown hue which presages failure to heal is something which is impossible to predict reliably. The patient's own 'track record' is a useful pointer: have they healed lesions or surgery on the contralateral foot?

The one circumstance in which a patent graft but an ischaemic extremity may possibly be corrected is when the graft is a proximal one (for example, to the groin or to the above-knee popliteal). If there is more

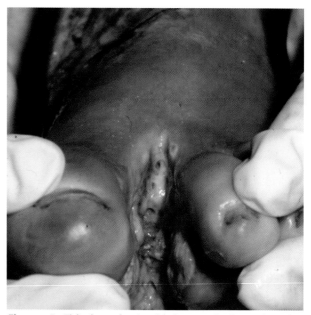

Figure 5. This is a foot which was ischaemic with infection between the web space of the toes. It was treated by toe amputation, at the same time as inserting a vein graft to the posterior tibial artery. The graft remained patent, but the infection recurred and a transtibial amputation was required, in the presence of a working bypass graft.

distal disease which can be treated by angioplasty or bypass, then that may well be worthwhile.

Surgery of the diabetic foot

This is the subject of Chapter 21, but at the risk of duplication, here are half a dozen tips:

- use of a 'bacteriological swab' (i.e. a long cotton bud) to explore sinuses avoids the risk of creating false tracks, which might occur with any metal instrument. This is a good way of showing where tracks go and whether bones or joints are involved during clinical examination;
- the adage "never let the sun set on undrained pus" (or gas) is vital for the diabetic foot;
- infusing methylene blue into a sinus at the time of operation can help to show its deep extent during debridement. This can avoid the complication of leaving small infected tracks unrecognised;
- surgery of the infected diabetic foot is not straightforward and requires experience. Some vascular surgeons delegate these cases to trainees because they seem to believe they are simple: just draining an abscess. Whereas set-piece procedures – like amputation of a toe which is healthy at its base – are simple and can be mastered quickly, dealing with sinuses or extensive sepsis needs a surgeon experienced in operating on the feet of diabetics and observing them thereafter;
- negative pressure wound therapy (VAC therapy) is worth considering for selected open wounds on diabetic feet;
- it is perhaps worth also including the general rule "never perform an amputation without a detailed arteriogram" which underpins the aim of salvaging every possible foot.

Major amputations

The main concerns when performing major amputation (most commonly transtibial amputation) on diabetic patients are infection and/or failure to heal.

Infection

If there is very extensive sepsis and oedema it is worth considering a guillotine amputation just above the ankle; allowing a number of days for the tissues to settle; and then performing a definitive transtibial amputation on healthy and non-oedematous tissues. This avoids the significant risk of complications if transtibial amputation is done in the presence of oedema and inflammation of the lower leg.

When doing an amputation in the context of extensive sepsis, or for revision of amputations which have been infected, I often insert gentamicin sponge into the depths of the wound, in addition to giving systemic antibiotic prophylaxis.

Gentamicin beads can be useful for treating deep but narrow sinuses which occasionally occur as a result of local infection after amputation. The beads produce a high local concentration of gentamicin throughout the sinus for about 2 weeks. The chain can be replaced every 2 weeks by progressively shorter chains (the chain can be kept in its packet, labelled in the patient's notes, for use bit-by-bit). The depths of the sinus gradually heal up as the chains of gentamicin beads get shorter. This can also be a useful technique in the diabetic foot.

Failure to heal and dehiscence

Transtibial amputations in diabetics can look entirely satisfactory for about a week and then gradually start to look red and unhealthy and to dehisce, for no discernable reason. With this spectre in mind, it is probably best to avoid the use of a 'stump shrinker' or any mobility aid on these stumps (residual limbs) for at least 10 days. If the wound looks even slightly red or imperfect, application of these should be delayed even longer.

Young fit diabetics who have major amputations need to be reminded frequently to take care: they can easily forget in the early stages that they have only one leg, so falling and damaging the stump.

Conclusions

In conclusion, diabetics present special challenges and risks of complications at all stages of their management. Good medical care, thoughtful interpretation of diagnostic tests, and meticulous technique during revascularisation procedures are all important. When limb salvage is not possible, then avoidance or early recognition of complications after amputation surgery are pivotal to rapid rehabilitation.

Acknowledgements

I thank Dr George Andros (Van Nuys, California), Professor Tony Watkinson (Exeter) and Mr Andrew Cowan (Exeter) for their advice during the preparation of this chapter. Tony Watkinson kindly provided illustrations.

Key points

- Both in the UK and worldwide, diabetes has become the leading cause of leg amputation, so optimal care of the feet and legs of diabetics is high on health care and political agendas.
- Diabetics often have multiple medical problems: avoiding complications involves recognising these and having a team approach to management, with a range of other specialists.
- Assessing the arteries of diabetics can be difficult because calcification may produce spurious Doppler pressure measurements: there is a risk from contrast arteriography, specifically with metformin treatment.
- Endovascular treatment is now possible for a wide range of arterial lesions in diabetics, but these pose risks (especially in small calcified arteries). Careful case selection and considerable expertise are necessary to minimise complications and to deal with them if they do occur.
- Surgery on calcified arteries in diabetics can be challenging. Use of vein is greatly preferable to prosthetic grafts for distal bypass, with a view to minimising the risks of both occlusion and infection.
- Major amputations in diabetics can be complicated by infection and by failure to heal. They require meticulous observation and care throughout the postoperative period.

References

1. Lange CP, Ploeg AJ, Lardenoye JW, Breslau PJ. Patient- and procedure-specific risk factors for postoperative complications in peripheral arterial vascular surgery. *Qual Saf Health Care* 2009; 18: 131-6.
2. Ihnat DM, Mills JL. Current assessment of endovascular therapy for infrainguinal arterial occlusive disease in patients with diabetes. *J Vasc Surg* 1020; 52: 92S-5.
3. Moxey PW, Gogalniceanu P, Hinchcliffe RJ, *et al*. Lower extremity amputations - a review of global variability in incidence. *Diabet Med* 2011 Mar 9. doi:10.1111/j.1464-5491.2011.03279.x.
4. National Institute for Health and Clinical Excellence. Diabetic foot problems - inpatient management (Nice Clinical Guideline 119), 2011. www.nice.org.uk/guidance/CG119.
5. Hertzer NR, Bena JF, Karafa MT. A personal experience with the influence of diabetes and other factors on the outcome of infrainguinal bypass grafts for occlusive disease. *J Vasc Surg* 2007; 46: 271-9.
6. Axelrod DA, Upchurch GR, De Monner S, *et al.* Perioperative cardiovascular risk stratification of patients with diabetes who undergo elective major vascular surgery. *J Vasc Surg* 2002; 35: 894-901.
7. Potier L, Abi Kalil C, Mohammedi K, Roussel R. Use and utility of ankle brachial index in patients with diabetes. *Eur J Vasc Endovasc Surg* 2011; 41: 100-6.
8. Campbell WB, Fletcher EWL, Hands LJ. Assessment of the distal lower limb arteries: a comparison of Doppler ultrasound and arteriography. *Ann R Coll Surg Engl* 1986; 68: 37-9.
9. Pomposelli F. Arterial imaging in patients with lower extremity ischaemia and diabetes mellitus. *J Vasc Surg* 2010; 52: 81S-91.
10. Nawaz S, Cleveland T, Gaines PA, Chan P. Clinical risk associated with contrast angiography in metformin treated patients: a clinical review. *Clin Rad* 1998; 53: 342-4.
11. Aspelin P, Aubry P, Fransson S-G, *et al*, for the NEPHRIC Study investigators. Nephrotoxic effects in high-risk patients undergoing angiography. *N Engl J Med* 2003; 348: 491-9.
12. DeRubertis BG, Pierce M, Ryer EJ, *et al*. Reduced primary patency rate in diabetic patients after percutaneous

intervention results from more frequent presentation with limb-threatening ischemia. *J Vasc Surg* 2008; 47: 101-8.

13. Richet HM, Chidiac C, Prat A, *et al.* Analysis of risk factors for surgical wound infections following vascular surgery. *Am J Med* 1991; 91 (Suppl 3B): 170S-2.

14. Josephs LG, Cordts PR, DiEdwardo CL, *et al.* Do infected inguinal lymph nodes increase the incidence of postoperative groin wound infection? *J Vasc Surg* 1993; 17: 1077-82.

15. Pomposelli FB, Freeman DV, Burgess AM, *et al.* Dorsalis pedis arterial bypass: durable limb salvage for foot ischemia in patients with diabetes mellitus. *J Vasc Surg* 1995; 21: 375-84.

16. Misare BD, Pomposelli FB, Gibbons GW, *et al.* Infrapopliteal bypasses to severely calcified, unclampable outflow arteries: two-year results. *J Vasc Surg* 1996; 24: 6-16.

17. Jackson AJ, Coats P, Orr DJ, *et al.* Pharmacotherapy to improve outcomes in infrainguinal bypass graft surgery: a review of current treatment strategies. *Ann Vasc Surg* 2010; 24: 562-72.

18. Rutherford RB, Jones DN, Bergentz S-E, *et al.* The efficacy of Dextran 40 in preventing early postoperative thrombosis following difficult lower extremity bypass. *J Vasc Surg* 1984; 1: 765-73.

19. Johnson BL, Glickman MH, Bandyk DF, Esses GE. Failure of foot salvage in patients with end-stage renal disease after surgical revascularization. *J Vasc Surg* 1995; 22: 280-6.

20. Wyatt MG, Kernick VFM, Clark H, Campbell WB. Femorotibial bypass: the learning curve. *Ann R Coll Surg Engl* 1995; 77: 413-6.

Chapter 5

Procedural thrombosis and the hypercoagulable state

Marc A. Bailey MB ChB BSc MRCS(Eng), Academic Clinical Fellow in Vascular Surgery
Michael J. Gough ChM FRCS, Professor of Vascular Surgery
The Leeds Vascular Institute, The General Infirmary at Leeds, Leeds, UK

Introduction

Thrombosis following vascular surgery is a significant cause of morbidity and mortality. Patients with a thrombotic tendency are at increased risk of vascular disease and are therefore likely to present to a vascular surgeon for treatment. They are also at increased risk of thrombosis following surgery and require careful peri-operative management.

Venous thrombo-embolism (VTE) is responsible for 60,000 deaths annually in the UK. This is five times as many patients as those who die as a consequence of nosocomial infections. The estimated annual cost to the NHS is in the region of £640 million (www.doh.gov). Vascular surgery is associated with significant risk of VTE and local prophylaxis strategies should be protocolised according to the recent National Institute for Health and Clinical Excellence (NICE) guidelines [1].

Thrombosis at the site of arterial reconstruction is arguably a more important clinical problem following vascular surgery. This can lead to symptom recurrence, re-operation, limb loss, stroke or death, dependent upon the artery involved. Mechanisms for graft occlusion/thrombosis and the recommendations for effective preventative strategies vary dependent upon the site and type of surgery performed.

The physiology of thrombus

Virchow's triad describes the key factors influencing thrombosis: hypercoagulability, endothelial injury or dysfunction and haemodynamic change. Each of these factors may activate the clotting cascade (Figure 1) via either the contact activation (intrinsic) or tissue factor (extrinsic) pathways. Both pathways converge ultimately on the final common pathway to produce thrombin. This facilitates the cleavage of fibrinogen to fibrin and cross-linkage of the fibrin clot in the presence of Factor XIIIa.

Hypercoagulable states

Some 30-40% of patients with unprovoked VTE will be found to have a thrombophilia. Similarly, patients known to have a thrombophilia are at high risk of thrombosis following any form of surgery, particularly to the vascular tree. Factor V Leiden and the prothrombin 20210 mutation are the most commonly encountered of these abnormalities [2]. Further, there is an association between many of the thombophilias and the development of peripheral arterial disease, independent of traditional cardiovascular risk factors [3]. Consequently, a significant number of patients with a diagnosed or

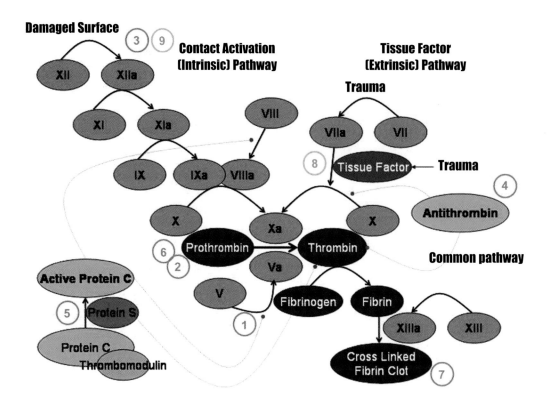

Figure 1. Graphical representation of the clotting cascade. The contact activation (intrinsic) pathway on the left and the tissue factor (extrinsic) pathway on the right combine at the point of Factor Xa production to form the common pathway. Pertinent inhibitors of the pathway, antithrombin and protein C and S are labelled in lilac. The site of interference of common thrombophilias is indicated by orange numbers: 1) Factor V Leiden; 2) Prothrombin 20210 polymorphism; 3) hyperhomocysteinaemia; 4) antithrombin III deficiency; 5) protein C/protein S deficiency; 6) antiphospholipid syndrome; 7) heparin-induced thrombocytopaenia. The areas of the pathway pertinent to graft failure are indicated by green numbers: 8) vein graft; 9) synthetic graft.

occult thrombophilia will present to vascular surgeons for intervention. Knowledge of the common thrombophilias (Table 1) and their safe peri-operative management is therefore essential.

Factor V Leiden

In this autosomal dominant condition, Factor V with the Leiden variant is resistant to inactivation by activated protein C, hence preventing regulation of thrombin formation (Figure 1: 1). The incidence in the general population is 2-10% although functional activated protein C resistance in patients with peripheral arterial disease is commoner at 11-22% [4]. The risk of unprovoked VTE is approximately 0.1% per year [5] in the general population, but patients with Factor V Leiden are at greater risk following surgical intervention and thus, if this anomaly is identified pre-operatively, additional VTE prophylaxis is essential.

Table 1. Risks associated with the common thrombophilias.

Thrombophilia	Incidence	Unprovoked VTE risk	Peri-operative prophylaxis	Recurrence risk	Duration of anticoagulation after DVT
Factor V Leiden	2-10%	RR 3	LMWH	Moderate	6/12-1yr*
Prothrombin 20210	2-4%	RR 1.7	LMWH	Moderate	6/12-1yr*
Hyperhomocysteineaemia	5-7%	OR 2.95	Folate LMWH	Moderate	3-6/12*
Antithombin III deficiency	1-2%	OR 5.0	Anti-thrombin III concentrate/FFP	High	Lifelong
Protein C deficiency Protein S deficiency	2%	OR 1.7	LMWH	Moderate	6/12-1yr*
Antiphospholipid syndrome	3-4%	RR 2.2-5.6	LMWH	High	Lifelong

* These guidelines are based on the current evidence. In most cases the evidence supports treatment greater than 3 months but is very much patient-dependent with regards to the ultimate duration.

LMWH = low-molecular-weight heparin; RR = relative risk; OR = odds ratio

Patients who suffer VTE on a background of Factor V Leiden have a moderate recurrence risk (relative risk estimate 1.39) and require greater than 3 months of anticoagulation [6], although debate continues regarding the optimal duration of therapy.

Prothrombin 20210 polymorphism

Substitution of adenine to guanine at position 20210 of the prothombin gene promotes prothrombin production, leading to elevated thrombin levels and hypercoaguability (Figure 1: 2). The incidence in the general population is 2-4% [7], making it the second most common thrombophilia. These patients should be treated as high risk for VTE in the peri-operative period and given appropriate extended prophylaxis. Following an index VTE event there is a moderate risk of recurrence (relative risk estimate 1.20) and anticoagulation for at least 6 months to 1 year is suggested [6].

Hyperhomocysteinaemia

High levels of serum homocysteine relate to disordered methionine metabolism and may reflect deficiencies in folic acid (vitamin B9), pyridoxine (vitamin B6) or cyanocobalamin (vitamin B12). Hyperhomocysteinaemia is also a consequence of homocysteinuria or the methylene-tetrahydrofolate-reducatase polymorphism. High levels of serum homocysteine are thought to induce vascular endothelial damage (Figure 1: 3) and are commonly linked to the development of early cardiovascular disease and acute arterial thrombosis. Indeed, the incidence in vascular surgical patients may be as high as 33% [8]. Elevated serum homocysteine is also an independent risk factor for VTE which is most apparent in younger patients [9]. The mainstay of treatment is folic acid supplementation which reduces plasma levels of homocysteine. However, a long-term reduction in VTE or cardiovascular events is unproven [10].

Patients with hyperhomocysteinaemia may be identified pre-operatively if routine screening is performed in the vascular clinic. When this is the case, folic acid should be prescribed before surgery in an attempt to reduce the thrombosis risk [11]. Surprisingly, there is no good evidence linking hyperhomocysteinaemia to graft occlusion [12].

Antithrombin III deficiency

Antithrombin III is a potent inhibitor of the clotting cascade by inhibiting thrombin itself and the conversion of Factor X to Xa in the tissue factor pathway (Figure 1: 4). Antithrombin III deficiency is an autosomal dominantly inherited condition leading to reduced circulating levels of antithrombin III and an increased potential for thrombosis; the risk of VTE is approximately 1.7% per year [5], some five times greater than the normal population [13], making it the most potent of the thrombophilias. Appropriate anticoagulation at times of high risk is imperative. However, as heparin potentiates the anticoagulant effect of antithrombin, these patients are resistant to heparinisation. Although low-molecular-weight heparin can be used for initial treatment whilst loading with warfarin, careful monitoring of serum anti-factor Xa levels is required.

If surgery is being considered for a patient with known antithrombin III deficiency, peri-operative administration of antithrombin III concentrate or fresh frozen plasma at 20ml/kg can be used as thromboprophylaxis [14]. Given the high risk of recurrence, lifelong anticoagulation with warfarin should be considered after a single episode of thrombosis in this patient group.

Protein C/protein S deficiency

Activated protein C inhibits the conversion of Factor V to Factor Va, a critical step in the conversion of prothombin to thrombin to initiate the common pathway. Protein C also inhibits the conversion of Factor VIII to VIIIa which is required for conversion of Factor X to Xa in the final step of the contact activation pathway (Figure 1: 5). Protein S is a vitamin K-dependent cofactor for the activation of protein C

from its inactive complex with thrombomodulin. Protein S also has direct inhibitory effects on thrombin.

The incidence of protein C deficiency is approximately 1 in 500 of the world population [15]. Although the frequency of protein S deficiency is approximately 1 in 7000 in the community, this increases to 2% in patients with VTE [16]. The estimated odds ratio for VTE compared to patients without this abnormality is 1.7 [13], although conferring a high risk postoperatively and thus mandating thromboprophylaxis. Further, these patients have a high risk of recurrent VTE [16], although there is no definitive evidence for lifelong anticoagulation; following a single event, this would seem logical.

Antiphospholipid antibodies

Antiphospholipid syndrome is defined as the auto-immune production of antibodies against phospholipids including prothrombin (Figure 1: 6), the most common of which are the lupus anticoagulant and anticardiolipin; both can induce thrombosis and miscarriage. The precise incidence is unknown but is estimated at 3-4% of the population [16]. This leads to a relative risk of VTE in patients with systemic lupus of 5.6 in the presence of the lupus anticoagulant antibody, and 2.2 in patients with the anticardiolipin antibody [17]. In patients without systemic lupus, there is also an increased risk of VTE, which is again greater in the presence of the lupus anticoagulant antibody compared to the anticardiolipin antibody [18]. Patients with the antiphospholipid syndrome are at a high risk of postoperative thrombotic events, particularly after vascular reconstruction [19]. The high risk of recurrent thrombosis demands lifelong anticoagulation after a first thrombotic event, although further VTE can occur despite adequate anticoagulation [20].

Heparin-induced thrombocytopaenia

Heparin-induced thrombocytopaenia (HIT), the development of a low platelet count following the administration of heparin, is associated with high risk of thrombosis. This is due to heparin-dependent IgG antibodies that bind to a conformationally modified epitope on platelet Factor IV leading to platelet aggregation and so-called 'white clot' (Figure 1: 7). The use of warfarin in these patients is not advised due to the high risk of skin necrosis which is thought to be the result of an early transient procoagulant action (inhibition of natural anticoagulant protein C); lepirudin is a suitable alternative [21].

HIT is particularly pertinent in vascular surgery, given the frequent use of heparin during and after surgery. Thrombocytopaenia typically develops 5-10 days after heparin administration but can occur acutely. A high index of suspicion and early recognition is imperative, allowing cessation of heparinoids and prescription of a suitable alternative, such as a lepirudin infusion (recombinant hirudin, a highly specific direct inhibitor of thrombin derived from yeast cells) to prevent life-threatening thrombosis. If a patient has a known history of HIT it is mandatory to avoid further exposure to heparin.

Venous thrombo-embolism (VTE)

Historically, patients undergoing orthopaedic, gynaecological or cancer surgery had the highest risk of postoperative VTE. However, it is now clear that all hospital patients are at risk. Nevertheless, the approach to VTE risk assessment and prophylaxis in the UK has been haphazard. At the time of the House of Commons Inquiry on the prevention of venous thrombo-embolism in hospitalised patients in 2005 [22], it was estimated that 40% of orthopaedic patients were not receiving any VTE prophylaxis despite the lack of a contra-indication. Three key publications have presented similar guidelines for VTE prevention in hospitalised patients based on meta-analysis of more than 800 studies [23-25]. Despite the subsequent 2007 NICE publication (Figure 2), VTE thromboprophylaxis frequently fails because these guidelines are not adhered to by physicians, surgeons and the public [22]. In particular, risk assessment is highly variable and the approach to VTE thromboprophylaxis is inconsistent.

Low risk:	No LMWH
	Early mobilisation
	Avoidance of dehydration
Moderate risk:	LMWH prophylaxis
High risk:	LMWH prophylaxis AND
	Graduated compression stockings OR
	Intermittent pneumatic compression

Figure 2. Thromboprophylaxis regimens based on risk.

Patient risk factors for VTE

- Active cancer or cancer treatment

- Age over 60 years

- Dehydration

- Known thrombophilias

- Obesity (body mass index [BMI] over 30kg/m^2)

- One or more significant medical comorbidities (for example: heart disease; metabolic, endocrine or respiratory pathologies; acute infectious diseases; inflammatory conditions)

- Personal history or first-degree relative with a history of VTE

- Use of hormone replacement therapy

- Use of oestrogen-containing contraceptive therapy

- Varicose veins with phlebitis

Admission-related risk factors for VTE

- Surgical procedure with a total anaesthetic and surgical time of more than 90 minutes, or 60 minutes if the surgery involves the pelvis or lower limb

- Acute surgical admission with inflammatory or intra-abdominal condition

- Expected significant reduction in mobility

- Critical care admission

Figure 3. Patient and admission-related risk factors for thrombo-embolism.

In January 2010, NICE updated the VTE guidelines in conjunction with the Independent Expert Working Group on The Prevention of Venous Thromboembolism in Hospitalised Patients [1]. The key message was that each patient must have an individualised assessment of their VTE risk on admission including both patient- and admission-related risks of thrombosis and bleeding (Figure 3) to allow an individual prescription based on the risk-benefit balance.

VTE prophylaxis in vascular surgery

Compared to other surgical specialties, vascular surgical patients are often older, undergo lengthy operations which impair postoperative mobility and may have limb ischaemia, all of which are additional thrombotic risk factors [26]. Further, vascular endothelial injury and haemodynamic instability are common. Conversely, patients undergoing vascular surgery routinely receive intravenous heparin during arterial cross-clamping and often a period of heparinisation in the immediate postoperative phase to maintain graft patency. Since at least half of postoperative DVTs are initiated during surgery, the use of intra-operative heparin may be beneficial. Further, vascular patients usually receive long-term treatment with at least one antiplatelet agent. The concept that they are protected from post-procedural VTE was confirmed by a review of 1.4 million surgical patients which reported a 90-day VTE risk of 0.2-2.8% following vascular surgery, compared to 2.5-16.3% after gastro-intestinal surgery for malignancy [27].

In contrast, Fletcher and Batiste [28] reported an incidence of DVT of 9.1% following lower limb arterial reconstruction and 14.3% following amputation in a series of 142 patients receiving routine thromboprophylaxis. Hollyoak et al [29] found that 32% of patients undergoing vascular surgery without thromboprophylaxis developed a DVT within 30 days, whilst more recently, de Maistre et al [30] reported an incidence of VTE of 8.1% after elective AAA repair in 137 patients, despite routine thromboprophylaxis. Following EVAR, Eagleton et al [31] described an incidence of VTE of 6% in 50 patients who did not receive thromboprophylaxis. However, in the only contemporary randomised trial [32], thromboprophylaxis did not reduce DVT after aortic reconstruction.

These conflicting reports have led to further confusion and differing practice amongst vascular surgeons. Whilst the routine use of thromboprophylaxis in all vascular patients cannot be supported because of potential bleeding risks [25], it is clear that many vascular interventions confer a specific risk of VTE. This further endorses the view that patients should undergo personalised VTE risk assessment and receive an appropriate VTE prevention plan [1].

Treatment of post-procedural VTE

A key question following the first episode of VTE is the duration of subsequent oral anticoagulation therapy. Whilst an event with an obvious predisposing cause and no complicating factors would be treated with oral anticoagulation for 3 months, an unprovoked VTE or a provoked VTE with an underlying thrombophilia may require longer-term, or even lifelong treatment [1]. Further, the development of VTE following surgical intervention despite appropriate thromboprophylaxis is not a simple event and the optimal duration of anticoagulation is unclear. No definitive evidence exists, although an interesting randomised controlled trial by Agnelli et al [33] demonstrated that recurrence was not reduced by treating all idiopathic VTEs with 1 year of warfarin compared to 3 months. Although long-term anticoagulation can effectively reduce recurrence rates it carries a significant risk of haemorrhagic complications. Thus subjecting a patient to lifelong warfarin treatment requires careful consideration.

One factor that may make this decision easier is the increasing evidence that evaluation of the deep venous system (when there is a known DVT) can give an indication of patient-specific recurrence risk. Patients with persistent venous thrombus or partial or complete venous occlusion following 3 months of anticoagulation have a greater risk of recurrent DVT compared to those patients with total recanalisation of the affected vein [34]. Similarly, an elevated serum d-dimer after 3 months' therapy also predicts future risk of VTE [35]. Both these findings support the notion of an individualised approach to the duration of anticoagulation. Further studies are required before these approaches are adopted in routine practice.

Peri-operative arterial occlusion

Of potentially greater importance to vascular surgeons is the risk of peri-operative thrombosis of either a vascular graft or an endarterectomy site. Whilst this can occur with any arterial reconstruction, it is particularly pertinent following infra-inguinal bypass and carotid endarterectomy where it may result in irreversible limb ischaemia and amputation, or stroke and death. At the very least it will result in symptom recurrence if it follows lower limb surgery, which may subsequently require reintervention.

Infra-inguinal bypass

Following infra-inguinal arterial reconstruction, 5-10% of grafts fail within the first month [36]. In some patients it may be unclear why graft occlusion has occurred; technical error (10-25%) or poor patient selection (inadequate inflow, poor run-off) are important factors. Intra-operative assessment of the anastomoses, graft flow and the presence of residual venous valves with duplex ultrasound may identify abnormal flow patterns or stenoses that can be revised to avoid early graft failure. Alternatively, postoperative heparinisation might be considered if it is thought that graft revision is unlikely to improve flow. However, this should not be undertaken lightly because of the risk of postoperative bleeding. Duplex ultrasound has largely replaced peripheral resistance measurements or on-table angiography for graft assessment although the latter may be necessary to confirm a possible abnormality detected by ultrasound.

The risk of peri-operative thrombosis is also related to the type of graft used. Although vein grafts are less thrombogenic than synthetic materials they undergo initial de-endothelialisation before arterialisation takes place, when subjected to arterial pressure [36]. During this time, tissue factor expression is enhanced, activating the extrinsic pathway of the clotting cascade (Figure 1: 8) [37] placing the graft at most risk of thrombosis during this early phase of remodelling. Nevertheless, the risk of early graft occlusion is higher when a synthetic graft is implanted because the lack of an endothelial lining induces platelet aggregation and thrombosis via the contact activation pathway (Figure 1: 9) [38]. Finally, when no obvious reason for graft thrombosis can be identified, the possibility of an underling thrombophilia should be considered.

If peri-operative graft occlusion results in acute or critical limb ischaemia, then immediate revisional surgery will be required. On-table angiography is an important adjuvant to graft thrombectomy and should include imaging of the in-flow, the distal anastomosis and run-off vessels. This will dictate the appropriate action. Following early revisional surgery, peri-operative anticoagulation with heparin is usually advised. If long-term anticoagulation is thought appropriate, blood should be taken for a thrombophilia screen before commencing warfarin treatment, particularly if no clear cause was identified for the graft thrombosis.

Carotid endarterectomy

Stroke following carotid endarterectomy is rare (3.8% in the GALA trial [39]) and is usually a consequence of thrombo-embolic events. Much of the historical debate has revolved around patch angioplasty of the internal carotid artery following endarterectomy. The most recent update of the Cochrane review [40] supports routine patch closure which reduces the risk of ipsilateral stroke during the peri-operative period (OR 0.31; p<0.0001) and long-term follow-up (OR 0.32). Currently there is insufficient evidence to determine if any particular type of patch confers additional benefit [41].

When intra-operative stroke occurs this is often due to technical error, although cerebral hypoperfusion may also be important. Several authors have advised intra-operative quality assurance with angioscopy or duplex ultrasound to indentify anatomical abnormalities that may require revision.

Post-procedural carotid thrombosis may also be the result of poor surgical technique which seems to be less likely if patch angioplasty is performed. However, there is considerable evidence that this might be a consequence of a white platelet clot at the endarterectomy site [42]. Naylor and co-workers demonstrated that postoperative monitoring with transcranial Doppler could identify patients with sustained high embolisation rates who are at most risk of stroke. In their original studies this responded to targeted intervention with Dextran with impressive reductions in post-procedural stroke rates. More recently, the same group have demonstrated that dual antiplatelet therapy prior to surgery successfully reduced the post-procedural stroke rate and obviated the need for transcranial Doppler monitoring or supplemental Dextran [43].

Conclusions

Thrombosis following vascular surgical intervention is an important cause of morbidity and mortality. Post-procedural VTE is often avoidable if an appropriate VTE prevention strategy is instigated pre-operatively. However, a significant number of patients will suffer thrombosis at the site of arterial reconstruction or in the deep veins following vascular surgery. This may be promoted by the presence of a known or occult thrombophilia. Appropriate medical management (intra-operative anticoagulation, antiplatelet therapy, statins) and intra-operative quality assessment can help prevent graft thrombosis.

An unresolved issue following venous thrombosis is the optimal duration of anticoagulation. In the future, repeat duplex imaging and serum d-dimer levels following a 3-month course of warfarin may help estimate the risk of recurrence and the duration of anticoagulation, and thus lead to individualised therapy decisions.

Key points

◆ Patients undergoing vascular surgery should have an individual VTE risk assessment and thromboprophylaxis plan instituted pre-operatively.
◆ Patients with a known thrombophilia for whom surgery is planned require appropriately tailored VTE prophylaxis.
◆ Patients who develop postoperative VTE despite thromboprophylaxis should be investigated for an underlying thrombophilia.
◆ Following a single VTE event, the optimal duration of treatment depends on the individualised thrombus load and recurrence risk. Repeat duplex and/or d-dimer assays may prove useful for predicting this in the future.
◆ All patients undergoing infra-inguinal bypass grafting should receive a statin and single antiplatelet therapy to improve graft patency; the potential benefit of dual antiplatelet therapy requires further assessment.
◆ All patients undergoing carotid endarterectomy should receive dual antiplatelet therapy pre-operatively to reduce the risk of peri-procedural thrombo-embolic stroke.

References

1. The National Institute for Health and Clinical Excellence. Venous Thromboembolism: Reducing the Risk. NICE Clinical Guideline 92, 2010. www.nice.org.uk/guidance/CG92.
2. Santamaria MG, Agnelli G, Taliani MR, et al; Warfarin Optimal Duration Italian Trial (WODIT) Investigators. Thrombophilic abnormalities and recurrence of venous thromboembolism in patients treated with standardized anticoagulant treatment. Thromb Res 2005; 116: 301-6.
3. Sofi F, Lari B, Rogolino A, et al. Thrombophilic risk factors for symptomatic peripheral arterial disease. J Vasc Surg 2005; 41: 255-60.

4.   Donaldson MC, Belkin M, Whittemore AD, *et al*. Impact of activated protein C resistance on general vascular surgical patients. *J Vasc Surg* 1997; 25: 1054-60.

5.   Vossen CY, Conard J, Fontcuberta J, *et al*. Risk of a first venous thrombotic event in carriers of a familial thrombophilic defect. The European prospective cohort on thrombophilia (EPCOT). *J Thromb Haemost* 2005; 3: 459-64.

6.   Marchlori A, Mosena L, Prins MH, Pradoni P. The risk of recurrent venous thromboembolism amongst heterozygous carriers of Factor V Leiden or prothrombin G20210A mutation. A systemic review of prospective studies. *Haematologica* 2007; 92: 1107-14.

7.   Martinelli I, Bucciarell P, Margaglione M, *et al*. The risk of venous thromboembolism in family members with mutations in the genes of Factor V or prothrombin or both. *Br J Haematol* 2000; 111: 1223-9.

8.   Spark JI, Laws P, Fitridge R. The incidence of hyperhomocysteinaemia in vascular patients. *Eur J Vasc Endovasc Surg* 2003; 26: 558-61.

9.   Ray JG. Meta-analysis of hyperhomocysteinemia as a risk factor for venous thromboembolic disease. *Arch Intern Med* 1998; 158: 2101-6.

10. Ray JG, Kearon C, Yi Q, *et al*; Heart Outcomes Prevention Evaluation 2 (HOPE-2) Investigators. Homocysteine-lowering therapy and risk for venous thromboembolism: a randomized trial. *Ann Intern Med* 2007; 146: 761-7.

11. Myles PS, Chan MT, Forbes A, *et al*. Preoperative folate and homocysteine status in patients undergoing major surgery. *Clinical Nutrition* 2006; 25: 736-45.

12. de Borst GJ, Tangelder MJ, Algra A, *et al*; Dutch BOA (Bypass Oral anticoagulants or Aspirin) Study Group. The influence of hyperhomocysteinemia on graft patency after infrainguinal bypass surgery in the Dutch BOA Study. *J Vasc Surg* 2002; 36: 336-40.

13. Van der Meet FJM, Koster T, Vandenbroucke JP, *et al*. The Leiden thrombophilia study (LETS). *Thromb Haemost* 1997; 78: 631-5.

14. Rodgers GM. Role of antithrombin concentrate in treatment of hereditary antithrombin deficiency. An update. *Thromb Haemost* 2009; 101: 806-12.

15. Tait RC, Walker ID, Reitsma PH, *et al*. Prevalence of protein C deficiency in the healthy population. *Thromb Haemost* 1995; 73: 87-93.

16. Brouwer JL, Lijfering WM, Ten Kate MK, *et al*. High long-term absolute risk of recurrent venous thromboembolism in patients with hereditary deficiencies of protein S, protein C or antithrombin. *Thromb Haemost* 2009; 101: 93-9.

17. Wahl DG, Guillemin F, de ME, *et al*. Risk for venous thrombosis related to antiphospholipid antibodies in systemic lupus erythematosis - a meta-analysis. *Lupus* 1997; 6: 467-73.

18. Galli M, Luciani D, Bertolini G, Barbui T. Lupus anticoagulants are stronger risk factors for thrombosis than anticardiolipin antibodies in the antiphospholipid syndrome: a systematic review of the literature. *Blood* 2003; 101: 1827-32.

19. Ahn SS, Kalunian K, Rosove M, Moore WS. Postoperative thrombotic complications in patients with lupus anticoagulant:

increased risk after vascular procedures. *Vasc Surg* 1988; 7: 749-56.

20. Erkan D, Leibowitz E, Berman J, Lockshin MD. Perioperative medical management of antiphospholipid syndrome: hospital for special surgery experience, review of literature, and recommendations. *J Rheumatol* 2002; 29: 843-49.

21. Hirsh J, Heddle N, Kelton J. Treatment of heparin-induced thrombocytopenia: a critical review. *Arch Int Med* 2004; 164: 361-9.

22. House of Commons Health Committee. The prevention of venous thromboembolism in hospitalised patients. London, UK: The Stationary Office Ltd, 2005.

23. Nicolaides AN, Breddin HK, Fareed J, *et al*; Cardiovascular Disease Educational and Research Trust and the International Union of Angiology. Prevention of Venous Thromboembolism. International Consensus Statement. Guidelines compiled in accordance with the scientific evidence. *Int Angiol* 2001; 20: 1-37.

24. Baglin T, Barrowcliffe TW, Cohen A, Greaves M. The British Committee for Standards in Haematology. Guidelines on the Use and Monitoring of Heparin. *Br J Haematol* 2006; 133: 19-34.

25. Geerts WH, Bergqvist D, Pineo GF, *et al*. American College of Chest Physicians Evidence-Based Clinical Practice Guidelines, 8th ed. Prevention of Venous Thromboembolism. *Chest* 2008; 133: 381S-453.

26. Anderson FA Jr, Spencer FA. Risk factors for venous thromboembolism. *Circulation* 2003; 107: I9-16.

27. White RH, Zhou H, Romano PS. Incidence of symptomatic venous thromboembolism after different elective or urgent surgical procedures. *Thromb Haemost* 2003; 90: 446-55.

28. Fletcher JP, Batiste P. Incidence of deep vein thrombosis following vascular surgery. *Int Angiol* 1997; 16: 65-8.

29. Hollyoak M, Woodruff P, Muller M, *et al*. Deep venous thrombosis in postoperative vascular surgical patients: a frequent finding without prophylaxis. *J Vasc Surg* 2001; 34: 656-60.

30. de Maistre E, Terriat B, Lesne-Padieu AS, *et al*. High incidence of venous thrombosis after surgery for abdominal aortic aneurysm. *J Vasc Surg* 2009; 49: 596-601.

31. Eagleton MJ, Grigoryants V, Peterson DA, *et al*. Endovascular treatment of abdominal aortic aneurysm is associated with a low incidence of deep venous thrombosis. *J Vasc Surg* 2002; 36: 912-6.

32. Killewich LA, Aswad MA, Sandager GP, *et al*. A randomized, prospective trial of deep venous thrombosis prophylaxis in aortic surgery. *Arch Surg* 1997; 132: 499-504.

33. Agnelli G, Prandoni P, Santamaria MG, *et al*; Warfarin Optimal Duration Italian Trial Investigators. Three months versus one year of oral anticoagulant therapy for idiopathic deep venous thrombosis. Warfarin Optimal Duration Italian Trial Investigators. *N Engl J Med* 2001; 345: 165-9.

34. Prandoni P, Prins MH, Lensing AW, *et al*; AESOPUS Investigators. Residual thrombosis on ultrasonography to guide the duration of anticoagulation in patients with deep venous thrombosis: a randomized trial. *Ann Int Med* 2009; 150: 577-85.

35. Verhovsek M, Doulketis JD, Yi Q, et al. Systematic review: d-dimer to predict recurrent disease after stopping anticoagulant therapy for unprovoked venous thromboembolism. *Ann Int Med* 2008; 149: 481-90.

36. Darling RC, Chang BB, Shah DM, Leather RP. Choice of peroneal or dorsalis pedis artery bypass for limb salvage. *Sem Vasc Surg* 1997; 10: 17-22.

37. Muluk SC, Vorp DA, Severyn DA, et al. Enhancement of tissue factor expression by vein segments exposed to coronary arterial hemodynamics. *J Vasc Surg* 1998; 27: 521-7.

38. Nielsen TG, Hesse B, Eiberg J, et al. Scintigraphic assessment of focal platelet accumulations following infrainguinal bypass surgery in humans. *Clin Physiol* 1997; 17: 545-55.

39. Lewis SC, Warlow CP, Bodenham AR, et al, for the GALA Collaborative group. General anaesthesia versus local anaesthesia for carotid surgery (GALA): an open, multicentre, randomised trial. *Lancet* 2008; 372: 2132-42.

40. Rerkasem K, Rothwell PM. Patch angioplasty versus primary closure for carotid endarterectomy. *Cochrane Database Syst Rev* 2009; 4: CD000160.

41. Rerkasem K, Rothwell PM. Patches of different types for carotid patch angioplasty. *Cochrane Database Syst Rev* 2010; 3: CD000071.

42. Naylor AR, Hayes PD, Allroggen H, et al. Reducing the risk of carotid surgery: a 7-year audit of the role of monitoring and quality control assessment. *J Vasc Surg* 2000; 32: 750-9.

43. Sharpe RY, Dennis MJS, Nasim A, et al. Dual antiplatelet therapy prior to carotid endarterectomy reduces post-operative embolisation and thromboembolic events: post-operative transcranial Doppler monitoring is now unnecessary. *Eur J Vasc Endovasc Surg* 2010; 40: 162-7.

Chapter 6

The management of haemorrhage in vascular surgery

Russell W. Jamieson MChir MRCS(Ed), Specialist Registrar in Vascular Surgery
Roderick T. A. Chalmers MD FRCS(Ed), Consultant Vascular Surgeon
Edinburgh Vascular Surgical Service, Royal Infirmary of Edinburgh, Edinburgh, UK

Introduction

"All bleeding stops eventually" – although this may be true, modern surgery dictates a more structured, scientific approach to the control of vascular haemorrhage. Many of the recent advances in the control of vascular haemorrhage are the fruit of work in conflict environments with battlefield surgery dictating rapid control and stabilisation of bleeding. Topics such as hypotensive resuscitation, tourniquets, haemostatic dressings, 1:1 transfusion and damage control surgery [1] will not be discussed in this chapter, which is geared towards the hospital-based vascular surgeon. Here we seek to identify emerging and established peri-operative techniques that afford control over haemorrhage and the disastrous consequences of uncontrolled bleeding. These techniques fall into four main categories: minimising the impact of haemorrhage, analysis and targeted treatment of coagulopathy, adjuncts to clot formation and non-surgical control of bleeding vessels.

Minimising the impact of haemorrhage

Autologous transfusion

Transfusion is a frequent accompaniment to major vascular procedures. Banked blood is poor quality and can act as a vector for transmission of bacterial and viral infection. Cross-matching is time consuming and transfusion reactions and the opportunity for error are always a possibility.

Autologous transfusion has long been seen as a good alternative, whether it be in pre-operative autologous banked blood, or intra-operative transfusion. Cell-saving systems have been available for many years and are becoming increasingly sophisticated (Figures 1, 2 and 3). Captured blood spill is mixed with anticoagulant, collected, washed, separated and returned for re-infusion as a red cell concentrate. Autologous transfusion has become routine for procedures involving massive haemorrhage, but there is less evidence for its use in routine elective vascular surgery. For infrarenal aortic surgery, the first meta-analysis of randomised trials suggested the evidence for cell salvage was lacking with small trials and divergent results [2]. Subsequent meta-analysis, after the publication of two larger randomised trials, did find in favour of cell saving for aortic surgery [3]. A more recent trial from Serbia, looking at the clinical and financial outcomes of 90 patients in three subgroups (occlusive disease, aneurysmal disease and ruptures) undergoing aortic surgery with or without cell salvage, concluded that in all groups the need for transfused allogenic blood was less [4]. In particular, the rupture subgroup benefited from the early availability of matched blood and with

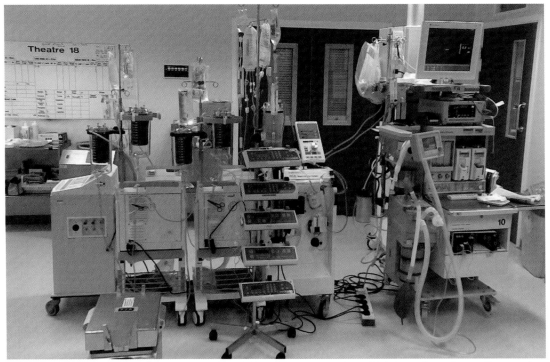

Figure 1. The calm before the storm – the twin cell saver and rapid infuser together with a series of infusion pumps waiting for a thoraco-abdominal aortic aneurysm repair.

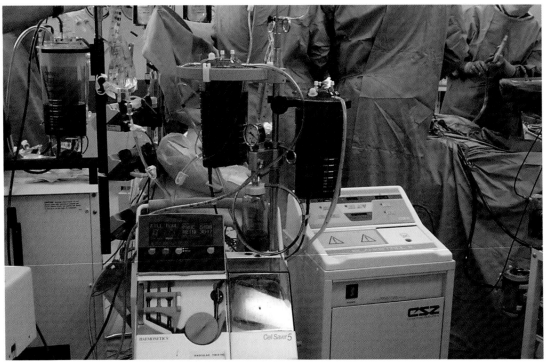

Figure 2. The cell saver in action. Blood is salvaged, mixed with anticooagulant, collected, washed, separated and returned for re-infusion as a red cell concentrate.

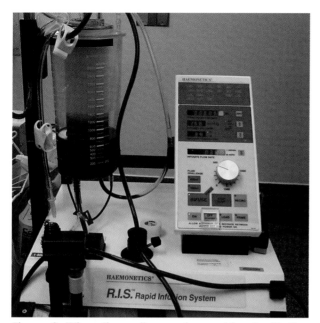

Figure 3. When the cell saver is combined with the rapid-infusion system, up to 1.5 litres per minute of blood can be returned at critical stages in the operation.

higher blood losses, made the most use of cell salvage. From a cost-benefit analysis cell salvage was deemed cost-effective if more than three units of autologous blood could be re-infused. There was no difference in clinical outcome noted between the groups. Similar studies across a range of surgical specialties have led to a recent review suggesting that the cost of cell salvage is between £150-190 per case based on a volume of 50 cases per year [5]. With a unit of donated blood costing approximately £135 it follows that, if greater than 1.5 units of blood can be re-infused, cell salvage is cost neutral in units performing over 50 cases per year. For many units including our own, the cell saver is employed routinely for all open aortic procedures.

Analysis and targeted treatment of coagulopathy

Near-patient testing

Haemoglobin estimation

The assessment of haemorrhage by weighing swabs and measuring blood loss is an inexact science. Near-patient testing of haemoglobin has been available for many years, yet in vascular surgery is not routinely reported [6]. Our unit uses a Hemocue® B-haemoglobin photometer (Hemo-Cue AB, Sweden) to estimate haemoglobin levels intra-operatively without the need to wait for formal laboratory analysis. With results available in under a minute, delays in detecting significant anaemia are avoided and transfusion can be initiated.

Thrombo-elastography

It is often assumed that conventional coagulation tests (INR and APPT) reflect the coagulation state of the patient. These tests, however, monitor only the initial phase of coagulation and it is possible to have normal values yet abnormal clotting [7]. Thrombo-elastography is a visco-elastic measure of the whole of the haemostatic cascade and development of clot in a whole blood sample. The two most commonly used thrombo-elastographs are the TEG® system (Haemoscope Corp., USA) and the ROTEM® system (TEM International GmbH, Germany) (Figure 4). They discriminate between surgical bleeding and a haemostasis disorder, hyperfibrinolysis, the extent of dilutional coagulopathy, requirement for fibrinogen or platelet substitution, and allow heparin and protamine dosage monitoring. Both utilise an oscillating pin in a sample cup of citrated whole blood. The resistance during the oscillation is translated into a thrombo-elastogram, from which the lag time to the start of clot formation, the kinetics of clot formation, the strength of the clot and finally the dissolution of clot or fibrinolysis can be derived. Thrombo-elastography has found application in near-patient monitoring of haemostasis in major trauma surgery, cardiac surgery, and liver transplantation. The current European guidelines for the management of bleeding following major trauma [8] and during cardiothoracic surgery [9] advise that thrombo-elastography now be considered to assist in characterising the coagulopathy and guide haemostatic management. In the case vignette on p76 we demonstrate the utility of ROTEM® analysis in guiding correction of coagulopathy. We now routinely use ROTEM® to monitor our aortic surgery patients, in particular our thoraco-abdominal cases where major blood loss and coagulopathy can be anticipated.

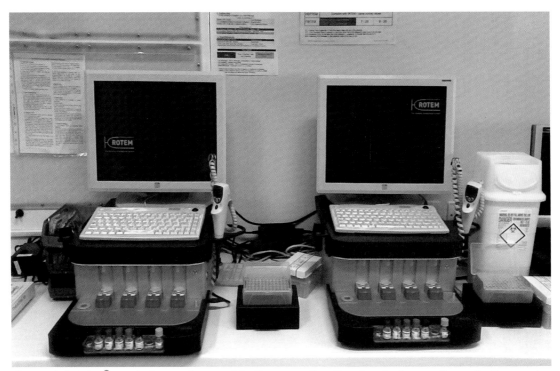

Figure 4. ROTEM® analysis can be used in the operating theatre during aortic and other major surgery to monitor coagulation.

Platelet function

Many vascular patients presenting for intervention are now on one or more antiplatelet agents. Frequently, coronary interventions dictate that such agents should only be stopped in cases where bleeding risk outweighs the risk of ischaemic events. In emergency cases one does not have the luxury of stopping these drugs far enough in advance. Bleeding in patients on dual antiplatelet agents tends to be a steady generalised oozing that can be difficult to stop. Assessment of platelet function is an emerging field in near-patient testing [10] with studies supporting the use of platelet function analysis to guide antiplatelet dosing, particularly in relation to coronary disease and cardiac surgery. Platelet aggregometry can be used to determine the effect of aspirin, clopidogrel and other antiplatelet agents. Impedance aggregometry is based on the principle that blood platelets are non-thrombogenic in their resting state, but expose receptors on their surface when they are activated, which allow them to attach on vascular injuries and artificial surfaces. Activated platelets stick to sensor wires enhancing the electrical resistance between them which is continuously recorded. For the vascular surgeon faced with generalised ooze, assessment of platelet function can be useful in confirming the cause of bleeding and assessing response to intervention. We now routinely use a Multiplate® (Verum Diagnostica GmbH, Germany) impedence aggregometry to assess platelet function during cases with diffuse bleeding. The case vignette on p74 demonstrates the use of such near-patient testing to gain control over vascular haemorrhage.

Adjuncts to clot formation

Local haemostatic agents

Local haemostatic agents are proving increasingly useful adjuncts to traditional surgical techniques and packing in the context of vascular haemorrhage [11]. They are especially useful in cases with difficult access, a lack of a defined bleeding point and anastomotic suture line bleeding between synthetic vascular grafts. These agents fall into three main categories – topical haemostats, adhesives and sealants.

Topical haemostats

Topical haemostats are most widely used in the context of diffuse, often venous bleeding where direct pressure is not possible or ongoing ooze is anticipated. Collagen-based haemostatic agents promote a degranulation of platelets and platelet aggregation. The collagen backbone provides a matrix for a haemostatic plug to develop and by impregnation of procoagulants, such as thrombin, a firm clot can be produced. These agents are widely used in the setting of diffuse bleeding and a randomised trial has shown they reduce time to haemostasis in the setting of cardiac, orthopaedic and liver surgery [12]. Where cell salvage is utilised, caution in the use of such agents is advised, given the potential for the collagen fibrils to pass through cell-salvage filters and be re-infused with micro-embolic consequences [13]. Gelatin-based haemostatic agents rely more on physical effects than direct platelet degranulation to encourage clot formation. They swell on contact with blood encouraging tamponade and can be combined with procoagulant to produce clot which typically takes 4-6 weeks to degrade. Cellulose-based haemostatic agents have numerous properties to trigger clot formation with activation of platelets and both the intrinsic and extrinsic clotting pathways. Surgicel® (Ethicon, UK) is probably the best known cellulose-based haemostat and has been used for many years, although the evidence base to support it is limited [11]. Although absorbable, the manufacturer advises removal once haemostasis has been obtained; failure to do so can result in granuloma formation which is radiologically difficult to distinguish from more sinister pathology [14].

Adhesives

BioGlue® (Cryolife, Georgia, USA) was introduced to the European market in 1998 and is formed by the covalent bonding of its two separate components, albumin and glutaraldehyde, with proteins on the surface of human tissue. It forms a rapid bond that is independent of the coagulation status of the patient. In a prospective randomised controlled clinical trial, BioGlue® proved very effective in reducing suture line bleeding in a range of vascular procedures (cardiac, aortic and peripheral), reinforcing the suture line and reducing the need for pledgets [15]. One limitation of BioGlue® is the requirement for a relatively dry field prior to application. Our unit frequently deploys BioGlue® to reduce suture line bleeding especially between two synthetic grafts and around visceral patches during thoraco-abdominal aneurysm repairs.

Fibrin-based sealants

Fibrin-based sealants have been available for over 30 years. All contain a source of fibrinogen together with thrombin and, in some cases, antifibrinolytic agents. Sealants with higher fibrinogen to thrombin ratios have stronger clots but these clots take longer to stabilise [16]. For most sealants the two components are freeze dried and require thawing and reconstitution prior to application typically via a pressurised double-barrel spray gun designed to mix the two components in a jet. On contact with the bleeding tissue, fibrin is formed and interacts with Factor VIII to encourage clot formation. Fibrin sealants have been shown to reduce total blood loss and transfusion requirement with a Cochrane Database Review establishing a 37% relative risk reduction in the need for transfusion where sealant was used based on 18 trials involving 1406 patients [17]. The mean reduction in blood loss noted in 14 trials was 161ml. Although widely studied in the field of urology, liver surgery and ENT surgery, trials of fibrin sealants in vascular surgery are limited.

Recently a randomised, controlled clinical trial evaluated the safety and haemostatic effectiveness of a fibrin sealant (EVICEL™ Fibrin Sealant [Human]) during vascular surgery [18]. This new sealant from Johnson & Johnson™ is a pure mix of human fibrinogen and thrombin without any antifibrinolytic agents. It seeks to replace CROSSEAL™ (QUIXIL™ in Europe) which contained tranexamic acid as it had been linked to neurotoxicity if introduced into cerebrospinal fluid. The trial randomised patients undergoing PTFE bypass procedures to control of anastomotic bleeding by either application of the sealant or standard manual pressure. The primary endpoint of haemostasis at 4 minutes saw 85% controlled with sealant in comparison to only 39% with manual pressure. Similar significant improvement was noted at 7 and 10 minutes and there were no major safety concerns in the sealant group. This trial involved PTFE anastomoses to arteries at either the groin, or in the upper extremities, where access is

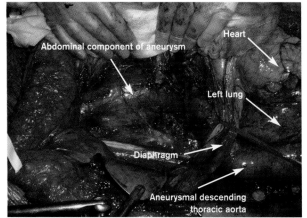

Figure 5. During a thoraco-abdominal aortic aneurysm repair, the medial visceral rotation generates a vast raw surface – we routinely spray this area with EVICEL™ Fibrin Sealant (Human) (Johnson & Johnson) to gain haemostasis.

usually good. The real value of such fibrin sealant is likely to be where access is problematic, where rapid haemostasis is vital (visceral patch in clamp and go thoraco-abdominal aneurysm repairs), or where native vessel quality is poor (calcified, splitting aortic necks). In such cases one could argue over the relative merits of fibrin sealant over Bioglue®, although to our knowledge there has yet to be a comparative trial. Our unit routinely uses BioGlue® in this setting with fibrin sealant reserved for larger areas when obtaining a dry field is unrealistic. We spray the sealant onto the raw surface exposed by medial visceral rotation during thoraco-abdominal aortic aneurysm repair (Figure 5). Much like the use of fibrin sealant in liver surgery [19], here the sealant acts on a large oozing surface with impressive rapid haemostasis.

Antifibrinolytics

To reduce peri-operative blood loss, antifibrinolytic drugs (aprotinin [Trasylol™, Bayer, USA], tranexamic acid [TXA], and ε-aminocaproic acid [EACA]) have been widely used, especially in the field of cardiac surgery. Aprotinin is a non-specific, serine protease inhibitor, derived from bovine lung, with antifibrinolytic properties [20]. It acts as an inhibitor of several serine proteases, including trypsin, plasmin, plasma kallikrein and tissue kallikrein. Aprotinin also inhibits the contact phase activation of coagulation that both initiates

coagulation and promotes fibrinolysis. It was withdrawn from the market in 2008 following concerns that its use resulted in excess mortality and serum creatinine rise [21]. TXA and EACA are synthetic analogue derivatives of the amino acid lysine that act principally by blocking the lysine binding sites on plasminogen molecules, inhibiting the formation of plasmin and therefore inhibiting fibrinolysis. Tranexamic acid is about ten times more potent than ε-aminocaproic acid. A very recent update of the Cochrane Database Review on "Antifibrinolytic use for minimising perioperative allogeneic blood transfusion" now reflects the removal of aprotinin from the market [22]. The review examined data from 252 randomised control trials with over 25,000 participants. Aprotinin reduced the need for blood transfusion (relative risk 0.66). Comparative trials between aprotinin and the lysine analogues were slightly in favour of aprotinin (relative risk 0.9). In contrast to the non-randomised trials published prior to the withdrawal of aprotinin, the review found that when compared to no treatment, patients given aprotinin were not at increased risk of myocardial infarction, renal impairment or death. When compared directly with either or both lysine analogues, however, aprotinin was associated with a significant increase in mortality (relative risk 1.39). From this review it is clear that little evidence for the use of antifibrinolytic drugs in vascular surgery is available. Only two trials of aprotinin, one trial of TXA and none involving EACA were included in the data analysed. The current European guidelines for the management of bleeding following major trauma suggests that antifibrinolytic agents should be considered and that, if used, their effects should be monitored by thrombo-elastography if possible [8]. Our unit does not use any of these agents at present.

Pro-coagulants

Desmopressin

Desmopressin (1-desamino-8-D-arginine vasopressin, DDAVP) is a synthetic analogue of arginine vasopressin, a naturally occurring anti-diuretic hormone. One of the many effects of vasopressin is the stimulation of release of von Willibrand Factor by the Weibel-Palade body of endothelial cells which enhances platelet adhesion to wound sites. Desmopressin has been successfully used to facilitate haemostasis in a range of inherited bleeding disorders (von Willibrand's disease, haemophilia A and some platelet function defects) [23]. The use of desmopressin in elective surgery where major bleeding is anticipated has been reviewed by the Cochrane Database group [24]. They found no convincing evidence that desmopressin reduces the need for transfusion in the peri-operative period in patients without a congenital bleeding disorder and although total blood loss was less, it was not felt to be clinically significant. The views of the Cochrane Database group are echoed by the current European guidelines for the management of bleeding following major trauma which suggest desmopressin should not be used routinely [8]. As in the case vignette on p74, the guidelines suggest desmopressin may prove useful in microvascular bleeding in patients treated with antiplatelets.

Recombinant activated Factor VII (rFVIIa)

Initially developed to treat haemorrhage in haemophilia patients with neutralising auto-antibodies to Factors VII and IX, recombinant activated Factor VII (rFVIIa) (NovoSeven®, Novo Nordisk A/S, Denmark) is increasingly under investigation as an aid to haemostasis in cases of massive haemorrhage in non-haemophilic patients. From experimental use in military surgery [25], rFVIIa has entered clinical practice with impressive results in randomised controlled trials in both blunt and penetrating abdominal trauma [26]. Particularly in blunt trauma, where bleeding tends to be a more generalised oozing, rFVIIa has led to significantly less blood transfusion and a 19% reduction in the need for massive transfusion. The use of rFVIIa in vascular surgery has been reported in a number of small case series, but in 2008 two publications provided a review and meta-analysis of the use of rFVIIa in major bleeding during vascular and urological cases [27, 28]. In the vascular patient group, 75% of cases involved aortic surgery with rFVIIa being used in both open and endovascular procedures [28]. Although the numbers were small, significant differences were noted in the red cell transfusion requirement [28] and 73% of patients given rFVIIa had a reduction in bleeding and a survival benefit [27]. Very recently, a meta-analysis identified 26 randomised controlled trials up to January 2010 (14

prophylactic use and 12 treatment) which compared rFVIIa against placebo in any patient population, except those with haemophilia [29]. The conclusion was that rFVIIa led to a reduction in blood loss, less blood transfusion, fewer patients receiving transfusion and, in the treatment trials, led to a non-significant reduction in mortality. Because this meta-analysis looked at disparate patient groups and interventions, extrapolation to the use of rFVIIa in vascular surgery is not possible. In press at present is a study on the use of rFVIIa in patients undergoing open ruptured abdominal aortic aneurysm repair, Type III or Type IV thoraco-abdominal aortic aneurysm repair [30]. This study collected prospective data in the above patient groups treated with rFVIIa when bleeding was found to be intractable despite standard adjuncts including cell salvage, best practice blood product administration, antithrombolytics and desmopressin. Blood loss, transfusion requirements, arrest of haemorrhage and survival were compared to matched historical controls treated in a similar manner, but not given rFVIIa. The results show that rFVIIa successfully reduced blood loss and transfusion of blood and products postoperatively. Haemostasis was obtained in 87.5% of patients in the rFVIIa group which importantly translated into a 30-day mortality of 12.5% in comparison to 81% in the historical controls.

Non-surgical control of bleeding vessels

Balloon occlusion catheters

Most vascular surgeons will be happy using balloon occlusion catheters in the elective setting to obtain vessel control in situations where clamping is not possible or desirable. The use of balloon occlusion in the presence of life-threatening exsanguination is thankfully a procedure that most surgeons will have limited experience with. Occlusion balloon catheters are intended for temporary occlusion of large blood vessels. They range from dedicated endovascular catheters (Coda™ Occlusion Catheter (Cook Medical Inc., Indiana) to the large Occlusion Balloon Catheter™ (Boston Scientific, Massachusetts), the smaller Standard Berenstein Occlusion Balloon Catheter™ and the Standard Occlusion Balloon

Catheter™ (Boston Scientific, Massachusetts). All are highly compliant to accommodate a wide range of vessel diameters and adjust to the shape of the vessel in which they are inflated. Once the balloon reaches the vessel diameter it elongates without undue radial force. Inflation is volume-driven and generally gauged with fluoroscopy; longitudinal expansion in the presence of a stable diameter indicates that occlusion has probably been achieved.

In the setting of major haemorrhage, a simple Fogarty or even Foley catheter is more than adequate. Since the original case report [31] of a Fogarty balloon catheter inserted in a lumbar vein at laparotomy to control massive haemorrhage (the catheter was simply cut off and left in the patient!), most literature regarding the control of haemorrhage in the emergency setting through the use of occlusion balloons is limited to case series. The Department of Surgery at Emory University, Georgia, USA, have recently published their experience over 10 years [32]. They identified 44 cases of occlusion catheter use and noted that survival was linked to the length of time the balloon was deployed (81% if <6 hours; 52% if ≥6 hours). Liver, abdominal vascular and facial/pharyngeal injuries often required prolonged occlusion times. Mean indwelling times for iliac, liver, and carotid injuries were 31 hours, 53 hours, and 78 hours, respectively, with 93% of cases initially achieving successful tamponade.

High intensity focused ultrasound (HIFU)

High intensity focused ultrasound is emerging as a valuable clinical tool [33]. By the tight focusing of a beam of high energy ultrasound into a small target volume, HIFU is capable of thermal ablation of tissues. Research is exponential as more clinical applications for non-invasive cellular destruction emerge. Oncology is benefiting from HIFU treatment to both destroy and limit perfusion to tumours through coagulation of tissues with abdominal, gynaecological, liver, prostatic and brain cancers all targeted. Recently, work has emerged on the use of HIFU in delivering acoustic haemostasis and haemorrhage control [34]. HIFU can deliver energy to deep regions of tissue where haemorrhage is occurring, allowing cauterization at depth of parenchymal tissues, or in difficult-to-access anatomical regions, while causing no or minimal biological effects in the intervening and surrounding tissues. By combining image-guiding ultrasound (such as B mode and colour Doppler) with HIFU it has been possible, in a pig model of penetrating pelvic bleeding, to treat a 4cm deep partial transection injury (a 0.5cm long arteriotomy) of the internal iliac artery [35]. After induction of bleeding under ultrasound guidance with a penetrating scalpel, HIFU treatment was applied transcutaneously and bleeding completely arrested within approximately 70 seconds leaving a patent vessel. By adjusting the settings, vessel occlusion can also be obtained [36]. Although clearly still an experimental tool, the pace of progress is rapid and it would appear entirely reasonable to envisage the vascular surgeon of the future controlling haemorrhage using HIFU.

Conclusions

The control of vascular haemorrhage is no longer restricted to firm pressure, packing and fast suturing. Vascular surgeons currently have at their disposal a range of increasingly sophisticated techniques to minimise the impact of haemorrhage, analyse and treat coagulopathy, encourage clot formation and control bleeding vessels. Haemostatic technology is rapidly advancing and not confined to bleeding during vascular surgery. Indeed much of our current practice is not supported by direct evidence in the field of vascular surgery. This is something which should be addressed by properly constructed randomised controlled trials. Intra-operative bleeding from heavily diseased arteries in patients on antiplatelet agents and loaded with heparin should intuitively pose a different challenge to the general venous ooze from a cirrhotic liver in a patient with a prolonged prothombin time. Undoubtedly different solutions are required.

Key points

◆ Autologous transfusion is probably cost-effective if greater than 1.5 units of blood are re-infused and over 50 cases are performed annually.

◆ Near-patient testing is very useful in monitoring coagulopathy and guiding management. Thrombo-elastography in particular, is emerging as a vital assessment tool in cases of major haemorrhage.

◆ Local haemostatic agents are of value; adhesives and fibrin-based sealants have evidence to support their use in vascular surgery, particularly for anastomotic bleeding. Antifibrinolytics have little direct evidence to support their use in vascular surgery but undoubtedly have a role to play in haemostasis during major surgery.

◆ Desmopressin does not have a routine role during vascular surgery but may be of use in patients loaded with antiplatelet agents.

◆ Data are emerging to suggest that recombinant activated Factor VII may have an important role in the future in arresting major vascular haemorrhage.

◆ Non-surgical control of haemorrhage with balloon occlusion catheters is possible, although the evidence is limited and their use is typically reserved for emergency cases. High intensity focused ultrasound is emerging as a potential tool in the vascular surgeon's armoury to control bleeding at depth.

◆ Haemostatic technology is rapidly advancing but little evidence is available in vascular surgery. Extrapolation from other surgical fields may not be appropriate and randomised controlled trials are required.

References

1. D'Alleyrand JC, Dutton RP, Pollak AN. Extrapolation of battlefield resuscitative care to the civilian setting. *J Surg Orthop Adv* 2006; 19: 62-9.

2. Alvarez GG, Fergusson DA, Neilipovitz DT, *et al*. Cell salvage does not minimize perioperative allogeneic blood transfusion in abdominal vascular surgery: a systematic review. *Can J Anaesth* 2004; 51: 425-31.

3. Takagi H, Sekino S, Kato T, *et al*. Intraoperative autotransfusion in abdominal aortic aneurysm surgery: meta-analysis of randomized controlled trials. *Arch Surg* 2007; 142: 1098-101.

4. Markovic M, Davidovic L, Savic N, *et al*. Intraoperative cell salvage versus allogeneic transfusion during abdominal aortic surgery: clinical and financial outcomes. *Vascular* 2009; 17: 83-92.

5. Kuppurao L, Wee M. Perioperative cell salvage. *Continuing Education in Anaesthesia, Critical Care & Pain* 2010; 10: 104-8.

6. Lardi AM, Hirst C, Mortimer AJ, *et al*. Evaluation of the HemoCue for measuring intra-operative haemoglobin concentrations: a comparison with the Coulter Max-M. *Anaesthesia* 1998; 53: 349-52.

7. Levrat A, Gros A, Rugeri L, *et al*. Evaluation of rotation thrombelastography for the diagnosis of hyperfibrinolysis in trauma patients. *Br J Anaesth* 2008; 100: 792-7.

8. Rossaint R, Bouillon B, Cerny V, *et al*. Management of bleeding following major trauma: an updated European guideline. *Crit Care* 2010; 14: R52.

9. Dunning J, Versteegh M, Fabbri A, *et al*. Guideline on antiplatelet and anticoagulation management in cardiac surgery. *Eur J Cardiothorac Surg* 2008; 34: 73-92.

10. Ferreiro JL, Sibbing D, Angiolillo DJ. Platelet function testing and risk of bleeding complications. *Thromb Haemost* 2010; 103: 1128-35.

11. Seyednejad H, Imani M, Jamieson T, *et al*. Topical haemostatic agents. *Br J Surg* 2008; 95: 1197-225.

12. CoStasis Multi-center Collaborative Writing Committee. A novel collagen-based composite offers effective hemostasis for multiple surgical indications: results of a randomized controlled trial. *Surgery* 2001; 129: 445-50.

13. Robicsek F, Duncan GD, Born GV, *et al*. Inherent dangers of simultaneous application of microfibrillar collagen hemostat and blood-saving devices. *J Thorac Cardiovasc Surg* 1986; 92: 766-70.

14. Sandhu GS, Elexpuru-Camiruaga JA, Buckley S. Oxidized cellulose (Surgicel) granulomata mimicking tumour recurrence. *Br J Neurosurg* 1996; 10: 617-9.

15. Coselli JS, Bavaria JE, Fehrenbacher J, *et al*. Prospective randomized study of a protein-based tissue adhesive used as a hemostatic and structural adjunct in cardiac and vascular anastomotic repair procedures. *J Am Coll Surg* 2003; 197: 243-52; discussion 52-3.

16. Busuttil RW. A comparison of antifibrinolytic agents used in hemostatic fibrin sealants. *J Am Coll Surg* 2003; 197: 1021-8.

17. Carless PA, Henry DA, Anthony DM. Fibrin sealant use for minimising peri-operative allogeneic blood transfusion. *Cochrane Database Syst Rev* 2003; 1. Available from: http://www.mrw.interscience.wiley.com/cochrane/clsysrev/articles/CD004171/frame.html.

18. Chalmers RT, Darling Iii RC, Wingard JT, *et al.* Randomized clinical trial of tranexamic acid-free fibrin sealant during vascular surgical procedures. *Br J Surg* 2010; 97: 1784-9.

19. Schwartz M, Madariaga J, Hirose R, *et al.* Comparison of a new fibrin sealant with standard topical hemostatic agents. *Arch Surg* 2004; 139: 1148-54.

20. Fritz H, Wunderer G. Biochemistry and applications of aprotinin, the kallikrein inhibitor from bovine organs. *Arzneimittelforschung* 1983; 33: 479-94.

21. Mangano DT, Miao Y, Vuylsteke A, *et al.* Mortality associated with aprotinin during 5 years following coronary artery bypass graft surgery. *JAMA* 2007; 297: 471-9.

22. Henry DA, Carless PA, Moxey AJ, *et al.* Anti-fibrinolytic use for minimising perioperative allogeneic blood transfusion. *Cochrane Database Syst Rev* 2011; 1: CD001886.

23. Franchini M. The use of desmopressin as a hemostatic agent: a concise review. *Am J Hematol* 2007; 82: 731-5.

24. Carless PA, Henry DA, Moxey AJ, *et al.* Desmopressin for minimising perioperative allogeneic blood transfusion. *Cochrane Database Syst Rev* 2004; 1: CD001884.

25. Kenet G, Walden R, Eldad A, *et al.* Treatment of traumatic bleeding with recombinant factor VIIa. *Lancet* 1999; 354(9193): 1879.

26. Boffard KD, Riou B, Warren B, *et al.* Recombinant factor VIIa as adjunctive therapy for bleeding control in severely injured trauma patients: two parallel randomized, placebo-controlled, double-blind clinical trials. *J Trauma* 2005; 59: 8-15; discussion -8.

27. von Heymann C, Jonas S, Spies C, *et al.* Recombinant activated factor VIIa for the treatment of bleeding in major abdominal surgery including vascular and urological surgery:

28. Warren OJ, Alcock EM, Choong AM, *et al.* Recombinant activated factor VII: a solution to refractory haemorrhage in vascular surgery? *Eur J Vasc Endovasc Surg* 2008; 35: 145-52.

29. Lin Y, Stanworth S, Birchall J, *et al.* Use of recombinant factor VIIa for the prevention and treatment of bleeding in patients without hemophilia: a systematic review and meta-analysis. *CMAJ* 2011; 183: E9-19.

30. Koncar IB, Davidovic LB, Savic N, *et al.* Role of recombinant factor VIIa in the treatment of intractable bleeding in vascular surgery. *J Vasc Surg* 2011: 53: 1032-7.

31. Davidson AT, Sr. Direct intralumen balloon tamponade: a technic for the control of massive retroperitoneal hemorrhage. *Am J Surg* 1978; 136: 393-4.

32. Ball CG, Wyrzykowski AD, Nicholas JM, *et al.* A decade's experience with balloon catheter tamponade for the emergency control of hemorrhage. *J Trauma* 2011; 70: 330-3.

33. ter Haar G, Coussios C. High intensity focused ultrasound: past, present and future. *Int J Hyperthermia* 2007; 23: 85-7.

34. Vaezy S, Zderic V. Hemorrhage control using high intensity focused ultrasound. *Int J Hyperthermia* 2007; 23: 203-11.

35. Vaezy S, Shi X, Martin RW, *et al.* Real-time visualization of high-intensity focused ultrasound treatment using ultrasound imaging. *Ultrasound Med Biol* 2001; 27: 33-42.

36. Burgess S, Zderic V, Vaezy S. Image-guided acoustic hemostasis for hemorrhage in the posterior liver. *Ultrasound Med Biol* 2007; 33: 113-9.

Case vignette — Challenging carotid endarterectomy bleeding – near-patient platelet function analysis

Russell W. Jamieson MChir MRCS(Ed), Specialist Registrar in Vascular Surgery
Roderick T. A. Chalmers MD FRCS(Ed), Consultant Vascular Surgeon
Edinburgh Vascular Surgical Service, Royal Infirmary of Edinburgh, Edinburgh, UK

A 45-year-old man presented with a single episode of transient left-sided monocular blindness. His carotid duplex revealed a 90% stenosis of his left internal carotid artery and his referring neurologist started him on aspirin 75mg and clopidogrel 75mg daily. He underwent a semi-urgent carotid endarterectomy under local regional block. He was fully heparinised intra-operatively (5000IU intravenously) and underwent an uncomplicated endarterctomy and bovine pericardial patch repair. He had significant, constant suture hole bleeding and a generalised ooze from the tissues. Protamine reversal of the heparinisation did little to stem the ooze. A near-patient platelet function assay was performed using a Multiplate® Platelet Aggregometer (Verum Diagnostica GmbH, Germany). In comparison to a normal control sample (Figure 1), the patient was found to have significant inhibition of platelet function from both aspirin and clopidogrel (Figure 2). This persisted after the administration of one pool of banked platelets (Figure 3). The patient was treated with intravenous desmopressin to enhance von

Case vignette Challenging carotid endarterectomy bleeding – near-patient platelet function analysis

Figure 1. Multiplate® platelet impedence aggregometry analysis of a normal control specimen.

Figure 2. Multiplate® platelet impedence aggregometry analysis performed when protamine reversal of heparinisation failed to improve the generalised ooze and suture line bleeding. The profoundly depressed curves in both the ADP Test and ASPI Test reflect the inhibition of platelet aggregation by clopidogrel and aspirin, respectively.

Figure 3. Multiplate® platelet impedence aggregometry analysis performed after one pooled unit of platelets had been given. No significant improvement was noted clinically or on testing.

Willebrand levels and encourage platelet function, which resulted in a very rapid cessation of ooze and a slight improvement in platelet aggregation (Figure 4). When a subsequent platelet transfusion was given, near normal platelet function was obtained (Figure 5).

Figure 4. Multiplate® platelet impedence aggregometry analysis performed after desmopressin (DDAVP) had been administered. A rapid clinical improvement in the bleeding status was noted with some improvement in the platelet aggregometry.

Figure 5. Multiplate® platelet impedence aggregometry analysis performed 90 minutes after an additional pooled unit of platelets had been administered. The patient had minimal blood in his drain, no evidence of a neck haematoma and was clinically well. His platelet aggregometry was almost normal.

Case vignette

Thrombo-elastography during thoraco-abdominal aortic aneurysm repair

Russell W. Jamieson MChir MRCS(Ed), Specialist Registrar in Vascular Surgery
Roderick T.A. Chalmers MD FRCS(Ed), Consultant Vascular Surgeon
Edinburgh Vascular Surgical Service, Royal Infirmary of Edinburgh, Edinburgh, UK

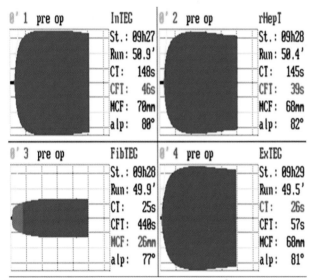

Figure 1. Pre-operative ROTEM® analysis demonstrating near normal coagulation.

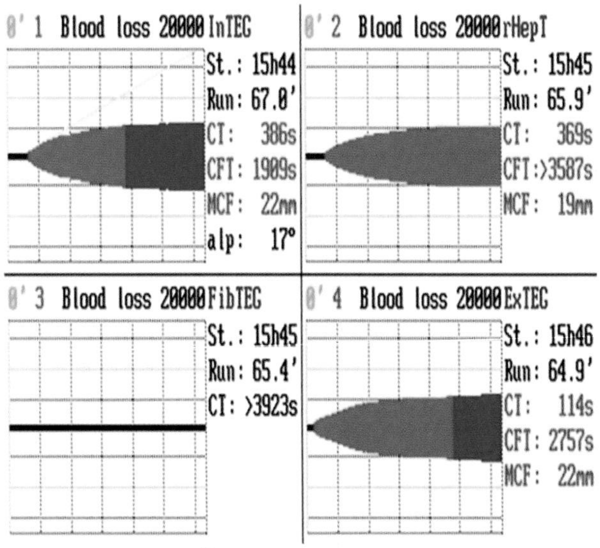

A 72-year-old lady, previously fit and well with only mild treated hypertension and some breathlessness on exertion underwent a Type II thoraco-abdominal aortic aneurysm repair. Coagulopathy was anticipated given the potential for large blood loss and visceral ischaemia/reperfusion. A pre-operative ROTEM® analysis was performed (Figure 1). Following visceral reperfusion, this, together with significant blood loss, resulted in a multifactorial coagulopathy (Figure 2). Formal bloods were sent to the laboratory but results were not available until almost 2 hours later. These results confirmed the ROTEM® analysis but such a delay negates their use acutely. On the basis of the ROTEM® analysis, clotting factors were administered immediately and the bleeding profile of the patient improved dramatically. The ROTEM® reading normalised (Figure 3) and the subsequent formal blood tests confirmed a near normal clotting status.

Figure 2. ROTEM® analysis taken after visceral reperfusion demonstrating the multifactorial coagulopathy. Formal blood results, available much later, confirmed the multifactorial coagulopathy.

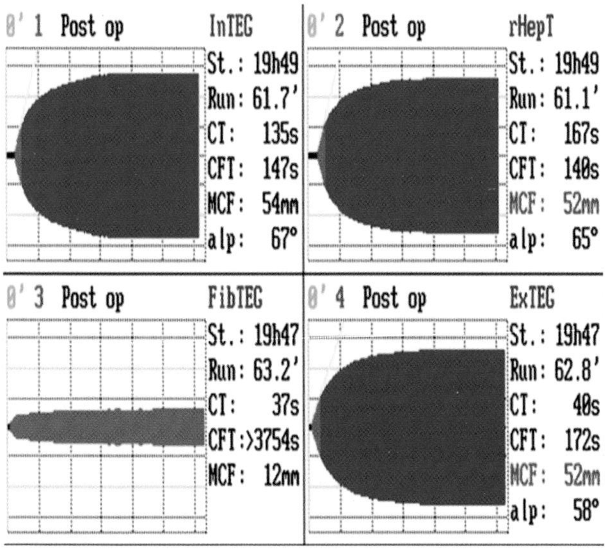

Figure 3. Based solely on the results of the near-patient ROTEM® analysis, clotting factors were administered immediately and coagulation corrected as shown.

Chapter 7

How to prevent and manage major postoperative vascular infections

A. Ross Naylor MD FRCS, Professor of Vascular Surgery
Leicester Royal Infirmary, Leicester, UK

Introduction

Prosthetic graft infection, though rare, can be one of the most challenging vascular surgical problems. The incidence of graft infection varies according to the nature of the graft (cavitary/extra-anatomic) and location (carotid/femoral). The incidence of aortic graft infection (after open surgery) is 2-3%, falling to 1% after endovascular aneurysm repair. Axillobifemoral bypasses carry a higher incidence of infection (up to 8%), approximately 5-8% of prosthetic infra-inguinal bypasses will become infected, while carotid patch infection has a much lower incidence (<1%).

Classification

Graft infections are classified as early, if they present within 4 months of surgery, or late, if they occur thereafter. The Szilagyi classification of vascular infections is based on the extent of the infection [1]:

- grade 1 (wound only);
- grade 2 (wound and underlying subcutaneous tissues); and
- grade 3 (infection involving the vascular prosthesis).

The Szilagyi classification is, however, a little rudimentary and a more clinically oriented classification has been devised by Bunt [2] (Table 1).

Aetiology

Vascular patients are prone to infection because of the following:

- they tend to be elderly;
- many present with chronic wounds in association with hospital/nursing home care prior to admission;
- they have impaired immunity (diabetes, steroid therapy, renal impairment, malignancy);
- the use of groin incisions;
- prolonged operation times (blood loss/ hypothermia);
- prosthetic conduits (Dacron® is more susceptible to micro-organism adherence than PTFE);
- problems with wound healing (diabetes, renal impairment, reperfusion oedema); and
- antiplatelet agents and intra-operative heparin can predispose towards wound haematomas.

Most graft infections probably start with contamination at the time of surgery, hence the need for a meticulous approach to prevention (see later).

Table 1. The Bunt classification of prosthetic graft infections [2].

Peripheral graft infection

P0: Infection of a cavitary graft (e.g. abdominal/thoracic aorta, iliofemoral)

P1: Infection of a graft whose entire location is non-cavitary (e.g. axillofemoral, femoropopliteal)

P2: Infection of a non-cavitary segment of graft whose origin is cavitary (e.g. groin infection in aortofemoral bypass)

P3: Infection of a prosthetic patch (e.g. carotid, common femoral)

Graft enteric erosion

Graft enteric fistula

Aortic stump sepsis after excision of an infected aortic graft

Factors increasing the risk of intra-operative contamination include:

- the nature of the surgery (higher risk with emergency procedures);
- the location of the operation (higher risk with groin wounds);
- the presence of open wounds (distal limb necrosis/gangrene which predispose to lymphatic contamination);
- infected aneurysm thrombus;
- chyle leaks;
- redo surgery; and
- any concurrent bowel surgery.

Secondary haematological seeding can occur via bacteraemia related to infections involving cardiac valves, intestinal tract, urinary tract, or dental manipulation. Grafts can also become infected via

Table 2. Temporal changes in micro-organisms involved with vascular graft infections.

1985 [3, 4]	2000 [5]
Staphylococcus epidermidis	MRSA
Staphylococcus aureus	Coliforms
Streptococcus faecalis	Methicillin-sensitive *Staphylococcus aureus*
Escherichia coli	*Streptococcus milleri*
Klebsiella	Assorted skin flora
Pseudomonas	*Pseudomonas*
Corynebacterium	
Proteus	
Citrobacter	
Serratia	

Micro-organisms

There have been important changes in the micro-organisms responsible for prosthetic graft infection over the last two decades. Table 2 summarises the commonest cultured micro-organisms from studies published around 1985 [3, 4], compared with bacteria cultured during a 1-year prospective audit of graft infections carried out by the Joint Vascular Research Group (JVRG) in 2000 [5]. The biggest single change was the emergence of methicillin-resistant *Staphylococcus aureus* (MRSA) and by 2000, MRSA was the commonest single organism involved in Type II (40%) and Type III (33%) Szilagyi infections in the United Kingdom [6]. Nasim subsequently observed that the prevalence of MRSA-positive swabs (contamination/infection) increased from 1% in 1994 to 7% in 2000 [6] and a similar increase in MRSA vascular infections has been reported in other health systems [7].

Clinical impact of complex wound and graft infections

In the JVRG audit, 24% of Szilagyi Type II wound infections progressed on to overt graft infection [5]. MRSA was cultured in 40% of Type II wound infections and led to a significant increase in hospital stay (32 vs. 20 days). Type II Szilagyi wound infections were associated with an overall mortality of 11% and a death/amputation rate of 22% [5].

In the JVRG audit of patients with overt graft infection (at all locations), MRSA was the commonest single infecting organism (33%). Overall, 33% of patients with a graft infection died, while 65% either died or required a major limb amputation (79% of all limb amputations involved MRSA). MRSA infections were associated with significant increases in hospital stay (46 vs. 20 days) [5]. Other studies have also reported devastating outcomes following MRSA-related graft infections. In London, 15 MRSA-infected prosthetic infra-inguinal bypasses were treated

between 1995-1997; four (26%) died, while ten (66%) either died or underwent amputation [8]. In Leicester, 17 patients with MRSA graft infection were reported by Nasim [6]. One of three MRSA-infected carotid patches suffered a disabling stroke (following a massive haemorrhage), all six patients with MRSA aortic graft infection died, while all eight patients with an MRSA-infected infra-inguinal bypass required amputation.

These extreme examples of high morbidity and mortality associated with MRSA served as a major wake up call to vascular surgeons around the world and triggered increasing interest into how and why the infection occurred. In Leicester (UK), Scriven [9] demonstrated, in a consecutive series of 100 vascular in-patients, that 4% were MRSA-positive on screening following admission. However, by the time of discharge, no fewer than 16% acquired MRSA at some time during their stay (exit from theatre [n=1], exit from ITU [n=6], on the vascular ward [n=9]).

There are recognised risk factors for developing MRSA infections which include:

- previous MRSA infection;
- immunosuppression;
- type I diabetes;
- chronic open wounds;
- antibiotic use within the last 90 days;
- central venous catheterisation;
- residence in a long-term care facility;
- prolonged hospitalisation;
- admission to ITU;
- lower limb bypass;
- dialysis;
- advanced age; and
- hospitalisation before onset of infection [10, 11].

Preventive strategies

Table 3 summarises a preventive strategy against vascular graft infections, divided into general pre-operative issues, theatre practice and also methods for dealing with MRSA. Experience suggests that, in addition to these measures, vascular surgeons must assume a leadership role in the prevention of infection.

Table 3. Strategies for preventing vascular graft infections.

General (pre-operative)

Minimise pre-operative stay, pre-operative shower with antibacterial solutions
Reconsider operative strategies if there are open wounds (can they be improved?)
Reconsider operative strategies if there are no autologous conduits available
Reconsider whether an endovascular option might be available
Identify 'high-risk' patients before surgery and consider extended antibiotic cover
Maintain a strict infection control policy, even if pressurised to compromise standards because of bed pressures

General (theatre)

Remove hair immediately before the operation using an electric razor
Prophylactic antibiotics should be administered at least 30 minutes before making the skin incision
Use adhesive plastic drapes to minimise contact between skin/wound edges and any prosthesis
Avoid direct contact between prosthesis and skin or any other contaminated surfaces
Avoid concurrent operative procedures (especially those involving the gastrointestinal tract)
Consider using antibiotic/silver-bonded prostheses, or gentamycin-impregnated sponges
Employ meticulous surgical technique

Pre-operative MRSA precautions

Pre-operative showering with antiseptic solutions plus nasal mupirocin
Screen for MRSA in elective patients, consider cancelling non-urgent procedures if MRSA-positive
Eradicate MRSA in elective patients found to be positive on screening
Screen for MRSA in emergency admissions and only transfer to vascular unit when proven negative
Only allow MRSA-negative patients onto the main vascular ward
MRSA-positive vascular patients need to be nursed in single rooms with meticulous infection control precautions
Do not allow standards to be compromised

In St. George's Hospital London, a change in isolation policy was instituted in 2003, wherein vascular patients were rigorously segregated according to their predicted risk of acquiring MRSA. In addition, any patient undergoing a prosthetic reconstruction was isolated and antibiotic policies were changed. This was associated with a decline in the rate of hospital-acquired MRSA colonisation from 10.6% to 1.4% [11].

In Leicester, similar radical changes in practice were introduced in 2006. All elective vascular patients were screened for MRSA in the pre-assessment clinic. If patients were found to be positive, non-urgent procedures were postponed until they had three negative MRSA screens. MRSA status was reviewed at the weekly ward meeting prior to the patient's admission. At the pre-assessment clinic, elective vascular in-patients were provided with a supply of nasal mupirocin and Stellisept® shower washes to be started 3 days prior to admission; these were continued daily in hospital until discharge. A consultant microbiologist participated on a weekly ward round and reviewed antibiotic use with the junior medical staff and on-call consultant. All emergency vascular admissions were admitted to the Surgical Admissions Unit (rather than the Vascular Unit) where they were screened for MRSA. No patient (including emergency transfers) was allowed to be admitted onto the Vascular Unit (unless to a single room) except if they were negative for MRSA. In the event that an unscreened vascular patient was transferred into a single room in the Vascular Unit, they were considered to be MRSA-positive until proven otherwise, and they were barrier nursed until their MRSA status was determined. All patients with suspected/proven MRSA or *Clostridium difficile* were isolated and barrier nursed. Surgical wounds and any open wounds were swabbed repeatedly during admission and anyone developing diarrhoea was placed immediately in an isolation room and barrier nursed until a stool sample result was available. Finally, and perhaps most important, there was an agreement with senior management that the Duty Bed Manager could not admit unscreened, non-vascular patients into the Vascular Unit, even in times of bed crises.

Within 6 months of introducing this policy in 2006, an internal audit revealed that antibiotic costs had fallen by 50%. This was almost certainly the consequence of having a consultant microbiologist on the ward round to scrutinise antibiotic prescribing practices. More importantly, the new policy was associated with near complete abolition of any new infections or positive cultures of MRSA or *C. difficile* (<1% for 2006-2008, 0% for 2009 and 2010).

Management of prosthetic graft infection

The management of graft infection is based upon four key principles: control of haemorrhage, eradication of infection, minimising morbidity and mortality, and optimising distal perfusion. These aims seem straightforward; however, they can be challenging, and the actual choice of management will depend upon mode of presentation and the overall fitness of the patient. The challenges encountered in planning and treating patients with prosthetic infection will be illustrated by reviewing management strategies of patients with carotid patch infection, aortic graft infection and prosthetic infra-inguinal bypass infection.

Carotid patch infection

Prevalence

Everyone knows about carotid patch infection, but only 75 cases have been reported in 27 studies since 1962.

Microbiology

Staphylococci and *Streptococci* comprise 90% of micro-organisms cultured.

Table 4. Mode of presentation in carotid patch infection (75 cases).

Presentation	<2 mths	2-6mths	>6mths	Total
Wound infection/abscess	12	0	4	16
Patch rupture	6	1	1	8
False aneurysm	3	3	12	18
Sinus	4	0	19	23(*)
Sinus + false aneurysm	0	1	4	5
TIA/stroke	1	0	1	2
Neck mass (not pulsatile)	0	0	3	3
Total	26 (35%)	5(7%)	44(59%)	75

(*) 2 patients also suffered TIA/stroke

Presentation

Table 4 summarises the bimodal distribution of presenting symptoms in the 75 published cases. Approximately one third presented within 2 months of their operation and were highly likely to present with overt wound infections/abscesses or patch rupture (massive haemorrhage). By contrast, 59% presented after 6 months had elapsed. Here the most common presentations were chronic sinus formation and false aneurysm. Only two patients presented with either a TIA or stroke.

Investigation

A duplex scan can be supplemented by CT angiography. There is rarely any need for intra-arterial angiography and MR probably adds little to duplex/CT. The aims of investigation are to determine the extent of peri-arterial induration/inflammation, the upper limit of infection, the presence of a false aneurysm (Figure 1), patency of the carotid arteries and to establish whether the upper (normal) internal carotid artery (ICA) can be accessed easily. It is also helpful to review the original operation note and to answer the following questions:

◆ were there any problems encountered with distal access?

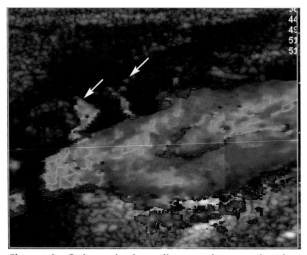

Figure 1. Colour duplex ultrasound scan showing several discrete jets of blood flow from an infected carotid patch into a false aneurysm (arrows).

◆ was the procedure performed under locoregional anaesthesia?
◆ did the patient suffer a neurological deficit (will they tolerate ligation)?
◆ and how high up the ICA did the patch angioplasty extend (a 2cm patch is easier to treat than a 4cm patch)?

From a practical point of view, no-one should incise an abscess overlying a carotid wound without a vascular surgeon being present. Another practical issue (which is professionally sensitive) is to ensure that the surgeon is comfortable with accessing the upper limits of the ICA before starting to operate on an infected carotid patch. If not, then it would be safer to either refer the patient to someone with greater experience or to arrange for a more experienced surgeon to assist. Redo carotid surgery for infected carotid patches can be extremely challenging.

Management

A number of management strategies have been described and these can be divided into the following:

◆ debridement +/- postoperative antibiotic irrigation, sternomastoid flap coverage and postoperative oral antibiotics;
◆ no debridement plus systemic/oral antibiotics or insertion of a covered stent; or
◆ debridement plus patch excision in conjunction with carotid ligation, vein patch closure/vein bypass, prosthetic reconstruction or primary closure.

The key message from the 75 published cases is that patch excision followed by reconstruction with prosthetic material carries a universally bad outcome (most will develop reinfection). A few patients in the world literature (<5) have been treated with a covered stent, but there are no long-term follow-up data to indicate whether these were prone to reinfection. Insertion of a covered stent could, however, be an ideal strategy in frail or very high-risk patients with a false aneurysm. It is probably not appropriate to insert a covered stent as a bridging procedure, pending a more definitive surgical intervention, because it will then be very difficult to access the ICA above the stent at a later date and perform a safe reconstruction.

The available evidence suggests that the patch should be excised and then replaced with autologous vein (patch/bypass). This strategy (adopted in 45/75 patients in the world literature) was associated with the lowest rates of long-term reinfection (90% freedom from operative death/reinfection at 2 years [12]). All patients should be warned that redo surgery for patch infection carries a significant procedural risk (5-10% death/stroke, 10% risk of cranial nerve injury).

If there is a possibility that the distal ICA may need to be explored (perhaps up to the skull base), this must be anticipated in advance, especially if mandibular subluxation is being considered. An alternative surgical approach allows for exposure of the upper reaches of the ICA by extending the incision anterior to the ear and mobilising the parotid gland superomedially (with the assistance of an ear, nose and throat surgeon) [13]. This facilitates excellent distal exposure (see vignette) and has the additional advantage that it can still be used once the operation is underway.

Aortic graft infection

Prevalence

The prevalence of aortic graft infection is 2-3% following open abdominal aortic aneurysm repair and/or surgery for occlusive surgery, and 1% after endovascular procedures. The incidence increases in patients undergoing ruptured aneurysm surgery and in operations involving groin anastomoses.

Microbiology

In the 1980s, the commonest infecting organisms were *Staphylococcus epidermidis*, *Staphylococcus aureus* and *Streptococcus faecalis* (*Enterococcus*), *Pseudomonas*, *Proteus* and *Escherichia coli*. These are still encountered in contemporary practice, but have been joined by MRSA (see above).

Presentation

Aortic graft infections present with a spectrum of symptoms ranging from the hyper-acute (aorto-enteric fistula [AEF]) to the more chronic (sinus leakage). Early infections tend to present with signs of overt sepsis (pyrexia, septicaemia, abscess formation, anaemia, purulent wound discharge or haemorrhage) (Figure 2). Late infection may have a more insidious presentation (discomfort, malaise, weight loss, anorexia [especially with MRSA] and anaemia), although wound discharge, haemorrhage and false aneurysm formation can still occur. Other presentations include chronic sinus formation, septic emboli and graft thrombosis.

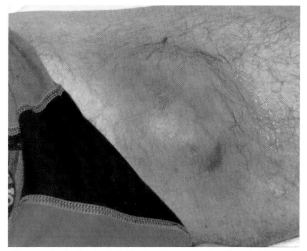

Figure 2. Infected false aneurysm in the left groin after an aortobifemoral bypass.

On a practical point, a diagnosis of aorto-enteric fistula must be considered in any patient with gastrointestinal bleeding (acute or chronic) in the presence of an aortic graft. Unfortunately, patients can still languish on acute medical units before this vital association is finally considered.

Investigation

Any investigative strategy will be influenced by the urgency of presentation. Massive gastrointestinal haemorrhage (secondary to an AEF) mandates urgent treatment and access to imaging may, therefore, be limited. However, any patient with a suspected AEF should undergo CT angiography in order to determine suitability for insertion of a covered stent (see below). All other patients will benefit from a more thorough battery of investigations.

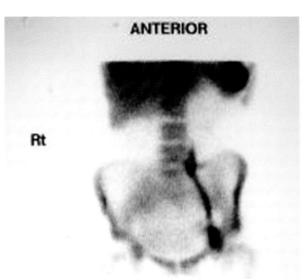

ANTERIOR

Rt

Figure 3. Labelled white cell scan showing increased uptake along the length of the left limb of an aortobifemoral bypass. A negative scan does not exclude infection, but a positive scan is highly suggestive of underlying infection.

Table 5. Strategies for treating aortic graft infection.

Less invasive strategies

Antibiotic therapy
Cavity/wound irrigation

Endovascular options

Lining existing grafts with covered stents
Placement of coils to occlude bleeding fistulae

Partial/total graft excision plus

♦   closure of arteriotomies with autologous vein
♦   oversew aortic stump with:
     – delayed revascularisation as necessary
     – primary amputation
     – extra-anatomic bypass
♦   *in situ* replacement with:
     – unbonded prosthesis
     – rifampicin-bonded prosthesis
     – silver-coated prosthesis
     – cryopreserved allograft
     – superficial femoral vein

The aims of CTA are to identify peri-graft fluid collections, air/fluid interfaces, evaluate graft patency and the proximity of any anastomoses to important structures (renal arteries, etc). Where possible, a CT or ultrasound-guided aspiration of fluid may allow the infecting organism to be identified. This will influence the choice of treatment (see below) as well as allowing appropriate antibiotics to be started.

There is rarely any need for intra-arterial angiography, but labelled white cell scans may be helpful in patients in whom there is uncertainty about the diagnosis. A negative white cell scan may not exclude infection, but a positive scan (Figure 3) is strongly supportive of the graft being infected.

Management

Aortic graft infection is one of the more difficult conditions to treat in vascular surgery and is associated with a high morbidity and mortality. Most publications mention total graft excision (TGE) and secondary revascularisation as being the standard. However, this may be too much for frail, debilitated patients. In that situation, a lesser intervention becomes ideal. The choice of management strategy will always be a trade-off between avoiding excessive procedural risks and reinfection. Accordingly, the actual choice of management will depend on:

♦   the mode of presentation,
♦   comorbidity; and
♦   whether an endovascular option is available.

The options are summarised in Table 5.

Less invasive strategies

Antibiotic therapy (alone) should only be considered in patients with localised, low-grade infections, or in those deemed unfit for more radical interventions. Selected patients can be managed by systemic antibiotics in combination with irrigation of cavities/wounds with antibiotics or aqueous iodine. Irrigation catheters can be inserted after local debridement or via ultrasound/CT guidance.

Endovascular options

The endovascular era has provided a number of innovations that offer a less invasive alternative to the more radical surgical strategies, especially in frail patients. Simple solutions involve percutaneous insertion of aortic balloon catheters to arrest haemorrhage while the patient is being stabilised. Other examples include percutaneous insertion of coils, etc., within chronically bleeding fistulae or the insertion of covered stents. The latter strategy can be of immense value in the treatment of a haemodynamically compromised patient with massive haemorrhage from an aorto-enteric fistula (Figure 4). However, while the insertion of a covered stent seems to be an attractive solution to a difficult problem, anyone considering this must also determine whether this is to be a final solution or a bridge to a more definitive surgical procedure when the patient has recovered from the acute episode. In a recent Greek multicentre audit, AEF treated by a covered stent were associated with much lower mortality and morbidity rates (than open surgery), but most ultimately became reinfected, and attempts to surgically remove the original graft and covered stent

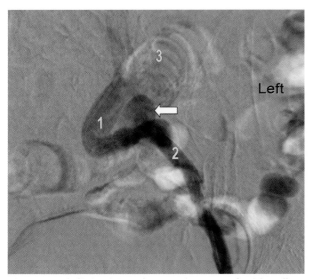

Figure 4. Digital subtraction angiogram of a bleeding aorto-enteric fistula: 1) left aortic graft limb; 2) left external iliac artery; 3) loop of small bowel into which the false aneurysm (white arrow) is bleeding. This was treated by insertion of a covered stent to exclude the fistula. This patient had an extremely hostile abdomen and was not considered for a definitive secondary surgical procedure.

following presentation with recurrent sepsis or haemorrhage, almost invariably resulted in the patient's death [14]. That has also been our anecdotal experience in Leicester.

Accordingly, less fit patients with a bleeding AEF will probably benefit from insertion of a covered stent with most never being considered for secondary open surgery. By contrast, younger fitter patients should be considered for a definitive surgical procedure (e.g. TGE + revascularisation) some months after insertion of a covered stent. This issue must be discussed with the patient (following full recovery) and not when they present at a later date in extremis.

Surgical strategies

Options include partial graft excision (PGE) or TGE, combined with some form of revascularisation. A good example of adopting the former strategy is to perform PGE plus an obturator bypass to the distal profunda/superficial femoral artery in patients with an aortofemoral infection confined to the groin.

TGE plus revascularisation, however, tends to be the preferred treatment option wherever possible. TGE can be performed either through the traditional direct approach to the aorta, or via a right medial visceral rotation. Here, the right colon and duodenum are mobilised medially (the approach used for harvesting the right kidney for transplantation) and the juxtarenal aorta is exposed at the level of the left renal vein.

Following TGE, surgical options include:

♦ oversewing the aortic stump followed by delayed revascularisation as necessary (not generally advisable), extra-anatomic bypass (axillobifemoral or bi-axillofemoral bypass) or primary amputation; or
♦ *in situ* replacement with either an unbonded prosthesis (not recommended), a rifampicin or silver-bonded prosthesis (both probably have similar outcomes), a homograft (less commonly used in the UK but an artery biobank is now available for use) or superficial femoral vein.

Each of these strategies has their supporters and detractors.

TGE + oversewing the aortic stump + extra-anatomic bypass is probably the most commonly employed strategy in the UK, with options being to perform the axillofemoral bypass 2-3 days before TGE (not generally recommended because of the higher risk of reinfection), immediately before or immediately after TGE. The author's preference is to perform the extra-anatomic bypass immediately before removing the graft, the advantage being that lower limb perfusion is maintained throughout what is otherwise a long and physiologically challenging procedure. In a literature review of 688 cases treated between 1990-2004 [15], the 30-day mortality rate was 20%, the 30-day amputation rate was 10%, and the prevalence of aortic stump 'blowout' was about 5%. One-year survival was 63%, but 27% suffered graft occlusion at some point in their follow-up and 15% of extra-anatomic bypasses became reinfected.

TGE + *in situ* replacement with either a silver or rifampicin-bonded prosthesis is a quicker procedure than any of the alternatives (the new graft is laid into the same bed as the old one). It carries a 30-day mortality rate of 6-16% and offers excellent long-term patency rates (i.e. amputations are rare). It is, however, vulnerable to late reinfection in 5-15% of patients [15].

TGE + *in situ* replacement with superficial femoral vein (harvested from one or both legs) has emerged as a very effective and durable surgical strategy in patients with an infected aortic graft. It is not, however, suitable in patients with an acutely bleeding AEF because the procedure takes far too long (5-8 hours). In addition, this strategy is contra-indicated in patients with a history of DVT and it is essential to preserve the deep profundal vein or there is a high risk of significant swelling and compartment syndrome postoperatively. In most situations, a bifurcated venous conduit is fashioned, with the alternative being a unilateral aortofemoral deep vein bypass with a femorofemoro extension. Low mortality and amputation rates have been reported in the literature (0-10% and 0-5%, respectively); 1-year survival exceeds 75% and fewer than 10% need to wear compression hosiery long term [16].

Prosthetic infra-inguinal bypass infection

Prevalence

The prevalence of prosthetic infra-inguinal bypass infection is 5-8% of patients (overall).

Microbiology

Approximately 50-60% will be *Staphylococci*. However, the femoral anastomosis is more prone to Gram-negative or other bowel-related organisms (due to proximity to the perineum) than the distal anastomosis.

Presentation

Apart from the general risk factors detailed earlier, specific risk factors for prosthetic infra-inguinal infections include: amputation within 4 weeks of performing the bypass, early re-operation after graft insertion, graft thrombosis and distal gangrene [17, 18].

Presentations include: abscess formation, wound discharge, systematic sepsis or evidence of a disrupted anastomosis (haemorrhage, false aneurysm). In Mertens' large series, the median time from bypass to developing overt graft infection was 3 months [18].

Management

As with aortic graft infection, the choice of management will depend on a number of clinical and other prognostic features (especially whether the infection is localised to one or both anastomoses) and ranges through systemic antibiotics, local drainage/irrigation (+/- sartorius or other muscle flap coverage), partial graft excision and total graft excision.

In one of the largest published series, the operative mortality was 18%, the early/delayed amputation rate was 40%, and 83% of those treated by partial graft excision required further operations for ongoing sepsis (compared with only 13% in patients undergoing total graft excision). The 5-year survival was 77% [18].

The most important conclusion is to avoid prosthetic material in infra-inguinal reconstructions wherever possible. In the modern era, angioplasty is now the first-line treatment for most patients with claudication or critical limb ischaemia. Where this is not practical (a relative minority in clinical practice), it is usually possible to harvest sufficient autologous vein (arm/leg) in order to perform a bypass. Accordingly, prosthetic conduits should really only be used as a last resort and patients must be warned about the risks of graft infection if they are required. Great caution should be exercised in proceeding with a prosthetic revascularisation in anyone who is MRSA-positive or who has distal gangrene.

Conclusions

Despite major technological advances over the last decade, vascular-related infections remain an important source of morbidity and mortality. The key is prevention, and surgeons must take on a leading role in infection control policies within their unit. Once a graft infection is suspected, it is important that a thorough investigative strategy is planned and implemented. If necessary, it may be appropriate to refer the patient to a more experienced colleague as these are not easy conditions to treat.

Key points

- Graft infection is one of the most feared complications in vascular surgery.
- Prevention is easier than treatment.
- Vascular surgeons must adopt a leadership role for enforcing preventive strategies.
- If you do not feel confident about treating a patient with graft infection, do not start! You can always find a colleague to help you.
- Never incise an abscess over a carotid wound unless a vascular surgeon is present.
- In carotid patch infections, the optimal treatment is patch excision and insertion of autologous tissue. Do not revascularise with prosthetic material.
- A diagnosis of aorto-enteric fistula should be considered in any patient who presents with gastrointestinal blood loss and a history of aortic surgery.
- If the plan is to insert a covered stent to treat an aorto-enteric fistula, the decision should be made whether this is a bridging procedure or not. Any definitive surgical procedure should be scheduled as soon as the patient has made a recovery after stent insertion.
- Prosthetic material should probably only be used for infra-inguinal bypasses if there is no endovascular alternative and no autologous vein. Anyone using prosthetic material must warn the patient about the risk of graft infection.

References

1. Szilagyi DE, Smith RF, Elliott JP, *et al*. Infection in arterial reconstruction with synthetic grafts. *Ann Surg* 1972; 176: 321-33.

2. Bunt TJ. Synthetic vascular graft infections: I graft infections. *Surgery* 1983; 93: 733-46.

3. Kaebnick HW, Bandyk DF, Bergamini TW, *et al*. The microbiology of explanted vascular prostheses. *Surgery* 1987; 102: 756-62.

4. Lorentzen JE, Nielsen OM, Arendrup H, *et al*. Vascular graft infection: an analysis of sixty-two graft infections in 2411 consecutively implanted synthetic vascular grafts. *Surgery* 1985; 98: 81-6.

5. Naylor AR, Hayes PD, Darke S, on behalf of the Joint Vascular Research Group. A prospective audit of complex wound and graft infections in Great Britain and Ireland: the emergence of MRSA. *Eur J Vasc Endovasc Surg* 2001; 21: 289-94.

6. Nasim A, Thompson MM, Naylor AR, *et al*. The impact of MRSA on vascular surgery. *Eur J Vasc Endovasc Surg* 2001; 22: 211-4.

7.   Taylor MD, Napolitano LM. Methicillin-resistant *Staphylococcus aureus* infections in vascular surgery: increasing prevalence. *Surg Infect* 2004; 5: 180-7.

8.   Chalmers RTA, Wolfe JHN, Cheshire NJW, *et al.* Improved management of infra-inguinal bypass graft infection with methicillin-resistant *Staphylococcus. Br J Surg* 1999; 86: 1433-6.

9.   Scriven JM, Silva P, Swann RA, *et al.* The acquisition of methicillin-resistant *Staphylococcus aureus* (MRSA) in vascular patients. *Eur J Vasc Endovasc* 2003; 25: 147-51.

10. Bandyk DF. Vascular surgical site infection; risk factors and preventive measures. *Sem Vasc Surg* 2008; 21: 119-23.

11. Thompson MM. An audit demonstrating a reduction in MRSA infection in a specialised vascular unit resulting from a change in infection control protocol. *Eur J Vasc Endovasc Surg* 2006; 31: 609-15.

12. Naylor AR, Payne D, Thompson MM, *et al.* Prosthetic patch infection after carotid endarterectomy. *Eur J Vasc Endovasc Surg* 2002; 23: 11-6.

13. Naylor AR, Moir A. An aid to accessing the distal internal carotid artery. *J Vasc Surg* 2009; 49: 1345-7.

14. Kakkos SK, Antoniadis PN, Clonaris C, *et al.* Open or endovascular repair of aorto-enteric fistula? A multicentre comparative study. *Eur J Vasc Endovasc Surg* 2011: in press.

15. Naylor AR. Infection following aortic and carotid surgery. In: *Rare Vascular Disorders: a practical guide for the vascular specialist.* In: Earnshaw J, Parvin S, Eds. Shrewsbury, UK: tfm Publishing, 2005: 223-36.

16. Ehsan O, Gibbons CP. A ten-year experience of using femoro-popliteal vein for revascularisation in graft and arterial infections. *Eur J Vasc Endovasc Surg* 2009; 38: 172-9.

17. Brothers TE, Robison JG, Elliott BM. Predictors of prosthetic graft infection after infra-inguinal bypass. *Am J Coll Surg* 2009; 208: 557-561.

18. Mertens RA, O'Hara PJ, Hertzer NR, *et al.* Surgical management of infra-inguinal arterial prosthetic graft infections: review of a thirty-five year experience. *J Vasc Surg* 1995; 21: 782-91.

Case vignette   Carotid patch infection

A. Ross Naylor MD FRCS, Professor of Vascular Surgery
Leicester Royal Infirmary, Leicester, UK

An 83-year-old male, who had undergone an uneventful right carotid endarterectomy in 2002, presented in 2009 with a 6-month history of a swelling of the right side of his neck (Figure 1). Duplex ultrasound revealed disruption of the patch with a large, multiloculated and partially thrombosed false aneurysm (FA). The upper limit of the false aneurysm extended well under the mandible (Figure 1) and it was anticipated from the outset that a high distal exposure would be necessary. The procedure was undertaken as a joint operation with an ear, nose and throat surgeon.

The proximal common carotid artery was controlled (Figure 2) and an incision was made anterior to the ear to facilitate distal exposure (Figure 3). After mobilisation of the parotid gland superomedially and identification of the facial nerve, the distal ICA (above the false aneurysm) was controlled (Figure 4) without the need to disturb the main wound and risk major haemorrhage. The original incision was then reopened (Figure 5), exposing the inferior pole of the false aneurysm. It was then possible to excise the patch and the false aneurysm and insert a Pruitt Inahara shunt with a segment of reversed long saphenous vein over the distal limb (Figure 6). The external carotid artery was controlled with a Fogarty catheter and an interposition vein bypass performed (Figure 7). There were no postoperative complications and the patient has remained infection free for 18 months.

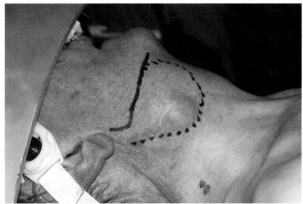

Figure 1.

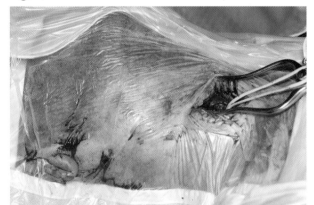

Figure 2.

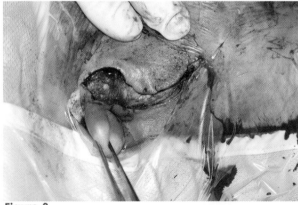

Figure 3.

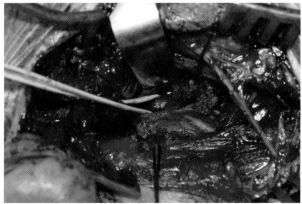

Figure 4.

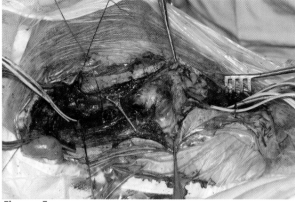

Figure 5.

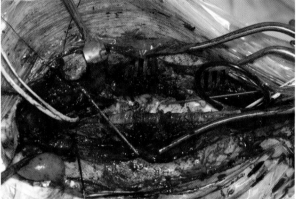

Figure 6.

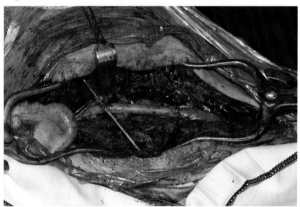

Figure 7.

Chapter 8   Drug-related complications in vascular patients

Ian Nordon MD FRCS, Specialist Registrar in Vascular Surgery
Cliff Shearman MS FRCS, Professor of Vascular Surgery
Department of Vascular Surgery, Southampton General Hospital, Southampton, UK

Introduction

Pharmacological therapy plays an essential role in both primary and secondary prevention of vascular disease. After many vascular interventions, patients are offered a number of therapeutic agents intended to optimise their outcome, prolong their life and enhance the durability of the procedure. However, while the risks of intervention are generally well recognised, the potential serious adverse effects associated with pharmacotherapy are often overlooked and rarely discussed with the patients. Vascular specialists must have a clear understanding of both the indications for initiating pharmacological therapy and complications associated with medicines in this vulnerable cohort of patients (Figure 1).

Antiplatelet agents

Main risk: bleeding.

Oral antiplatelet drugs are a cornerstone of modern pharmacotherapy in cardiovascular atherothrombotic diseases. The efficacy of aspirin, dipyridamole and clopidogrel in decreasing the risk of adverse events in vascular patients has been well established over the past 20 years.

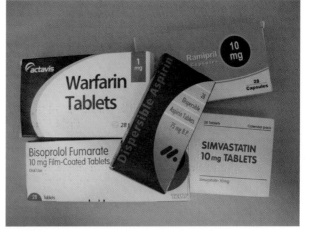

Figure 1. A range of medications is available for patients with peripheral arterial disease.

Aspirin has anti-inflammatory, antipyretic, analgesic and antiplatelet properties. It exerts its therapeutic effect through inhibition of cyclo-oxygenase-1 and disruption of prostanglandin synthesis. Despite its therapeutic benefits, the limiting factor for aspirin use has been its association with gastrointestinal complications, particularly peptic ulceration and gastrointestinal bleeding (Figures 2 and 3). After adjusting for other risk factors, regular aspirin use more than twice a week has been shown to confer a relative risk (RR) of gastrointestinal bleeding of 1.32

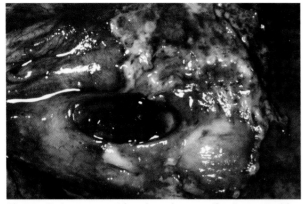

Figure 2. Large gastric ulcer in a patient on aspirin. *Courtesy of Dr P. Gallagher, Consultant Pathologist, Southampton General Hospital, Southampton, UK.*

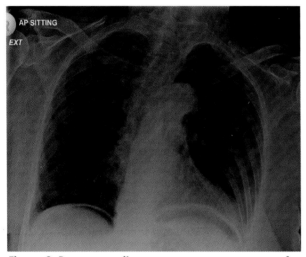

Figure 3. Pneumoperitoneum as a consequence of a perforated gastric ulcer.

(95% confidence interval [CI], 1.12-1.55) compared to matched controls [1]. The risk appears to be dose-dependent. Patients taking >200mg aspirin/day have a 2.69% chance of having a major gastrointestinal bleeding event compared to 0.97% in patients taking <100mg/day (p=0.001) [2]. Daily doses of 75mg, 150mg and 300mg of aspirin are associated with an odds ratio of bleeding of 2.3 (95% CI, 1.2-4.4), 3.2 (95% CI, 1.7-6.5) and 3.9 (95% CI, 2.5-6.3), respectively [3].

Patients on a combination of corticosteroids and aspirin have an increased risk of gastrointestinal bleeding. The RR of bleeding when taking combination therapy is 5.3 (95% CI, 2.9-8.8) [4]. A similar increased risk is described when aspirin and warfarin are combined to prevent graft thrombosis after infra-inguinal bypass. The increased incidence of major gastrointestinal bleeding with the combination of aspirin and warfarin compared to aspirin alone was 4.1% vs. 1.7% (95% CI, 0.1-4.6; p=0.06).

Clopidogrel, a thienopyridine, acts through antagonism of the P2Y12 receptor for adenosine diphosphate (ADP), and is seen as a safe alternative to aspirin. The CAPRIE (Clopidogrel versus Aspirin in Patients at Risk of Ischaemic Events) trial found that long-term clopidogrel was more effective and better tolerated than aspirin in the secondary prevention of cardiovascular events. Clopidogrel was associated with fewer gastrointestinal adverse events (abdominal pain, dyspepsia, ulceration) compared with aspirin (27.1% vs. 29.8%, respectively; p <0.001) [5]. Rare side effects of clopidogrel include life-threatening bone marrow suppression manifested as toxic bone marrow failure, aplastic anaemia, thrombocytopaenia, neutropaenia or pancytopaenia [6]. Clopidogrel has been reported to cause excessive bleeding during surgery. With increasing clopidogrel use, the number of patients needing urgent intervention (when clopidogrel cannot be stopped) will also increase. In some cases, platelet transfusion is necessary to control bleeding.

Dual antiplatelet medication may be indicated following coronary stent deployment or acute stroke. However, the potential benefit of dual therapy in peripheral arterial disease (PAD) has not yet been identified. The Clopidogrel for High Atherothrombotic Risk and Ischemic Stabilization, Management, and Avoidance (CHARISMA) trial was the largest and longest study of the risks of dual antiplatelet therapy. It provided data on the frequency of bleeding, risk factors and consequences of bleeding. Severe bleeding occurred in 1.7% of the clopidogrel and aspirin group versus 1.3% on aspirin alone (p=0.087); moderate bleeding occurred in 2.1% and 1.3%, respectively (p<0.001). The risk of bleeding was greatest in the first year of prescription. After multivariable analysis, a relationship between moderate bleeding and all-cause mortality was identified (hazard ratio [HR], 2.55; 95% CI, 1.71-3.80; p<0.0001), along with myocardial infarction (HR, 2.92; 95% CI, 2.04-4.18; p<0.0001) and stroke (HR, 4.20; 95% CI, 3.05-5.77; p<0.0001) [7].

A Cochrane systematic review reported similar findings. Compared with aspirin alone, the risk of having a major bleed during 1 year of treatment was higher in the clopidogrel plus aspirin group (OR 1.34, 95% CI, 1.14-1.57; p<0.01), with an absolute excess of 6 per 1000 patients treated with the combination for 1 year (25 vs. 19, risk difference 0.6%, 95% CI, 0-1) [8]. If dual therapy is considered in a patient with PAD, these risks should be discussed. The current lack of direct evidence of the benefit in PAD makes dual therapy questionable.

In patients undergoing elective vascular interventions, aspirin should usually be continued unless there are particular concerns about the risk of bleeding. The response of patients on clopidogrel (especially if also on aspirin) is less predictable and so if possible clopidogrel should be stopped 7-10 days prior to surgery. However, patients with coronary stents may need clopidogrel continuing. In these patients it is important to liaise with the cardiology team and plan the timing of surgery based on the urgency of the vascular procedure and the planned duration of dual antiplatelet therapy.

Recently the issue of resistance to antiplatelet agents, in particular aspirin and clopidogrel, has become apparent. Resistance refers to failure to achieve a therapeutically significant antiplatelet effect and may result in continued occurrence of ischaemic events despite apparently adequate therapy and compliance. The prevalence of resistance to aspirin appears to be low. In contrast, resistance to clopidogrel, which is mostly due to inefficient metabolism of the pro-drug to its active metabolite, is more common, and affects the clinical efficacy of the drug [9].

Anticoagulants

Main risk: bleeding.

Systemic anticoagulation is indicated in atrial fibrillation, deep vein thrombosis, venous thrombo-embolism, congestive cardiac failure, stroke and hypercoagulability. An increasing number of elderly people are treated with anticoagulation to prevent thrombo-embolic complications of their medical conditions. Anticoagulation is traditionally achieved by administration of heparins and coumarins.

Unfractionated heparin (UFH) potentiates the anticoagulant activity of Factors IX, X, XI, XII and antithrombin-III; it also suppresses platelet function. Low-molecular-weight heparin (LMWH) causes an antithrombin-dependent inhibition of Factor Xa. It has a longer half-life than UFH and has a lower potential for bleeding. The principal risk associated with heparin administration is haemorrhage; this risk is increased with concomitant antiplatelet or non-steroidal anti-inflammatory drug treatment.

Heparin-induced thrombocytopaenia (HIT) is the most important of the immune-mediated, drug-induced thrombocytopaenias. Recent data show that up to 8% of patients on heparin will develop the antibody associated with HIT and that approximately 1-5% of patients on heparin will progress to develop HIT with thrombocytopaenia, suffering from venous and/or arterial thrombosis in at least one third of cases [10]. Thrombocytopaenia usually occurs 5 to 10 days after the initial administration of the heparin. Bleeding is rare; the main complication of HIT is arterial thrombosis. Thrombosis in HIT is associated with a mortality rate of 20-30%, with an equivalent number of patients becoming permanently disabled by amputation, stroke or other arterial occlusions [11]. Prompt clinical and laboratory recognition is essential in order to stop heparin use immediately and commence an alternative anticoagulant.

Warfarin, a vitamin K antagonist, is the mainstay of long-term anticoagulation, for which it has become the second most common cause of adverse drug events in emergency departments. The overall risk of major bleeding with warfarin is 7-8% per year. In patients aged 40 to 84 years old who were newly treated with warfarin and with no prior history of bleeding, the overall rate of bleeding was reported to be 15.2 per 100 patient years during the initial 12 months. The rate of fatal bleeds, secondary to intracranial haemorrhage, was 0.6 per 100 patient years [12]. The incidence of intracranial haemorrhage appears to be related to the INR; the risk increased significantly above an INR of 3.5 [13] (Figure 4).

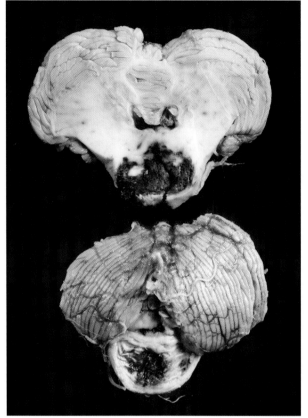

Figure 4. **Fatal intracranial bleed. Pontine haemorrhage in patient who had been taking warfarin.** *Courtesy of Dr P. Gallagher, Consultant Pathologist, Southampton General Hospital, Southampton, UK.*

Table 1. Complications from thrombolytic therapy[15].	
Complication	**Overall incidence (%)**
Death	<1
Haemorrhagic stroke	1-2.3
Major haemorrhage	<5.1
Minor haemorrhage	14.8
Catheter-related trauma (dissection/false aneurysm)	1.4
Compartment syndrome	2
Distal embolisation	<1

Patients with renal failure are a particular high-risk group and have an increased risk of both thrombotic and bleeding complications. A number of antithrombotic drugs undergo renal excretion. Therefore, estimation of renal function is necessary when prescribing anticoagulants to high-risk patients, such as the elderly and those with diabetes mellitus. Dose adjustment of anticoagulants may be indicated when the creatinine clearance falls below 30ml/minute. Unfractionated heparin and vitamin K antagonists generally do not require dose adjustment with renal dysfunction; however, smaller doses of warfarin may be required to achieve a therapeutic INR. LMWHs all undergo renal excretion, and lower doses may be advisable in patients with chronic renal failure [14].

Thrombolysis

Main risk: stroke.

Catheter-directed thrombolytic therapy is an effective complimentary therapy in patients with acute leg ischaemia, but is associated with risk. It is contra-indicated in any patient with a haemorrhagic disorder or an anatomical lesion that may bleed, such as recent surgery. Complications reported include severe internal bleeding, intracranial bleeding, and embolisation from a remote source (e.g. left ventricle) [15]. The risk of these complications is proportional to the duration of therapy. Complications occur in up to 4% of procedures requiring 8 hours thrombolytic therapy and up to 34% requiring 40 hours (Table 1, Figure 5).

Irrespective of the site, the management of severe bleeding during lysis is as follows: discontinue the thrombolytic agent and anticoagulants, replenish coagulation factors (fresh frozen plasma, cryoprecipitate), and transfuse blood as required. Any haematoma should only be evacuated for pressure on adjacent structures, or to repair a vascular injury that continues to bleed. Reversal of the fibrinolytic state with tranexamic acid is also often used but is less effective than cryoprecipitate, which restores fibrinogen levels. If an acute stroke occurs, thrombolytic treatment should be discontinued and a CT brain scan obtained to determine whether the

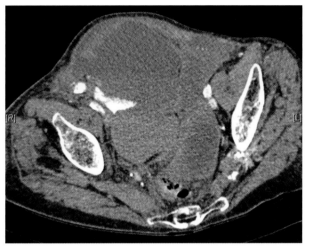

Figure 5. Large retroperitoneal bleed during thrombolytic therapy.

stroke is thrombotic or haemorrhagic [16]. There is an argument for continuing thrombolysis in the former.

Statin therapy

Main risk: muscle pain.

Statins have been shown clearly to improve outcomes both in patients with PAD and carotid artery disease [17, 18]. They are also associated with beneficial effects in patients undergoing open surgical or endovascular abdominal aortic aneurysm repair.

A large meta-analysis (n=90,056 patients; 14 randomised trials), the Cholesterol Treatment Trialists' Collaborators, showed that for each 1.0mmol/L (39mg/dL) decrease in low-density lipoprotein cholesterol, statin treatment was associated with a 12% reduction in all-cause mortality (RR, 0.88; 95% CI, 0.84-0.91; p <.0001) and a 19% reduction in cardiac death (RR, 0.81; 95% CI, 0.76-0.85; p <.0001) compared to placebo [19]. Despite these obvious outcome benefits, statins are associated with adverse effects including myopathy, rhabdomyolysis and hepatotoxicity.

Statins are well tolerated by most individuals but can produce a variety of muscle-related complaints or myopathies. The most serious risk is myositis with rhabdomyolysis. This risk was highlighted by the withdrawal of cerivastatin in August 2001, after the drug was associated with approximately 100 deaths from rhabdomyolysis. Clinically important rhabdomyolysis with other statins is rare, with an overall reported incidence of fatal rhabdomyolysis of 0.15 per 1 million prescriptions [20]. The incidence of less severe muscle complaints such as aching and discomfort is not well defined but may be as high as 5%. Although patients may be tried on a different statin there is no evidence to suggest any one statin is more or less likely to cause this complication which is usually dose-dependent.

Elevated hepatic transaminase activities have been reported in 0.5-2.0% of patients treated with a statin, and are dose-dependent [21]. There is no evidence that this leads to hepatotoxicity, and it is therefore not an indication for terminating therapy.

A meta-analysis (n=13 statin trials; 91,140 patients) on the association between statin use and the development of new diabetes mellitus concluded that statin use was associated with a slight increase in the risk (OR 1.09; 95% CI, 1.02-1.17) [22]. The beneficial effects of statins in individuals at high cardiovascular risk outweigh the risks associated with the drugs.

Beta-blockers

Main risk: worsening established cardiac failure.

Hypertension is one of the major risk factors for cardiovascular morbidity and mortality. It is clear that lowering blood pressure is beneficial; however, there are still some doubts regarding the long-term safety of some antihypertensive drugs.

Beta-blockers are indicated for use in coronary artery disease and hypertension. However, optimal therapy for patients with associated PAD remains controversial due to the presumed haemodynamic consequences of beta-blockers, leading to worsening symptoms of intermittent claudication. A recent Cochrane review, however, concluded that there is currently no evidence that beta-blockers adversely affect walking distance in people with intermittent claudication, and therefore they may be used when clinically indicated [23].

Contrast agents

Main risk: renal failure.

Contrast agents are administered routinely in cross-sectional imaging studies and angiography. Contrast-induced acute kidney injury (AKI) is a common cause of renal failure in hospitalised patients. Clinical manifestations can range from a mild, transient rise in serum creatinine levels, to renal failure requiring haemodialysis. Pre-existing renal dysfunction remains the most important risk factor for contrast-induced AKI and is independent of the type of contrast agent used (ionic or non-ionic), and the volume infused [24] (see also Chapter 3).

The physiological basis of contrast-induced AKI seems to be transient local ischaemia in the renal tubule. There is a relationship between the degree of renal insufficiency and the likelihood of developing contrast-induced AKI. Although it occurs in only 1-2% in patients with normal renal function, contrast-induced AKI occurs in up to 10% in patients with serum creatinine levels between 1.3 and 1.9mg/dL, and up to 62% in those with levels greater than 2mg/dL [25].

The principles behind protection against contrast-induced AKI include decreasing the concentration of the contrast and its contact time in the kidney. The use of anti-oxidants to scavenge the harmful reactive oxygen species may also be beneficial. Ensuring adequate intravenous hydration is the most effective preventive measure using 0.9% normal saline solution. There remains debate about whether N-acetylcysteine 600mg orally before and after the procedure is protective, but it does not seem to be associated with significant risks [26].

Gadolinium, the contrast used to facilitate magnetic resonance angiography (MRA), has a safer side-effect profile than iodinated contrast. However, its safety in patients with advanced renal failure has been challenged following reported association with nephrogenic systemic fibrosis, a potentially fatal condition [27].

Iloprost

Major hazard: intolerance.

Iloprost, a prostanoid, is a synthetic analogue of prostacyclin PGI2. Iloprost dilates systemic and pulmonary arterial vascular beds, and is usually used in patients with complicated vasospastic disorders and vasculitis. It is sometimes prescribed off license for the treatment of surgically non-reconstructable critical leg ischaemia in an attempt to relieve pain and avoid major amputation.

A recent Cochrane systematic review demonstrated that prostanoids were effective with regard to relief of rest pain (RR 1.32; 95% CI, 1.10-1.57), and ulcer healing (RR 1.54; 95% CI, 1.22-1.96). However, there was no statistically significant reduction in amputations (RR 0.89; 95% CI, 0.76-1.04) or mortality (RR 1.07; 95% CI, 0.65-1.75) [28]. The side effects of intravenous iloprost have a statistically significant ($p < 0.001$) dose response, the most frequent included headache (37%), flushing (22%), and nausea (20%).

Vasoactive drugs

Cilostazol, a phosphodiesterase III inhibitor, has been recently approved for the treatment of intermittent claudication, and has been shown to improve pain-free walking distance. The mechanism by which cilostazol exerts its beneficial effects in patients with PAD is not clear. Cilostazol acts on platelets, vascular smooth muscle cells, endothelial cells, cardiomyocytes, and adipocytes through an elevation in cyclic adenosine monophosphate levels by a combination of the inhibition of intracellular PDE-3A and extracellular adenosine uptake [29]. Adverse effects of cilostazol such as loose stools, diarrhoea, dizziness, palpitations, and particularly, headache, as a result of vasodilatory properties, occur in up to 32% of patients [30]. In controlled studies, up to 3.7% of patients discontinued therapy as a result of headache. There is no evidence of an increased risk of myocardial infarction or stroke related to this medication [31].

Naftidrofuryl, a 5-hydroxytryptamine 2 receptor blocker, is also licensed for the treatment of intermittent claudication. In randomised controlled trials, side effects such as headache and gastrointestinal disturbance were no different from placebo.

Conclusions

Drugs are essential tools in the management of vascular disease. The main risks associated with the majority of these therapies are increased bleeding and renal impairment. Close monitoring of these vulnerable patients is as important as precise surgery. Vascular specialists and their patients should be vigilant for early signs of drug-related complications and modify therapy accordingly. Many patients are on combinations of different agents for multiple maladies, and clinicians should remain vigilant against dangerous interactions. It is essential that patients receiving these medications are counselled about the potential side effects, as well as their benefits.

Key points

- The medical management of cardiovascular risk confers significant benefit to patients with PAD. However, most therapies do carry risk which must be balanced against the potential benefits. Any clinician who recommends or prescribes these medications must be aware of the potential risks and warn patients about the potential side effects.
- The risk of gastrointestinal bleeding due to antiplatelet agents is dose-dependent.
- The risk of significant bleeding complications with dual antiplatelet therapy is 1:50.
- The effects of clopidogrel in patients undergoing surgery are unpredictable and when possible the medication should be stopped prior to intervention. If this is not possible and excessive bleeding is encountered then platelet transfusion may be required.
- Contrast-induced AKI is more likely if base-line creatinine is elevated.
- Catheter-directed thrombolysis confers a 2% risk of stroke.
- Statins are generally very well tolerated, yet confer a risk of muscular pains, myositis and, very rarely, rhabdomyolysis.
- Vasoactive therapies for claudication do not carry increased risk of myocardial infarction or stroke.

References

1. Huang ES, Strate LL, Ho WW, *et al*. A prospective study of aspirin use and the risk of gastrointestinal bleeding in men. *PLoS One* 2010; 5: e15721.
2. Serebruany VL, Steinhubl SR, Berger PB, *et al*. Analysis of risk of bleeding complications after different doses of aspirin in 192,036 patients enrolled in 31 randomized controlled trials. *Am J Cardiol* 2005; 95: 1218-22.
3. Weil J, Colin-Jones D, Langman M, *et al*. Prophylactic aspirin and risk of peptic ulcer bleeding. *BMJ* 1995; 310(6983): 827-30.
4. Nielsen GL, Sorensen HT, Mellemkjoer L, *et al*. Risk of hospitalization resulting from upper gastrointestinal bleeding among patients taking corticosteroids: a register-based cohort study. *Am J Med* 2001; 111: 541-5.
5. Hirsh J, Bhatt DL. Comparative benefits of clopidogrel and aspirin in high-risk patient populations: lessons from the CAPRIE and CURE studies. *Arch Intern Med* 2004; 164: 2106-10.
6. Almsherqi ZA, McLachlan CS, Sharef SM. Non-bleeding side effects of clopidogrel: have large multi-center clinical trials underestimated their incidence? *Int J Cardiol* 2007; 117: 415-7.
7. Berger PB, Bhatt DL, Fuster V, *et al*. Bleeding complications with dual antiplatelet therapy among patients with stable vascular disease or risk factors for vascular disease: results from the Clopidogrel for High Atherothrombotic Risk and Ischemic Stabilization, Management, and Avoidance (CHARISMA) trial. *Circulation* 2010; 121: 2575-83.
8. Squizzato A, Keller T, Romualdi E, Middeldorp S. Clopidogrel plus aspirin versus aspirin alone for preventing cardiovascular disease. *Cochrane Database Syst Rev* 2011; 1: CD005158.
9. Cattaneo M. Resistance to anti-platelet agents. *Thromb Res* 2011; 127S3: S61-3.
10. Franchini M. Heparin-induced thrombocytopenia: an update. *Thromb J* 2005; 3: 14.
11. Warkentin TE. Heparin-induced thrombocytopenia: a clinicopathologic syndrome. *Thromb Haemost* 1999; 82: 439-47.

12. Hollowell J, Ruigomez A, Johansson S, *et al.* The incidence of bleeding complications associated with warfarin treatment in general practice in the United Kingdom. *Br J Gen Pract* 2003; 53(489): 312-4.

13. Pautas E, Gouin-Thibault I, Debray M, *et al.* Haemorrhagic complications of vitamin k antagonists in the elderly: risk factors and management. *Drugs Aging* 2006; 23: 13-25.

14. Dager WE, Kiser TH. Systemic anticoagulation considerations in chronic kidney disease. *Adv Chronic Kidney Dis* 2010; 17: 420-7.

15. van den Berg JC. Thrombolysis for acute arterial occlusion. *J Vasc Surg* 2010; 52: 512-5.

16. Thrombolysis in the management of lower limb peripheral arterial occlusion - a consensus document. *J Vasc Interv Radiol* 2003; 14(9 Pt 2): S337-49.

17. Paraskevas KI, Athyros VG, Briana DD, *et al.* Statins exert multiple beneficial effects on patients undergoing percutaneous revascularization procedures. *Curr Drug Targets* 2007; 8: 942-51.

18. Paraskevas KI, Hamilton G, Mikhailidis DP. Statins: an essential component in the management of carotid artery disease. *J Vasc Surg* 2007; 46: 373-86.

19. Baigent C, Keech A, Kearney PM, *et al.* Efficacy and safety of cholesterol-lowering treatment: prospective meta-analysis of data from 90,056 participants in 14 randomised trials of statins. *Lancet* 2005; 366(9493): 1267-78.

20. Thompson PD, Clarkson P, Karas RH. Statin-associated myopathy. *JAMA* 2003; 289: 1681-90.

21. Third Report of the National Cholesterol Education Program (NCEP) Expert Panel on Detection, Evaluation, and Treatment of High Blood Cholesterol in Adults (Adult Treatment Panel III) final report. *Circulation* 2002; 106: 3143-421.

22. Sattar N, Preiss D, Murray HM, *et al.* Statins and risk of incident diabetes: a collaborative meta-analysis of randomised statin trials. *Lancet* 2010; 375(9716): 735-42.

23. Paravastu SC, Mendonca D, Da Silva A. Beta blockers for peripheral arterial disease. *Cochrane Database Syst Rev* 2008; 4: CD005508.

24. Parfrey PS, Griffiths SM, Barrett BJ, *et al.* Contrast material-induced renal failure in patients with diabetes mellitus, renal insufficiency, or both. A prospective controlled study. *N Engl J Med* 1989; 320: 143-9.

25. Pomposelli F. Arterial imaging in patients with lower extremity ischemia and diabetes mellitus. *J Vasc Surg* 2010; 52: 81S-91.

26. Solomon R, Dauerman HL. Contrast-induced acute kidney injury. *Circulation* 2010; 122: 2451-5.

27. Hasebroock KM, Serkova NJ. Toxicity of MRI and CT contrast agents. *Expert Opin Drug Metab Toxicol* 2009; 5: 403-16.

28. Ruffolo AJ, Romano M, Ciapponi A. Prostanoids for critical limb ischaemia. *Cochrane Database Syst Rev* 2010; 1: CD006544.

29. O'Donnell ME, Badger SA, Sharif MA, *et al.* The vascular and biochemical effects of cilostazol in patients with peripheral arterial disease. *J Vasc Surg* 2009; 49: 1226-34.

30. Hiatt W. The US experience with cilostazol in treating intermittent claudication. *Atherosclerosis* 2006; 6: 21-31.

31. Robless P, Mikhailidis DP, Stansby GP. Cilostazol for peripheral arterial disease. *Cochrane Database Syst Rev* 2008; 1: CD003748.

Case vignette Drug-related complications in a vascular patient

Ian Nordon MD FRCS, Specialist Registrar in Vascular Surgery
Cliff Shearman MS FRCS, Professor of Vascular Surgery
Department of Vascular Surgery, Southampton General Hospital, Southampton, UK

A 62-year-old retired lawyer presented to the stroke physicians following a transient episode of right arm weakness. He was generally fit and well on no medicines. After appropriate examination and investigation he was diagnosed as having a transient ischaemic attack. At that stage he was commenced on aspirin, clopidogrel and simvastatin as was the policy at that time in the unit. Carotid duplex scanning diagnosed a 90% internal carotid stenosis on the symptomatic side and he was referred for acute carotid endarterectomy.

At surgery, haemostasis was difficult to obtain and he was described as being 'very oozy'. Within 2 hours of his surgery he had discharged 800ml of blood into his drain necessitating re-exploration and further bleeding control. The second operation found no obvious source of bleeding but with the benefit of haemostatic adjuncts and a two-pool platelet transfusion, haemostasis was obtained.

During his recovery the man described significant calf and thigh pains on walking within the confines of the ward. Further lower limb duplex identified iliac occlusive disease and he proceeded to iliac angioplasty. This procedure was described as difficult, requiring 120ml contrast, and resulted in a significant groin haematoma (Figure 1) requiring blood transfusion. Two days later he was found to be in acute renal failure (serum creatinine 196mmol/L)

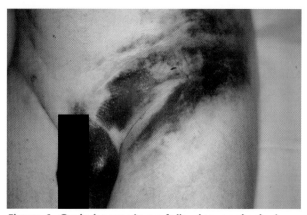

Figure 1. Groin haematoma following angioplasty.

and was diagnosed with contrast-induced AKI; this settled with intravenous fluids.

He was eventually discharged 15 days after his initial presentation. Surgical and endovascular intervention had been relatively straightforward but the main complications that occurred were due to the side effects of the medical treatments he had been given. The patient refused to continue antiplatelet medication despite the potential benefits being explained to him.

This case highlights how a patient may rapidly be exposed to a number of pharmacological therapies that although aimed at improving outcome expose them to significant risks.

Chapter 9

The prevention and treatment of peri-operative stroke and paraplegia after thoracic stenting

Rachel E. Clough MB BS BSc MRCS, NIHR BRC Clinical Training Fellow
Peter R. Taylor MA MChir FRCS, Professor of Vascular Surgery
Department of Vascular Surgery, NIHR Comprehensive Biomedical Research Centre of Guy's and St Thomas' NHS Foundation Trust and King's College London, and King's Health Partners, London, UK

Introduction

Endovascular repair is an attractive alternative to open surgical repair of the thoracic aorta and has become established as the first-line treatment for many aortic pathologies (Figures 1 and 2) [1, 2]. These include degenerative aneurysms, complicated acute Type B dissection, aortic transection, and aneurysms related to previous dissection, coarctation repair, vasculitis and infection. The results of registries and large cohort studies show a reduction in mortality and morbidity rates when compared to conventional open surgical repair [3, 4]. However, endovascular thoracic repair is still associated with stroke and paraplegia rates each in the region of 1-10%, and the aetiology is multifactorial [5-11].

This chapter identifies patients at high risk of developing stroke and paraplegia, prophylactic ways of reducing these and the treatment of patients with established neurological deficit.

Identification of high-risk patients

Stroke

Deliberate coverage of the arch vessels during thoracic aortic stenting increases the risk of stroke, as does concomitant occlusive disease of the carotid, vertebral and subclavian arteries. An incomplete circle of Willis will increase the risk of an ischaemic insult by limiting the contribution of the collateral circulation. Ishimaru identified anatomical limits for the proximal landing zone within the aortic arch:

- zone 0 includes the ascending aorta and the innominate artery;
- zone 1 the left common carotid artery;
- zone 2 the left subclavian artery;
- zone 3 the proximal descending thoracic aorta;
- zone 4 the distal descending thoracic aorta.

There is good evidence that the risk of stroke is highest with devices deployed in zone 0 and reduces the more distal the landing zone. Peri-operative strokes associated with thoracic endografting are almost always ischaemic in origin. Patients who have a heavy atherosclerotic burden in the aortic arch are at high risk of embolisation from guide wire manipulation and device insertion and deployment. The amount of thrombus in the arch can be identified on CT, and mobile thrombus visualised by echocardiography. Transcranial Doppler studies have shown that every part of the procedure can result in emboli to the middle cerebral arteries. This includes guide wire insertion, angiography and device placement and deployment. The vast majority are

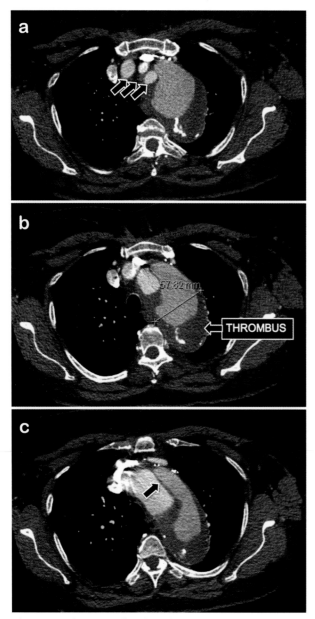

Figure 1. a) Large distal arch aneurysm related to a chronic dissection. The three arrows point to the innominate, left common carotid and left subclavian arteries from left to right. b) The distal arch aneurysm measures 5.7cm and there is thrombus in the false lumen (arrowed). c) The dissection flap extends across the arch from the ascending to the descending aorta.

clinically silent, but even a small embolus can have devastating consequences. Devices which conform to the aortic arch are now available and these may

reduce the incidence of embolisation during device insertion and deployment.

Paraplegia

Patients having thoracic aortic stenting are at particular risk of paraplegia if they have undergone previous infrarenal aortic aneurysm repair. The total length of aorta covered by thoracic devices also determines the risk of spinal cord ischaemia by increasing the number of occluded intercostal arteries. The artery of Adamkievicz is the most important artery supplying blood to the spinal cord, and it frequently arises from the lower thoracic aorta; it should be preserved if at all possible. The subclavian arteries also provide an important blood supply to the spinal cord. They give rise to the vertebral arteries which form the anterior spinal artery and other branches supply the upper intercostal arteries. Devices which deliberately occlude the left subclavian artery will therefore increase the risk of paraplegia. Finally, the internal iliac arteries also contribute to the blood supply to the distal spinal cord; deliberate occlusion of these vessels will increase the risk of spinal cord ischaemia.

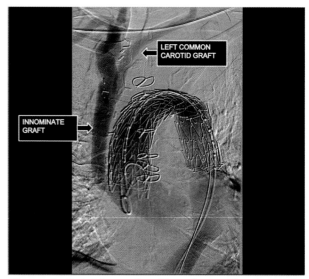

Figure 2. Hybrid repair with extra-anatomic grafts from the ascending aorta to the innominate artery with a branch to the left common carotid artery. The stent graft is deployed from the ascending aorta around the arch to the descending thoracic aorta.

Methods of reducing neurological problems

Stroke

Planned coverage of the brachiocephalic and the left common carotid arteries by the device requires prior revascularisation to reduce the incidence of stroke. This is not, however, universally accepted for the left subclavian artery [7, 12, 13]. A systematic review and meta-analysis found that left subclavian artery coverage, with or without revascularisation, was associated with an increased risk of stroke [12]. Deliberate occlusion of the left subclavian artery during thoracic endovascular repair increases the rate of vertebro-basilar ischaemia, and possibly anterior circulation stroke and spinal cord ischaemia, but the evidence is poor [14]. Other similar studies have not demonstrated an association between stroke and coverage of the left subclavian artery [13, 15]. The European Collaborators on Stent Graft Techniques for Aortic Aneurysm Repair (EUROSTAR) registry also found no significant increase in stroke with left subclavian coverage [7]. Carotid subclavian bypass to reduce the risk of stroke is not without risk. Complications include damage to the nerves of the brachial plexus and the phrenic nerve, damage to the thoracic duct and pneumothorax. Revascularisation of the left subclavian would not be indicated if the right vertebral artery was dominant or if the left vertebral artery was small or occluded. The recent recommendation by the Society for Vascular Surgery is to revascularise the left subclavian artery in all patients having deliberate occlusion, but the level of evidence is weak.

The use of a temporary extra-anatomic graft has been advocated by some to maintain cerebral perfusion during insertion of an endograft into the aortic arch [16]. This should also be an effective method of preventing emboli during deployment. Theoretically, distal protection devices used during carotid artery stenting could have a role in reducing the risk of carotid embolisation during thoracic stenting. However, at present they are not used as they would significantly increase the complexity and cost of the procedure.

Paraplegia

The perfusion of the spinal cord is a balance between the systemic blood pressure and the cerebrospinal fluid (CSF) pressure. Revascularising the left subclavian artery when it is deliberately covered has been shown to reduce the risk of paraplegia, as has treating stenoses or occlusions of both the left subclavian artery proximally and the internal iliac arteries distally. Keeping the systemic blood pressure high during the procedure may also help improve spinal cord perfusion and prevent paraplegia.

Prophylactic CSF drainage is the alternative means to prevent paraplegia and has been recommended by some authors in all patients having a thoracic endograft. However, it is not without risk including spinal cord compression from haemorrhage, subdural haemorrhage caused by excessive CSF drainage, dural fistula and infection. Ideally the procedure is performed under loco-regional anaesthesia, so that cord function can be assessed during the procedure. If general anaesthesia is used, then sensory and motor evoked potentials can demonstrate cord malfunction.

Patients with a neurological deficit

Stroke

Stroke is a devastating complication of thoracic endovascular aortic repair and is the major cause of death. Survivors have long-term disabilities which require in-patient rehabilitation and continued long-term support in the community. Magnetic resonance diffusion-weighted and CT imaging are able to identify the ischaemic penumbra, which is a salvageable area with reversible ischaemia surrounding the cerebral infarct [17, 18]. Acute neurological degeneration describes the increase in the size of the cerebral infarction due to the viability of the penumbra [19]. Early revascularisation of this area may help to reduce the size of the infarct and thus the neurological deficit.

New techniques are available to revascularise the penumbra in the acute scenario. Thrombolysis can be achieved with either intravenous or catheter-directed recombinant tissue plasminogen activator (rt-PA) [20, 21]. In the PROACT II trial of acute ischaemic stroke, complete flow in the middle cerebral artery was restored in 66% of patients [22]. However, in the peri-operative situation, thrombolysis is hazardous due to the risk of bleeding from the surgical wounds. New devices are approved for mechanical thrombectomy that can restore arterial patency. These include the Merci® retriever, which acts like a corkscrew to remove thrombus, and the Penumbra® aspiration catheter, both of which can recanalise an occluded vessel in up to 80% of patients [23, 24]. However, clinical recovery is disappointing and neuroradiological expertise may not be immediately available on site.

Paraplegia

The incidence of spinal cord ischaemia during thoracic endovascular repair is reported to range from 0-10%, with a figure of around 5% for larger series [10, 11, 25-29]. In patients with a thoracic aneurysm, the Gore Tag pivotal trial reported an incidence of 3% in a series of 139 patients; the clinical trial for the TX2 device showed an overall incidence of 6% [5, 6]. Others have described rates of 4% in a series of 326 procedures with mixed pathology. In the EUROSTAR Registry, the incidence was 2.5%, and was increased four-fold with coverage of the left subclavian artery [7, 26].

The contribution of the internal iliac artery to the distal spinal cord may be important and angioplasty of any ostial stenoses may permanently reverse paraplegia [30]. Longer endoluminal devices occlude more intercostal arteries and have been shown to be associated with paraplegia [31, 32].

It is very important that a CSF drain is inserted immediately the diagnosis of paraplegia is suspected. There should be no delay for imaging to confirm the diagnosis as this inevitably increases the duration of ischaemia, and may convert a potentially reversible deficit into a permanent one. The beneficial effect of reducing CSF pressure far outweighs the uncertainty of the underlying pathology. The CSF drain should be kept at 12cm of water/saline above the spinal column

and no more than 20-30ml of CSF should be drained per hour as the risk of subdural haemorrhage increases with excessive drainage. The drain should be clamped if this volume is exceeded and released the next hour. If the neurological deficit is not reversed with this protocol, the systemic blood pressure can be elevated and the CSF pressure reduced to 10cm of saline. There is no clinical benefit in reducing the CSF pressure below this level. The drain is kept in for 3 days after which it is clamped for 4 hours. If the neurological deficit continues to be reversed, the drain is removed. Recurrence of paraplegia on clamping suggests that the perfusion of the cord is inadequate. Angioplasty of any stenosis of the internal iliac or subclavian arteries should be undertaken and carotid subclavian bypass should be performed if the left subclavian is deliberately covered without revascularisation. Failure of the spinal drain to reverse paraplegia despite adequate systemic blood pressure suggests that the drain is not therapeutic and it should be removed to avoid complications such as infection or dural fistula.

Conclusions

Neurological complications of thoracic endoluminal stent repair remain an important risk, with an incidence of stroke and paraplegia each of up to 10%.

Certain patients can be identified who are at high risk of neurological complications. Consideration can be given to prophylactic measures against stroke such as revascularisation of the left subclavian artery when it is deliberately covered and CSF drainage to prevent paraplegia in patients who require a long device and those with a previous infrarenal AAA repair.

Removal of thrombus from the cerebral circulation in patients with stroke improves the arterial patency but the clinical results remain disappointing and radiological expertise may not be readily available. Cerebrospinal fluid drainage can reverse paraplegia if it is done as soon as the clinical signs are apparent.

Key points

♦ Stroke may be prevented by revascularisation of the left subclavian artery but this is not without risk of neurovascular complications.

♦ Paraplegia can be prevented by insertion of a CSF drain.

♦ Stroke can be treated with thrombolysis or mechanical thrombectomy but the clinical outcome does not correlate with vessel patency.

♦ Paraplegia can be treated with systemic hypertension and CSF drainage.

♦ In the presence of clinical signs of paraplegia, insertion of a CSF drain should not be delayed for confirmatory imaging.

References

1. Cho JS, Haider SE, Makaroun MS. Endovascular therapy of thoracic aneurysms: Gore TAG trial results. *Semin Vasc Surg* 2006; 19: 18-24.

2. Fattori R, Nienaber CA, Rousseau H, *et al*. Results of endovascular repair of the thoracic aorta with the Talent thoracic stent graft: the Talent Thoracic Retrospective Registry. *J Thorac Cardiovasc Surg* 2006; 132: 332-9.

3. Bavaria JE, Appoo JJ, Makaroun MS, *et al*. Endovascular stent grafting versus open surgical repair of descending thoracic aortic aneurysms in low-risk patients: a multicenter comparative trial. *J Thorac Cardiovasc Surg* 2007; 133: 369-77.

4. Makaroun MS, Dillavou ED, Wheatley GH, Cambria RP. Five-year results of endovascular treatment with the Gore TAG device compared with open repair of thoracic aortic aneurysms. *J Vasc Surg* 2008; 47: 912-8.

5. Makaroun MS, Dillavou ED, Kee ST, *et al*. Endovascular treatment of thoracic aortic aneurysms: results of the phase II multicenter trial of the GORE TAG thoracic endoprosthesis. *J Vasc Surg* 2005; 41: 1-9.

6. Matsumura JS, Cambria RP, Dake MD, *et al*. International controlled clinical trial of thoracic endovascular aneurysm repair with the Zenith TX2 endovascular graft: 1-year results. *J Vasc Surg* 2008; 47: 247-57; discussion 57.

7. Buth J, Harris PL, Hobo R, *et al*. Neurologic complications associated with endovascular repair of thoracic aortic pathology: incidence and risk factors. a study from the European Collaborators on Stent/Graft Techniques for Aortic Aneurysm Repair (EUROSTAR) registry. *J Vasc Surg* 2007; 46: 1103-10.

8. Amabile P, Grisoli D, Giorgi R, *et al*. Incidence and determinants of spinal cord ischaemia in stent-graft repair of the thoracic aorta. *Eur J Vasc Endovasc Surg* 2008; 35: 455-61.

9. Dake MD, Miller DC, Mitchell RS, *et al*. The 'first generation' of endovascular stent-grafts for patients with aneurysms of the descending thoracic aorta. *J Thorac Cardiovasc Surg* 1998; 116: 689-703.

10. Mitchell RS, Miller DC, Dake MD, *et al*. Thoracic aortic aneurysm repair with an endovascular stent graft: the 'first generation'. *Ann Thorac Surg* 1999; 67: 1971-4.

11. Bergeron P, De Chaumaray T, Gay J, Douillez V. Endovascular treatment of thoracic aortic aneurysms. *J Cardiovasc Surg (Torino)* 2003; 44: 349-61.

12. Cooper DG, Walsh SR, Sadat U, *et al*. Neurological complications after left subclavian artery coverage during thoracic endovascular aortic repair: a systematic review and meta-analysis. *J Vasc Surg* 2009; 49: 1594-601.

13. Kotelis D, Geisbusch P, Hinz U, *et al*. Short and midterm results after left subclavian artery coverage during endovascular repair of the thoracic aorta. *J Vasc Surg* 2009; 50: 1285-92.

14. Rizvi AZ, Murad MH, Fairman RM, *et al*. The effect of left subclavian artery coverage on morbidity and mortality in patients undergoing endovascular thoracic aortic interventions: a systematic review and meta-analysis. *J Vasc Surg* 2009; 50: 1159-69.

15. Woo EY, Carpenter JP, Jackson BM, *et al*. Left subclavian artery coverage during thoracic endovascular aortic repair: a single-center experience. *J Vasc Surg* 2008; 48: 555-60.

16. Sonesson B, Resch T, Allers M, Malina M. Endovascular total aortic arch replacement by *in situ* stent graft fenestration technique. *J Vasc Surg* 2009; 49: 1589-91.

17. Tong DC, Yenari MA, Albers GW, *et al*. Correlation of perfusion- and diffusion-weighted MRI with NIHSS score in acute (<6.5 hour) ischemic stroke. *Neurology* 1998; 50: 864-70.

18. Murphy BD, Fox AJ, Lee DH, *et al*. Identification of penumbra and infarct in acute ischemic stroke using computed tomography perfusion-derived blood flow and blood volume measurements. *Stroke* 2006; 37: 1771-7.

19. Thanvi B, Treadwell S, Robinson T. Early neurological deterioration in acute ischaemic stroke: predictors, mechanisms and management. *Postgrad Med J* 2008; 84(994): 412-7.

20. Tissue plasminogen activator for acute ischemic stroke. The National Institute of Neurological Disorders and Stroke rt-PA Stroke Study Group. *N Engl J Med* 1995; 333(24): 1581-7.

21. Barnwell SL, Clark WM, Nguyen TT, *et al*. Safety and efficacy of delayed intraarterial urokinase therapy with mechanical clot disruption for thromboembolic stroke. *AJNR Am J Neuroradiol* 1994; 15: 1817-22.

22. Furlan A, Higashida R, Wechsler L, *et al*. Intra-arterial prourokinase for acute ischemic stroke. The PROACT II study: a randomized controlled trial. Prolyse in Acute Cerebral Thromboembolism. *JAMA* 1999; 282(21): 2003-11.

23. Smith WS, Sung G, Saver J, *et al*. Mechanical thrombectomy for acute ischemic stroke: final results of the Multi MERCI trial. *Stroke* 2008; 39: 1205-12.

24. The penumbra pivotal stroke trial: safety and effectiveness of a new generation of mechanical devices for clot removal in intracranial large vessel occlusive disease. *Stroke* 2009; 40: 2761-8.

25. Greenberg RK, Lu Q, Roselli EE, *et al*. Contemporary analysis of descending thoracic and thoracoabdominal aneurysm repair: a comparison of endovascular and open techniques. *Circulation* 2008; 118: 808-17.

26. Feezor RJ, Martin TD, Hess PJ, Jr., *et al*. Extent of aortic coverage and incidence of spinal cord ischemia after thoracic endovascular aneurysm repair. *Ann Thorac Surg* 2008; 86: 1809-14.

27. Axisa BM, Loftus IM, Fishwick G, *et al*. Endovascular repair of an innominate artery false aneurysm following blunt trauma. *J Endovasc Ther* 2000; 7: 245-50.

28. Bell RE, Reidy JF. Endovascular treatment of thoracic aortic disease. *Heart* 2003; 89: 823-4.

29. Clough RE, Black SA, Lyons OT, *et al*. Is endovascular repair of mycotic aortic aneurysms a durable treatment option? *Eur J Vasc Endovasc Surg* 2009; 37: 407-12.

30. Bajwa A, Davis M, Moawad M, Taylor PR. Paraplegia following elective endovascular repair of abdominal aortic aneurysm: reversal with cerebrospinal fluid drainage. *Eur J Vasc Endovasc Surg* 2008; 35: 46-8.

31. Matsuda H, Fukuda T, Iritani O, *et al*. Spinal cord injury is not negligible after TEVAR for lower descending aorta. *Eur J Vasc Endovasc Surg* 2010; 39: 179-86.

32. Bicknell CD, Riga CV, Wolfe JH. Prevention of paraplegia during thoracoabdominal aortic aneurysm repair. *Eur J Vasc Endovasc Surg* 2009; 37: 654-60.

Case vignette
Neurological complications of thoracic endovascular repair

Rachel E. Clough MB BS BSc MRCS, NIHR BRC Clinical Training Fellow
Peter R. Taylor MA MChir FRCS, Professor of Vascular Surgery
Department of Vascular Surgery, NIHR Comprehensive Biomedical Research Centre of Guy's and St Thomas' NHS Foundation Trust and King's College London, and King's Health Partners, London, UK

Cerebral ischaemia caused by an aortic endograft reversed with a chimney stent to the origin of the brachiocephalic artery

A 76-year-old man presented with a hoarse voice caused by a left recurrent laryngeal nerve palsy related to a 5.5cm saccular aneurysm of the distal aortic arch (Figure 1). A right common carotid to left common carotid bypass was performed with an 8mm PTFE graft 5 days prior to endovascular repair. A covered tapered stent graft measuring 20cm long with a proximal diameter of 36mm and a distal diameter of 32mm was inserted without difficulty under loco-regional anaesthesia. Completion angiography showed continued filling of the aneurysm sac and the

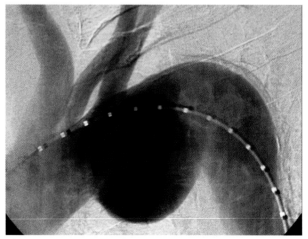

Figure 1. 5.5cm distal arch aneurysm causing aortovocal syndrome.

proximal left common carotid artery (Figure 2). Balloon dilatation of the proximal part of the stent graft successfully excluded the aneurysm but caused significant narrowing of the origin of the brachiocephalic artery, resulting in a progressive decrease in systemic blood pressure measured via a right radial arterial line (Figure 3). The patient started to complain of dizziness and lost consciousness when the systolic pressure fell below 60mmHg. The right brachial artery was punctured under ultrasound guidance and a 10mm self-expanding uncovered nitinol stent was retrogradely placed across the origin of the brachiocephalic artery (Figure 4). The blood pressure and consciousness returned to normal. At 4 years follow-up the aneurysm remains excluded and the patient has no neurological sequelae.

Inadvertent coverage of the origins of the great vessels of the aortic arch by an endovascular device may cause serious complications. These include stroke and myocardial infarction if the left subclavian is the origin of a coronary artery bypass using the left internal mammary artery. Rapid deployment of an uncovered chimney stent across the artery origin can reperfuse compromised vessels with good long-term results.

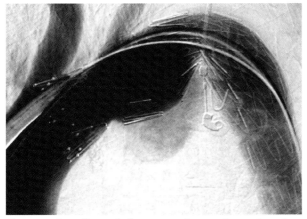

Figure 2. Completion angiography showing deliberate over-stenting of the brachiocephalic artery and continued filling of the aneurysm sac and proximal left common carotid artery.

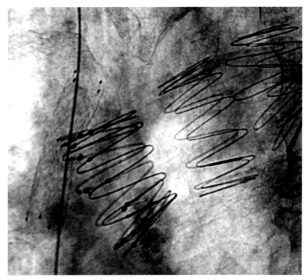

Figure 4. A nitinol uncovered chimney stent is retrogradely placed across the origin of the brachiocephalic artery with immediate reversal of the neurological deficit.

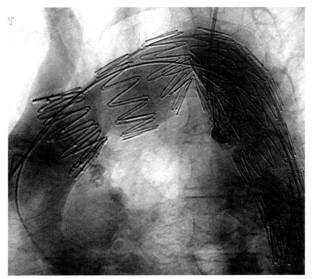

Figure 3. Balloon dilatation of the proximal stent graft excludes the aneurysm but causes significant narrowing of the origin of the brachiocephalic artery with progressive loss of consciousness.

Chapter 10   Complications related to the management of the acutely ischaemic limb

David Ratliff MD FRCP FRCS (Eng & Ed), Consultant Vascular Surgeon
Northampton General Hospital, Northampton, UK

Introduction

Acute limb ischaemia (ALI) is defined as a sudden decrease in limb perfusion that causes a potential threat to limb viability, manifest by ischaemic rest pain, ulcers and/or gangrene, in patients who present within 2 weeks of the acute event [1]. It may be caused by thrombosis in a diseased artery or bypass graft, or embolism from a proximal source. The clinical manifestations vary depending on the site and length of the occlusion.

Classification

The severity of ALI should be stratified according to the following categories (see Table 1) [2]:

Category	Description/prognosis	Findings		Doppler signals	
		Sensory loss	Muscle weakness	Arterial	Venous
I. Viable	Not immediately threatened	None	None	Audible	Audible
II. Threatened					
a. Marginally	Salvageable if promptly treated	Minimal (toes) or none	None	Inaudible	Audible
b. Immediately	Salvageable with immediate revascularisation	More than toes, associated with rest pain	Mild, moderate	Inaudible	Audible
III. Irreversible	Major tissue loss or permanent nerve damage inevitable	Profound, anaesthetic	Profound, paralysis (rigor)	Inaudible	Inaudible

Table 1. Clinical categories of acute limb ischaemia.

◆ I. *Viable* limbs are not immediately threatened. There is no sensory loss or muscle weakness, and both arterial and venous Doppler signals are audible;

◆ IIa. *Marginally threatened* limbs are salvageable with prompt treatment. Numbness and transient or minimal sensory loss is limited to the toes, there is no muscle weakness, arterial Doppler signals are inaudible and venous Doppler signals are audible;

◆ IIb. *Immediately threatened* limbs are salvageable with immediate revascularisation. Sensory loss involves more than the toes and is associated with rest pain. There is mild to moderate muscle weakness, arterial Doppler signals are inaudible and venous Doppler signals are audible;

◆ III. *Irreversibly (non-viable)* ischaemic limbs require major amputation regardless of treatment. There is profound sensory loss and muscle paralysis extending above the foot, absent capillary skin flow distally or evidence of more advanced ischaemia such as muscle rigidity or skin marbling and both arterial and venous Doppler signals are absent. Revascularisation may be appropriate to reduce the level of the amputation.

Complications of acute limb ischaemia

The major complications of ALI are amputation and death, and rates for both remain high despite intervention; they were 16% and 22%, respectively, in an audit published by The Vascular Society in 1998 [3]. Although more recent improvements to both surgical technique and pre/peri-operative management have reduced the rate of limb loss associated with ALI, the mortality still remains high [4]. Delay from symptom onset to surgery is a major determinant of outcome and attempts at improvement must be directed at early diagnosis and referral for a vascular opinion [4].

Patients presenting with ALI are frequently frail and elderly with multiple medical comorbidities, whose peripheral occlusion has often been precipitated by a myocardial event such as infarction, arrhythmia or decompensation [3-7]. Patients with acute myocardial infarction or poor cardiac output have an especially high mortality rate [8-9].

Additional complications of ALI include neurological symptoms in the limb, compartment syndrome, rhabdomyolysis and complications related to the method of treatment, such as wound complications after surgery and haemorrhagic complications after thrombolysis (see below).

Management

The management of ALI remains one of the most difficult challenges encountered by vascular specialists. Early diagnosis and rapid initiation of treatment are essential to achieve limb salvage. There is no one definitive treatment. Methods include anticoagulation, surgical embolectomy or thrombectomy and bypass grafting, thrombolysis and mechanical thrombectomy.

Complications related to anticoagulation

When the diagnosis of acute ischaemia is made, the patient should be resuscitated and immediately given a bolus of 5000U intravenous heparin, followed by a continuous intravenous infusion of 1000-1400U/hr according to body weight and local protocol. This prevents proximal and distal propagation of thrombus and preserves the microcirculation. Secondary thrombosis in distal vessels increases the risk of limb loss, particularly in patients with emboli.

Anticoagulation with heparin is the correct initial management of all patients with suspected ALI, as it stabilises and helps prevent deterioration of the limb whilst investigations (duplex/arteriography) are being arranged and treatment options considered. It may be the only treatment required in patients with acute on chronic ischaemia due to occlusion of the superficial femoral artery, where an adequate collateral circulation develops over the subsequent few days

(Class IIa). Acute arm ischaemia can also often be treated with heparin alone, as the collateral circulation is better than in the lower limb. Conservative management without brachial embolectomy can, however, result in a symptomatic cold hand and disability from forearm claudication [10].

Haemorrhage

The main complication of heparin is haemorrhage, usually from intravenous/arterial cannula sites and surgical incisions, although more major bleeding can also occur. This is often due to excessive anticoagulation.

All patients receiving intravenous heparin infusions should have their activated partial thromboplastin time (APTT) checked and the dose adjusted if necessary after 2-6 hours of therapy. If the dose is stable, this should be repeated at 24-hour intervals. The APTT should be kept in the range 42-72 seconds (1.5-2.5 normal APTT). When bleeding occurs, stopping the heparin infusion is usually sufficient. The APTT should be rechecked and the infusion restarted after 2 hours at a dosage determined by the APTT result. If the bleeding is severe, 1mg protamine should be given for every 100U heparin infused over the previous hour.

The risk of haemorrhage is increased in heparinised patients following recent surgery or in those with uraemia, thrombocytopaenia, a history of bleeding tendency, peptic ulcer or in elderly patients. Intramuscular injections are contra-indicated in patients receiving heparin.

Heparin-induced thrombocytopaenia

Clinically important heparin-induced thrombo-cytopaenia is immune-mediated and develops after 5-10 days; it can be complicated by thrombosis. The platelet count should be measured before treatment and monitored daily if heparin is given for longer than 4 days. Signs of heparin-induced thrombocytopaenia include a 50% reduction of the platelet count,

thrombosis or skin allergy. If heparin-induced thrombocytopaenia is suspected or confirmed, the heparin should be stopped and an alternative anticoagulant such as lepirudin or danaparoid prescribed.

Recurrent emboli despite anti-coagulation

Rarely, recurrent peripheral emboli may occur after successful embolectomy and adequate anticoagulation with heparin. This indicates an unstable source, such as a large volume of left atrial thrombus or an atrial myxoma. Repeat embolectomy may be performed, but the associated risk is high.

Debilitated patients with major comorbidity such as advanced cancer may also present with an acutely ischaemic limb. This can be due to spontaneous thrombosis of a healthy native vessel due to a procoagulant state, rather than to embolism. It is frequently a pre-morbid event.

Complications related to surgery

Surgical techniques for the treatment of ALI include balloon catheter embolectomy or thrombectomy, and bypass procedures. Occasionally, endarterectomy and patch angioplasty may be appropriate for an isolated occlusion of the common femoral artery. Intra-operative thrombolysis may be used as an adjunct to surgical revascularisation.

Wound complications

Wound complications include wound haematoma and dehiscence. They occur typically in the groin after embolectomy in association with anticoagulation initiated bleeding (Figure 1). Prevention depends on normal attention to careful dissection without undermining of the skin edges, meticulous haemostasis and wound closure. Incisions should be closed routinely with suction drainage in patients receiving postoperative anticoagulation.

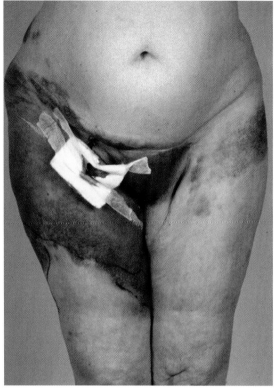

Figure 1. Severe bruising following femoral embolectomy.

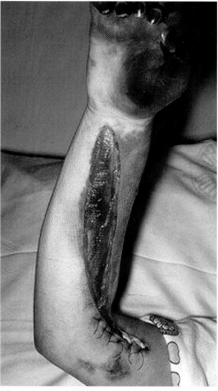

Figure 2. Volkmann's ischaemic contracture following acute arm ischaemia.

Limb oedema

Oedema is common after limb revascularisation and is due to ischaemia-reperfusion injury. It usually follows a benign course and progressively improves with patient mobilisation. Patients should be advised to elevate their leg when sitting, initially with the ankle at the level of the heart.

Neurological symptoms in the limb

Neurological symptoms include paraesthesia, burning discomfort and areas of reduced or altered sensation. They are caused by ischaemic neuropathy and can cause considerable morbidity. The patient should be reassured that they should resolve with time, but this may take several months. Gabapentin or amitriptyline may be beneficial and advice should be sought from the pain team.

Compartment syndrome

Severe oedema can occur following reperfusion of an acutely ischaemic limb and lead to an increased pressure within its closed fascial compartments This can be in the presence or absence of significant muscle necrosis. This compartment syndrome causes further ischaemia and later necrosis/fibrosis of muscle and may result in limb loss or permanent severe disability (Figure 2). It is more commonly seen after relief of ALI caused by trauma or the injection of crushed tablets by intravenous drug abusers, than after a thrombo-embolic event [11].

Symptoms of compartment syndrome include unexpected pain and paraesthesia in the distal extremity, which is often disproportionate to the magnitude of the initial injury. The pain responds poorly to analgesia and is typically not relieved by fracture immobilisation or reduction. Paraesthesia is caused by ischaemia of the nerves traversing the affected muscle compartment. On examination the affected compartment is tense, tender and swollen, with pain elicited by passive movement; the anterior compartment is the most frequently affected. Numbness may be present in the first dorsal web space, together with an inability to extend the toes or fully dorsiflex the ankle. This is due to impaired function in the deep peroneal nerve and may result subsequently in foot drop unless immediate action is taken.

Patients with compartment syndrome should undergo immediate fasciotomy. All four compartments of the leg should be widely opened by two incisions placed vertically on the posteromedial and anterolateral aspect of the limb [12] (Figure 3). This procedure is relatively simple and enables rapid

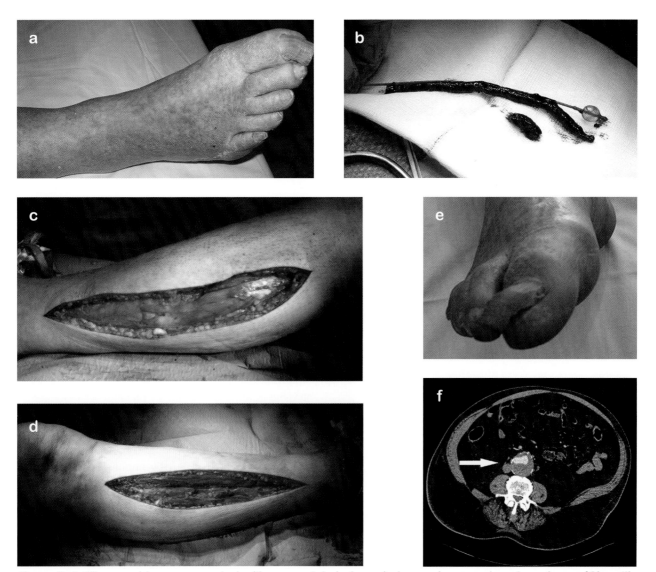

Figure 3. A 72-year-old man presented with an acutely ischaemic leg and compartment syndrome (Class IIb ischaemia) due to athero-embolism from a 5.5cm infrarenal aortic aneurysm. This was immediately revascularised by femoral embolectomy and a four-compartment fasciotomy. The fasciotomy incisions were closed primarily on the fifth postoperative day and the aneurysm was subsequently repaired. a) Immediately threatened limb (Class IIb ischaemia). b) Popliteal embolus removed by balloon catheter embolectomy. c) & d) Four-compartment fasciotomy. e) Pink foot after successful revascularisation, with superficial venous dilatation. f) CT scan of a 5.5cm aortic aneurysm containing a large amount of atheroma that caused the embolus.

decompression of the leg. Alternatively the four compartments can be decompressed by removing a segment of fibula, although this method is not in common practice (see also Chapter 11).

It is often difficult to predict the degree of postoperative swelling after limb revascularisation. Where this is likely to be severe, and typically where the degree and extent of the acute ischaemia at presentation is severe, it may be appropriate for a prophylactic early fasciotomy to be performed. Such situations include a prolonged ischaemic time (>6 hours), saddle embolus and proximal emboli, inadequate arterial collaterals, hypotension and poor back-bleeding from the distal arterial tree at embolectomy [13].

Compartment pressures may be measured as an adjunct to management. A normal intracompartment pressure (ICP) is <12mm Hg. Whilst absolute ICP measurements have been recommended [14], the threshold ICP for the diagnosis of compartment syndrome remains controversial. It is now considered good practice to use a dynamic ICP threshold related to the mean arterial pressure (MAP) or diastolic pressure. Fasciotomy is warranted if the difference between the ICP and MAP falls to <40mmHg, or the difference between ICP and diastolic pressure is <10mmHg [12].

In practice, fasciotomy is only necessary in 2-5% of patients who develop ALI after thrombo-embolic events. Nevertheless, prompt recognition and appropriate management is vital to optimise the chance of a full recovery and preserving a useful limb.

Rhabdomyolysis

Revascularisation of a severely acutely ischaemic limb can result in rhabdomyolysis, myoglobinuria, acute renal failure and hyperkalaemia. Rhabdomyolysis is the rapid breakdown of skeletal muscle due to injury to muscle tissue. The destruction of muscle leads to the release of the breakdown products of damaged muscle cells into the bloodstream, of which the most important is myoglobin. Myoglobin is present in muscle cells as a reserve of oxygen. This accumulates in the renal

tubules and then forms casts that obstruct the normal flow of fluid through the nephron. Iron released from the myoglobin damages kidney cells and causes acute tubular necrosis.

Clinically, damage to the kidneys may lead to oliguria or anuria, dark tea-coloured urine and acute renal failure, usually about 12-24 hours after the initial muscle damage. The diagnosis is confirmed by an elevated level of creatine kinase (CK) in the blood. Levels above five times the upper limit of normal indicate rhabdomyolysis. Depending on its extent, levels up to 100,000 units are not unusual [15]. The risk of acute renal failure is related directly to the initial and peak CK levels; the higher the CK, the more likely it is that kidney damage will occur [16].

The aim of treatment is to preserve kidney function by ensuring the patient is well hydrated and maintains a good urine output through the administration of generous amounts of intravenous fluids, and alkalinising the urine by adding bicarbonate to them. Acute renal failure due to myoglobinuria may require haemofiltration or haemodialysis until the kidney function improves, likely in 2-3 weeks.

Complications related to thrombolysis

Intra-arterial thrombolysis is an effective alternative to surgical treatment in selected patients with ischaemic but viable extremities (Class IIa ischaemia) [17]. Its usefulness is limited by the severity and duration of the ischaemia, and the length of time required to achieve dissolution of the thrombus. Several factors are important in determining whether surgical revascularisation or thrombolytic therapy is the most appropriate treatment. These include:

- ◆ the duration of symptoms;
- ◆ the presumed aetiology (embolism versus thrombosis);
- ◆ the suitability of the patient for surgery;
- ◆ the location and length of the lesion on angiography;
- ◆ the availability of autologous vein for reconstructive surgery.

Thrombolysis is particularly indicated when the surgical options are poor and the run-off vessels in the leg appear occluded [18]. A meta-analysis of the available trials in 2000 suggested that thrombolysis was most effective in short-duration ischaemia (<14 days) and for occluded grafts [19].

Results

The results of surgery versus thrombolysis for the initial management of ALI have been analysed in a Cochrane Review [20]. Five trials with a total of 1283 participants were included. There was no significant difference in limb salvage or death at 30 days, 6 months or 1 year between initial surgery and initial thrombolysis. Complications, however, were higher in the thrombolysis group:

- stroke was significantly more frequent at 30 days with thrombolysis (1.3%) than surgery (0%);
- major haemorrhage was more likely at 30 days with thrombolysis (8.8%) than surgery (3.3%);
- distal embolisation was more likely at 30 days after thrombolysis (12.4%) than surgery (0%).

The authors concluded that the higher risk of complications must be balanced against the risk of surgery in each patient.

In two further Cochrane Reviews, the infusion techniques for thrombolysis and efficacy of fibrinolytic agents were reviewed [21-22]. Thrombolysis with intra-arterial recombinant tissue plasminogen activator (rt-PA) appeared to be most effective with the angiographic catheter placed within the thrombus. Although high dose and forced infusion techniques achieve vessel patency in less time than low-dose infusion, there were more bleeding complications and no increase in patency rates or improvement in limb salvage at 30 days [21].

Stroke

1-2% of patients develop a stroke during thrombolysis, either due to infarction secondary to embolism or haemorrhage, in approximately equal proportions [20, 23-26]. Following a stroke, the heparin infusion should be stopped until the result of an emergency CT scan is known. If the diagnosis is cerebral infarction rather than haemorrhage, the infusion may be continued depending on individual patient factors.

Haemorrhage

Haemorrhage during thrombolysis may be clinically obvious, but is most dangerous when it is occult such as into the retroperitoneum or the gastrointestinal tract. If a patient develops hypotension or shock during thrombolysis, bleeding must be assumed until proven otherwise. Occasionally patients may not be bleeding and the hypotension is due to reperfusion of the ischaemic limb. Minor bleeding is common following arterial puncture in the groin. It is rarely necessary to stop the infusion and the outcome is not usually affected, although some dramatic bruising may occur. Local pressure and compression should be applied over an expanding haematoma.

Major haemorrhage can reduce limb salvage and may be fatal (Figure 4). The infusion should be stopped and the patient should be resuscitated and examined to determine the cause. Tenderness or a mass in the iliac fossa suggests a retroperitoneal haematoma necessitating an urgent CT. In cases of continuing haemorrhage, the thrombolytic therapy can be reversed with cryoprecipitate containing

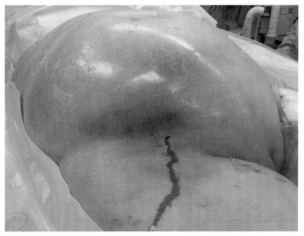

Figure 4. Massive retroperitoneal haematoma following thrombolysis.

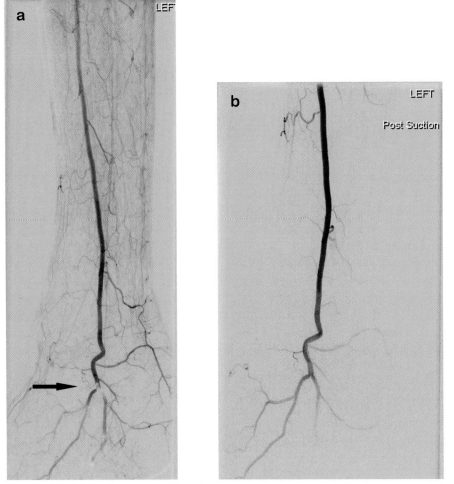

Figure 5. a) Distal embolisation (arrow) during thrombolysis. b) Successful removal by suction aspiration.

fibrinogen, fresh frozen plasma and antifibrinolytic drugs such as aprotinin or tranexamic acid.

Unfortunately, haematological monitoring does not accurately predict haemorrhagic complications during thrombolysis. Patients should be carefully monitored in a high dependency area with frequent review by experienced staff who are alert to this potential complication. The risk of haemorrhage can be minimised by avoiding invasive procedures and intramuscular injections during treatment. Retrograde puncture of the femoral artery contralateral to the occlusion should be performed whenever possible to access the artery for lysis, rather than antegrade puncture of the ipsilateral ischaemic limb.

Distal embolisation

Distal embolisation due to small fragments of lysing thrombus may occur in up to 30% cases of thrombolysis. This is clinically apparent as a sudden deterioration of the limb during an otherwise uneventful infusion. A further angiogram should be performed to establish the situation. The thrombus may be amenable to percutaneous aspiration (Figure 5) and the catheter advanced down the limb to continue thrombolysis. Lysis of remaining distal thrombus and patency can usually be restored by continuing the infusion and providing adequate analgesia; embolectomy is rarely necessary.

Rarely, massive embolisation threatens the viability of the limb. This occurs most frequently during lysis of thrombosed popliteal aneurysms and is probably the result of a large volume of thrombus being lysed. Urgent surgical treatment is required to salvage the limb.

Conclusions

Successful management of ALI remains a considerable challenge that depends on an accurate initial assessment and selection of the optimal treatment for each individual patient. This requires a multidisciplinary approach with close collaboration between vascular specialists working as a team, increasingly in vascular centres with a full range of the available therapeutic options.

Acknowledgements

My thanks to Professor Jonathan Beard for supplying Figures 1, 2 and 4 and to Mr John Thompson for Figure 5.

Key points

◆ All patients with ALI should be resuscitated and receive intravenous heparin.
◆ Patients should be stratified according to the severity of their ischaemia.
◆ Amputation and death rates remain high despite improved peri-operative management.
◆ As soon as compartment syndrome is diagnosed, it should be treated by a four-compartment fasciotomy.
◆ Major complications are greater with thrombolysis than surgery.

References

1. Norgren L, Hiatt WR, Dormandy JA, *et al*. Inter-Society Consensus for the Management of Peripheral Arterial Disease (TASC II). *J Vasc Surg* 2007; 45 Suppl S: S5.
2. Rutherford RB, Baker D, Ernst C, *et al*. Recommended standards for reports dealing with lower extremity ischaemia: Revised version. *J Vasc Surg* 1997; 26: 517-38.
3. Campbell WB, Ridler BMF, Szymanska TH. Current management of acute leg ischaemia: results of an audit by the Vascular Surgical Society of Great Britain and Ireland. *Br J Surg* 1998; 85: 1498-503.
4. Morris-Stiff G, D'Souza J, Raman S, *et al*. Update of experience for acute limb ischaemia in a district general hospital - are we getting any better? *Ann R Coll Surg Engl* 2009; 91: 1478-83.
5. Ouriel K, Veith FJ. Acute lower limb ischaemia: determinants of outcome. *Surgery* 1998; 124: 336-41.
6. Braithwaite BD, Davies B, Birch PA, *et al*. Management of acute leg ischaemia in the elderly. *Br J Surg* 1998: 85: 217-20.
7. Clason AE, Stonebridge PA, Duncan AJ, *et al*. Morbidity and mortality in acute lower limb ischaemia: a 5-year review. *Eur J Vasc Surg* 1989; 3: 339-43.
8. Jivegard L, Arfvidsson B, Frid I, *et al*. Cardiac output in patients with acute lower limb ischaemia of presumed embolic origin - a predictor of severity and outcome? *Eur J Vasc Surg* 1990; 4: 401-07.
9. Ljungman C, Adami HO, Bergqvist D, *et al*. Risk factors for early lower limb loss after embolectomy or acute arterial occlusion: a population-based case-control study. *Br J Surg* 1991; 78: 1482-85.
10. Earnshaw JJ. Acute arm ischaemia. In: *Rare Vascular Disorders - a Practical Guide for the Vascular Specialist*. Earnshaw JJ, Ed. Shrewsbury, UK: tfm Publishing, 2005: 149-56.
11. Partanen TA, Vikatmaa, Tukiainen E, *et al*. Outcome after injections of crushed tablets in intravenous drug abusers in the Helsinki University Central Hospital. *Eur J Vasc Endovasc Surg* 2009; 37: 704-11.
12. Modrall JG. Compartment syndrome. In: *Rutherford's Vascular Surgery*, 7th ed. Cronenwett JL, Johnston KW, Eds. Saunders 2010: 2412-21.
13. Papalambros EL, Panayiotopoulos YP, Bastounis E, *et al*. Prophylactic fasciotomy of the legs following acute arterial occlusion procedures. *Int Angiol* 1989; 8: 120-4.
14. Matsen FA, Winquist RA, Krugmire RB. Diagnosis and management of compartment syndromes. *J Bone Joint Surg* 1980; 62: 286-91.
15. Vanholder R, Sever MS, Erek E, *et al*. Rhabdomyolysis. *J Am Soc Nephrol* 2000; 11: 1553-61.
16. De Meijer AR, Fikkers BG, de Keijzer MH, *et al*. Serum creatine kinase as predictor of clinical course in

rhabdomyolysis: a 5-year intensive care survey. *Intensive Care Med* 2003; 29: 1121-5.

17. Hirsch AT, Haskal ZJ, Hertzer NR, *et al*. ACC/AHA 2005 Practice Guidelines for the Management of Patients with Peripheral Arterial Disease (lower extremity, renal, mesenteric, and abdominal aortic) a Collaborative Report. *Circulation* 2006; 113: e463.

18. Earnshaw JJ. Acute ischaemia: evaluation and decision making. In: *Rutherford's Vascular Surgery*, 7th Ed. Cronenwett JL, Johnston KW, Eds. Saunders 2010: 2389-98.

19. Palfreyman SJ, Booth A, Michaels JA. A systematic review of intra-arterial thrombolytic therapy for acute leg ischaemia. *Eur J Vasc Endovasc Surg* 2000; 19: 143-57.

20. Berridge DC, Kessel DO, Robertson I. Surgery versus thrombolysis for initial management of acute limb ischaemia. *Cochrane Database Syst Rev* 2002; Issue1.

21. Kessel DO, Berridge, Robertson I. Infusion techniques for peripheral arterial thrombolysis. *Cochrane Database Syst Rev* 2004; Issue 1.

22. Robertson I, Kessel DO, Berridge DC. Fibrinolytic agents for peripheral arterial occlusion. *Cochrane Database Syst Rev* 2010; Issue 3.

23. Braithwaite BD. Setting the 'gold standard' for peripheral thrombolysis. *Br J Surg* 1996; 83: 558-9.

24. Dawson K, Armon A, Braithwaite BD, *et al*. Stroke during intra-arterial thrombolysis: a survey of experience in the UK. *Br J Surg* 1996; 83: 568.

25. Braithwaite BD, Tomlinson MA, Walker SR, *et al*. Peripheral thrombolysis for acute-onset claudication. *Br J Surg* 1999; 86: 800-04.

26. Plate G, Jansson I, Forssell C, *et al*. Thrombolysis for acute lower limb ischaemia - a prospective randomised multicentre study comparing two strategies. *Eur J Vasc Endovasc Surg* 2006; 31: 651-60.

Chapter 11

Ischaemic reperfusion, compartment syndrome and multi-organ failure in vascular patients

Alex B. Watson MSc FRCS, Specialist Registrar in Vascular Surgery
Peter M. Lamont MD FRCS, Consultant Vascular Surgeon
Bristol Royal Infirmary, Bristol, UK

Introduction

There are two main groups of vascular patients at risk of ischaemia reperfusion injury: those undergoing open abdominal aortic aneurysm (AAA) surgery, elective or emergency, and those with acute limb ischaemia. Elective AAA repair is undoubtedly a successful operation but still carries a mortality of between 3-10%, with cardiac events accounting for most of the deaths [1]. Studies investigating the morbidity and mortality of AAA repair have found that a significant number of patients die postoperatively from single- or multiple-organ failure; those who survive organ failure often have prolonged stays in critical care, at considerable cost. The systemic inflammatory response syndrome and ischaemia reperfusion injury following aortic cross-clamping have been implicated in the development of organ failure after AAA repair. The same mechanisms are thought to underpin both local and systemic complications following surgery for acute limb ischaemia.

Establishing the cause of mortality

A number of studies have attempted to establish the causes of death after AAA repair. Sayers *et al*

looked at 671 patients who underwent AAA repair and found that although some patients died intra-operatively from cardiac collapse or failure to control bleeding, many patients died postoperatively from single- or multiple-organ failure [2]. A significant number of patients who develop multi-organ failure do not survive [3]. Patients who developed acute renal failure following ruptured AAA had an overall mortality rate of 75%. Other independent variables that predicted death included pre-operative vascular disease, requirement for re-operation and failure of additional organ systems (usually cardiac or respiratory) [4].

Early detection and treatment of organ dysfunction may prevent progression from single- to multiple-organ failure, and death [5]. The prevention of organ dysfunction is therefore a primary goal in major aortic surgery. It has been postulated that organ dysfunction and failure following AAA repair occurs as a result of ischaemia reperfusion injury and the development of a systemic inflammatory response syndrome. Theories regarding the pathogenesis of organ failure in response to inflammatory insults concentrate around the host's response to the initial insults and the magnitude and timing of these insults [6].

Systemic inflammatory response syndrome (SIRS)

All surgery leads to the development of an inflammatory response, which has four main components at the tissue/microcirculation level:

- vasodilatation;
- increased vascular permeability;
- intravascular white cell adhesion and activation; and
- coagulation.

Upregulation of adhesion molecules facilitates endothelial-white cell interaction to enable migration into the tissues. Neutrophils undergo a respiratory burst, releasing lysosomal enzymes, oxidants and free radicals, which are involved in the killing of invading micro-organisms [7]. This process occurs under the control of inflammatory mediators (cytokines, TNFα and the interleukins). These are produced by a number of different cells in the inflammatory response such as macrophages, neutrophils and endothelial cells, and have a variety of effects including adhesion molecule upregulation, chemotaxis and activation of other inflammatory pathways (coagulation, complement, kinins and fibrinolysis). This is a normal and beneficial response that is essential for survival and is an important aspect of tissue repair and wound healing [8]. Patients who develop major complications after AAA repair are known to exhibit an exaggerated interleukin-6 response after the surgery but before the complications become clinically evident, suggesting the involvement of an underlying pro-inflammatory process [9].

When the inflammatory response escapes its local control mechanisms, it may result in a systemic inflammatory response syndrome [10]. SIRS is characterised by high levels of circulating cytokines and activated neutrophils, and is clinically defined by changes in temperature, heart rate, respiratory rate and white cell count (Table 1).

This inflammatory state, with endothelial injury, leucocyte adhesion and increased vascular permeability, causes organ damage at the cellular level and this may progress to single- or multiple-organ failure. Studies looking at the relationship between SIRS, organ failure and mortality have shown that SIRS and organ failure are common following AAA repair, and that the development of multi-organ failure is significantly associated with mortality [11, 12]. SIRS occurs concurrently with, or even before, any organ failure in most cases and its resolution is a prognostic indicator of a successful outcome [11].

It should also be noted, however, that using SIRS as a means of predicting multi-organ failure is unreliable [13]. Conditions such as anxiety, pain and slight hypovolaemia (which frequently occurs following surgery), may lead to an increase in heart and respiratory rates in the absence of true SIRS [14-16]. Theories about why some of these patients develop SIRS and organ failure indicate that it is probably secondary to ischaemia-reperfusion injury [17].

Table 1. SIRS is defined by the presence of two or more of the four criteria listed here.

White cell count >12,000cells/mm^3, or <4,000 cells/mm^3, or >10% immature forms

Temperature >38°C or <36°C

Heart rate >90 beats/minute

Respiratory rate >20 breaths/minute, or PaCO$_2$ <4.3kPa

Ischaemia reperfusion injury (IRI) and multi-organ failure

During acute limb ischaemia, whether due to aortic cross-clamping or to other reasons such as trauma, embolism or acute thrombosis, the resultant hypoxia leads to a reduction in ATP levels, and xanthine dehydrogenase is converted to xanthine oxidase. The tissue pH levels fall, potassium levels rise and in severe cases of ischaemia, muscle tissue damage releases myoglobin. Following restoration of blood flow, oxygen-rich blood reperfuses the ischaemic limbs. Xanthine oxidase drives the reaction between oxygen and hypoxanthine to produce superoxide and other toxic free radicals. These free radicals and toxic products are then washed through the circulatory system. They therefore not only produce local damage, but exert distant effects as well, producing endothelial cell injury mainly by lipid peroxidation of the endothelial cell membrane [18-20].

This IRI causes widespread changes in the microcirculation, with increased production of vasoconstrictors such as thromboxane and endothelin, and decreased amounts of vasodilators (prostacyclin). Inflammatory pathways are also triggered. Damaged endothelial cells interact with neutrophils facilitated by adhesion molecules, which leads to neutrophil migration into tissues. The whole response is driven by cytokine mediators including TNFα, interleukins-1, - 6 and -10, thus resulting in a systemic inflammatory response syndrome, and compounding the damage [21].

Following excessive blood loss, additional insults include hypotension, acidosis, blood transfusion and hypothermia, which cause further widespread activation of the inflammatory pathways and probably account for the progression to multiple-organ failure in many patients. This is termed the two-hit hypothesis [11, 22].

Ischaemia reperfusion injury and the viscera

Cardiac events account for most of the mortality following AAA repair [1]. Myocardial ischaemia and damage, arrhythmias and cardiac arrest can all occur, and are thought to be due to a combination of IRI and hypoxic, acidotic and hyperkalaemic blood returning to the systemic circulation following clamp removal [23].

Acute lung injury following aortic cross-clamping also occurs secondary to IRI [24-26]. The clinical presentation is one of progressive hypoxia, non-cardiogenic pulmonary oedema and adult respiratory distress syndrome, which has a high mortality.

Acute renal failure complicating both elective and emergency aortic aneurysm repair is also associated with a high mortality [27, 28]. The cause of this is multi-factorial with marked changes in renal haemodynamics, IRI and rhabdomyolysis of ischaemic skeletal muscle causing myoglobinuria.

Gastrointestinal complications are also common after AAA repair and carry increased mortality and morbidity. Complications range from prolonged ileus, ischaemic colitis and bowel infarction, to acute pancreatitis and liver failure [29]. They not only occur as a result of direct mesenteric ischaemia but also because of IRI. Indeed studies have shown structural and functional changes of the intestine following lower limb ischaemia [30].

Reducing operative morbidity and mortality

Ischaemia reperfusion injury and multi-organ failure are clearly linked. It seems logical that if IRI could be minimised or prevented, subsequent organ dysfunction and failure would be reduced, thus decreasing the operative morbidity and mortality.

In simple terms this involves both reducing tissue ischaemia by minimising ischaemic time and reducing the local and systemic impact of toxic free radicals.

Reducing ischaemic time

When dealing with acute limb ischaemia there is little that can be done about the delay before presentation. However, the time taken to achieve revascularisation can be affected at many steps. The acutely ischaemic limb can be tolerated for up to 6 hours before the risk of compartment syndrome after revascularisation mandates fasciotomy, so the earlier the patient can safely be brought to theatre for surgery within this time limit, the better. Ensuring rapid referral, vascular review, diagnostic investigation and admittance to the operating theatre are all areas that may be targeted with local education, guidelines and admission protocols. In major aortic surgery requiring aortic cross-clamping, it is obvious that any vascular surgeon will try to minimise the cross-clamp time. Here, preparation and anticipation are the keys. Surgery is a team effort and a well-briefed and rehearsed operating team can greatly improve time efficiency. The kidneys may tolerate only 30 to 45 minutes of warm ischaemic time and this tolerance needs to be remembered when using a suprarenal clamp. Potential difficulties should be anticipated. For example, making the decision early that a renal artery may have to be reimplanted to secure a proximal anastomosis allows for a jump graft to be anastomosed to the aortic graft prior to suprarenal clamping, meaning one fewer anastomosis and less renal ischaemia.

Reducing tissue ischaemia

Endoluminal techniques

The benefits of endoluminal repair are threefold: it avoids the need for laparotomy, avoids the cardiac strain associated with cross-clamping and may reduce the distal ischaemia and subsequent IRI associated with open repair. Clinical studies have shown that the ischaemia reperfusion response associated with conventional open aneurysm surgery may largely be negated by endovascular techniques [31]. However, despite avoiding aortic cross-clamping completely, multi-organ dysfunction and failure are still a problem. There are also specific potential problems associated with endovascular surgery such as persistent postoperative pyrexia, arterial access, instrumentation injuries and endoleaks, with an increased need for secondary procedures.

Bypass techniques

Various bypass techniques have been used during AAA surgery, although the majority of studies in the literature involve thoraco-abdominal aneurysms. Unlike endoluminal repair, bypass techniques are augmentations of standard open repair techniques. A laparotomy is still required; however, bypass techniques mainly aim to decrease the distal ischaemia caused by cross-clamping and to a lesser extent to reduce the cardiac strain associated with temporary aortic occlusion.

Jacobs *et al* performed retrograde aortic perfusion by means of a left atrium-femoral bypass in 33 patients undergoing thoracic AAA repair. In some cases there was also selective perfusion of the coeliac trunk, superior mesenteric and both renal arteries using an octopus catheter. They found that retrograde and selective perfusion was a safe technique which prevented ischaemic renal and intestinal damage during cross-clamping of the aorta [32]. Critics point to the increased morbidity related to complications at bypass sites, potentially negating any systemic advantages.

Ischaemic preconditioning

Ischaemic preconditioning is a physiological mechanism whereby brief exposure to non-lethal ischaemia in one tissue confers protection against prolonged ischaemia in a distant tissue [33]. Observations from canine models some 20 years ago first suggested that following a brief period of ischaemia with reperfusion, a mechanism was triggered which prevented loss of intracellular ATP during subsequent ischaemic insults [34]. Further work has shown that a range of tissues can successfully be preconditioned and that the effects are transferrable to humans [35]. It was subsequently confirmed that ischaemia in distant vascular beds would confer protection to the heart. As skeletal muscle ischaemia can easily be induced by means of a tourniquet and is relatively resistant to ischaemic damage itself, it has become a target for ischaemic preconditioning to confer protection in multiple organs. This is known as remote ischaemic preconditioning (RIPC). The exact mechanism by which this works is unclear and theories include the activation of neural pathways, humoral effects of released blood factors and a suppression of inflammation and apoptosis in cells reducing the SIRS response [33]. Studies using RIPC in the context of cardiac surgery have shown reductions in cardiac damage but did little to reduce length of critical care stay [36]. With regards to major vascular procedures, however, Ali *et al* showed significant reductions in postoperative myocardial infarctions and duration of critical care [37]. In their study, 82 patients undergoing open AAA repair were randomised to RIPC by sequentially clamping the iliac arteries for 10 minutes of ischaemia then reperfusing for 10 minutes prior to aortic clamping. This small study provides encouraging evidence that RIPC could help reduce operative morbidity and mortality with a technique that is cheap and straightforward.

Free radical scavengers

IRI is associated with the production of superoxides and toxic free radicals which damage end organs as they are washed through the circulation. A number of studies have focused on whether this damage can be ameliorated by scavengers and antioxidants. One such study randomised patients undergoing elective open AAA repair to receive standard therapy with, or without the peri-operative administration of multi-antioxidants (vitamins E and C, allopurinol, N-acetylcysteine and mannitol) [38]. Significant reductions in leucocyte sequestration and oxidative stress were seen in association with reduced creatine kinase levels, suggesting reduced muscle injury.

Mannitol, an osmotic diuretic and weak renal vasodilator, has also been studied in isolation for its positive effects on IRI by acting as a free radical scavenger. Experimental studies have shown significant reductions in xanthine oxidase activity with attenuation of IRI-induced lung injury and cardiac damage [39, 40]. A single clinical trial examined the effect of mannitol on renal reperfusion injury during infrarenal aortic aneurysm surgery, and showed a reduction in subclinical renal injury [41]. Mannitol has also been shown to reduce skeletal muscle reperfusion injury and subsequent compartment pressures after revascularisation for leg ischaemia, through both its hyperosmolar effects reducing post-ischaemic oedema and free radical scavenger mechanisms reducing necrosis [42].

Whilst other studies have shown evidence of the anti-apoptotic and anti-inflammatory actions of other antioxidants in relation to IRI, there is little to recommend their use in current practice; however, mannitol is a familiar and relatively safe agent, and may have a place after major aortic surgery.

Blood transfusion

Peri-operative blood conservation is an important issue in major vascular surgery. A reduced requirement for heterologous blood transfusion through the use of cell salvage has been shown to be beneficial [43]. Acute normovolaemic haemodilution has been shown in some animal models to limit reperfusion injury and in clinical practice, it preserves renal function. However, it has not been possible to demonstrate significant savings on bank blood requirements, and in one study normovolaemic haemodilution had no impact on the systemic inflammatory response or clinical outcome when compared to cell salvage alone for AAA repair [44]. It is agreed that cell salvage should be available for all major aortic procedures.

Abdominal compartment syndrome (ACS)

Abdominal compartment syndrome can be defined as organ dysfunction secondary to raised intra-abdominal pressure. It occurs in about 20-30% of patients following ruptured AAA repair and is associated with a mortality of up to 70% [45]. The abdominal cavity including the pelvis is enclosed with a relatively fixed volume. Any increase in volume results in increased intra-abdominal pressure. This has deleterious effects on many organs within the abdomen, but also on the cardiorespiratory system (Table 2).

When the abdomen can no longer distend, pressure rises rapidly. The hollow viscera collapse resulting in decreased venous drainage and potential thrombosis. Further oedema and fluid release compound the situation and oxygen delivery is impaired resulting in ischaemia-related vasodilatation and capillary leakage. Once again, SIRS triggered by the initial insult, or secondary to the ACS, compounds the situation. Gut bacteria are translocated and the diaphragm becomes splinted impairing respiratory function. Restricted caval blood flow reduces venous return and cardiac output. If unrecognised or left untreated, death usually results (Figure 1).

These patients are often critically ill due to the primary pathology, and are often intubated and ventilated. There should be a high index of suspicion following any major aortic or abdominal surgery, particularly in the emergency setting. The onset of ACS may be characterised clinically by some or all of the following:

◆ increasing abdominal distension which is palpably tight (or difficult closure after surgery);
◆ tachypnoea, dyspnoea or increasing ventilatory requirements – classically increasing ventilatory pressures and decreased tidal volumes;
◆ poor urine output;
◆ decreasing cardiac output/increased inotrope requirement;
◆ high nasogastric tube outputs.

Table 2. Aetiology of abdominal compartment syndrome.
Primary
◆ Haemorrhage – intra/retroperitoneal, e.g. ruptured AAA
◆ Abdominal trauma
◆ Pelvic fracture
◆ Pancreatitis
◆ Ischaemic bowel
◆ Bowel obstruction/ileus
◆ Ascites
Secondary
◆ Sepsis
◆ Hypoproteinaemia
◆ Burns
◆ Packing/high tension abdominal closure

Intra-abdominal pressure can be measured indirectly by connecting a pressure transducer to an

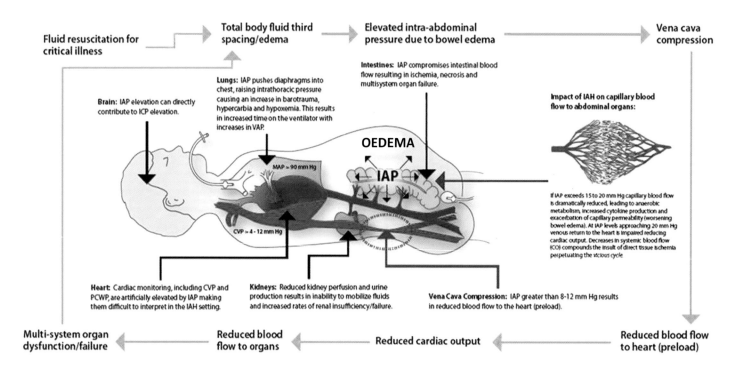

Figure 1. Pathophysiology of abdominal compartment syndrome. *Reproduced with permission from AbViser Medical.* © AbViser Medical.

indwelling urinary catheter since intravesical pressure correlates with intra-abdominal pressure. Most clinicians accept that intra-abdominal pressure ≥30cm H_2O as being diagnostic. Others have reported that improved outcomes have been observed in patients with signs of ACS but lower intravesical pressures, so erring on the side of caution and being guided clinically may be more pragmatic. Abdominal perfusion pressure (APP) (mean arterial pressure minus intravesical pressure) has been found to be a better predictor of end-organ injury than lactate, pH, urine output or base deficit [46]. If the cause is uncertain, or intra-abdominal haemorrhage is suspected, a CT may be helpful.

Prevention is better than cure. Prediction of the potential for ACS allows for early and regular measurement of intravesical pressure. If ACS is suspected, preventive strategies can be implemented. These include: bowel decompression with a nasogastric tube or colonoscopy in severe cases, improving abdominal wall compliance with analgesia, sedation and muscle relaxants, and avoiding excessive fluid resuscitation particularly with pure crystalloids. Abdominal perfusion can be improved by maintaining mean arterial pressure with goal-directed fluid resuscitation and inotropes, if necessary. The World Society of the Abdominal Compartment Syndrome advises decompressive laparostomy if intravesical pressure is over 25mmHg (and/or APP <50mmHg) and new organ dysfunction/failure is

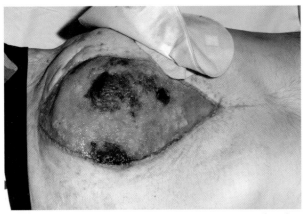

Figure 2. One month post-laparostomy – healing by secondary intention with negative pressure therapy. The abdominal contents have been completely covered by granulation tissue.

present and the ACS is refractory to medical management. Adequate resuscitation is vital before abdominal decompression to compensate for the sometimes dramatic drop in systemic vascular resistance, and potential for subsequent IRI.

Many techniques for managing the resulting laparostomy have been described, most famously the Bogata bag. Topical negative pressure wound dressings are now in common use; the subsequent management and methods of abdominal closure are outside the remit of this chapter (Figure 2).

Acute limb ischaemia and compartment syndrome

Following prolonged ischaemia, restoration of blood flow and reperfusion of ischaemic tissues not only causes a systemic IRI but may also result in an acute compartment syndrome. The muscles of the limbs are separated into compartments by myofascial layers. These effectively confine the muscles and associated nerves and vessels in an enclosed space with a relatively fixed volume. Ischaemia results in swelling and capillary leakage which is exacerbated on reperfusion. The resulting increase in muscle and interstitial volume increases the intra-compartmental pressure. Initially, venous pressure increases as outflow is restricted; it overcomes capillary perfusion pressure and oxygen delivery to the tissue ceases. The resulting hypoxia damages cells further, with increased release of vasoactive mediators and increased endothelial permeability. Autoregulation is lost and eventually all blood flow into the compartment can cease. Irrecoverable damage occurs to nerves and muscles as necrosis is established and myoglobin is released (Figure 3). The commonest cause of compartment syndrome is revascularisation for the treatment of acute ischaemia, but it can occur following crush and burn injuries, fractures, intra-arterial or compartmental drug injection or infusion, and extrinsic compression.

Compartment syndrome may affect any of the myofascial compartments in the arms or legs, although from a vascular point of view the lower leg compartments are most frequently involved.

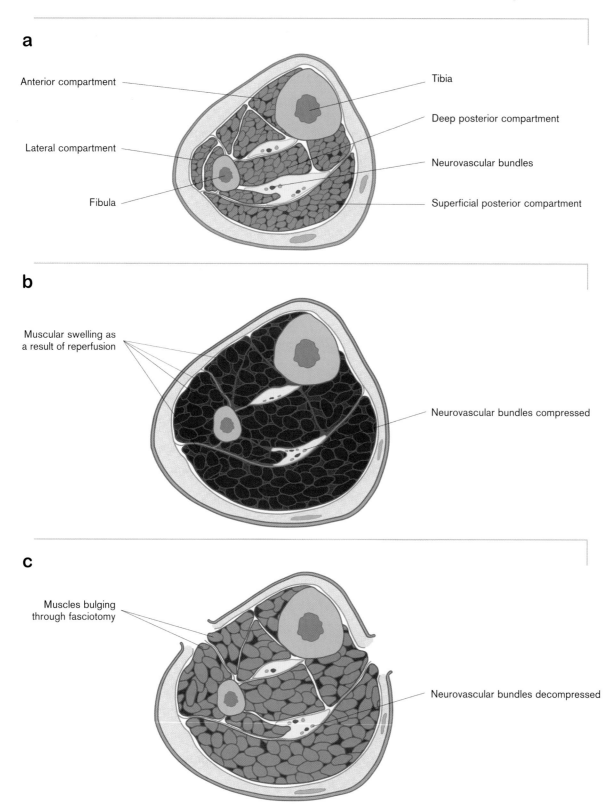

Figure 3. Lower leg cross-sections showing the development of a compartment syndrome and its decompression by fasciotomy. a) Cross-section through normal calf. b) Compartment syndrome: swelling of muscles causing compression of nerves and blood vessels. c) Post-fasciotomies. *Illustrations kindly provided by Michael Byrne.*

Classically, patients with compartment syndrome will have been treated for acute leg ischaemia, and then develop excessive muscular tenderness made worse by passive movement, and leg swelling. Sensory impairment, paralysis and loss of peripheral pulses are late signs and it is important to maintain a high index of suspicion in any patient who had prolonged warm ischaemia for several hours before revascularisation. Although imaging may help identify an underlying cause, it is not helpful in the diagnosis. If compartment syndrome is suspected, compartment pressures can be measured directly using the pressure transducers found on most anaesthetic machines (see Chapter 10).

If a compartment syndrome is suspected, or anticipated following revascularisation, management is as follows:

- oxygen administration increases the partial pressure of oxygen slightly. Hyperbaric oxygen has been shown to be beneficial but is usually not practical [47];
- correct hypovolaemia to maintain limb perfusion pressure;
- avoid leg elevation which reduces mean arterial perfusion pressure without significant reduction in compartment pressure;
- urgent surgical fasciotomy.

Lower leg fasciotomy

The lower leg is divided into four fascial compartments (Figure 3). For most patients with compartment syndrome after revascularisation of acute leg ischaemia, all four compartments should be decompressed. A two-incision technique is preferred: one sited anterolaterally approximately halfway between the fibula and the tibial crest, and the other posteromedially approximately 2cm posterior to the medial edge of the tibia (Figure 4).

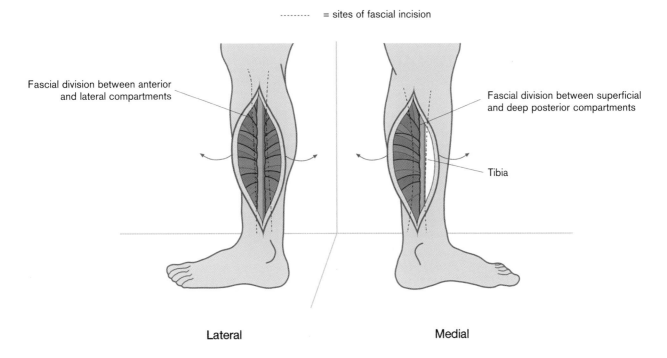

--------- = sites of fascial incision

Fascial division between anterior and lateral compartments

Fascial division between superficial and deep posterior compartments

Tibia

Lateral

Medial

Figure 4. Sites of skin and fascial incisions for four-compartment decompression in the lower leg. *Illustrations kindly provided by Michael Byrne.*

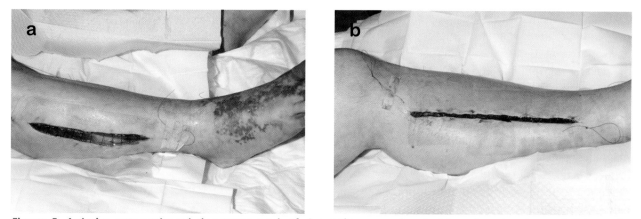

Figure 5. Anterior compartment decompressed. a) A running non-absorbable suture has been left loose to facilitate delayed closure. Note the severity of skin damage in the revascularised foot. b) Running suture pulled closed after 3 days to facilitate healing.

Following a long skin incision of at least 15cm, the septum dividing the anterior and lateral compartments is identified and the fascia opened vertically either side of it using blunt tipped scissors. Great care should be taken in order not to damage the peroneal nerves, crural arteries and tendons. The remaining two compartments (superficial and deep posterior) can be decompressed via the posterior-medial incision. On opening the superficial compartment close to the tibia as above, the deep compartment can be reached by incising the fascia over flexor digitorum longus. This will require release of some of the soleal bridge proximally. On this side care must be taken not to injure the long saphenous vein and its nerve.

To complete the procedure, a subcutaneous non-absorbable suture can be inserted loosely and secured (Figure 5a). This can then be pulled taut after a few days if it is possible to close the wounds, or at least reduce the area needed to heal by secondary intention (Figure 5b). Persistent muscle bulging which prevents delayed primary wound closure may require subsequent split-skin grafting to accelerate wound healing.

If anticipated and avoided, or treated promptly, then long-term sequelae of compartment syndrome are minimal. Foot drop secondary to compartment syndrome in the leg may persist for many months while the nerves recover and may lead to permanent disability through joint contractures. Delayed treatment or missed diagnosis can result in severe ischaemic contracture, renal failure as a result of rhabdomyolysis, amputation and potentially death.

Conclusions

Aortic cross-clamp-induced ischaemia reperfusion injury has been shown to cause organ damage [22, 24, 30, 48-50]. Postoperative organ dysfunction and failure, especially cardiac, is associated with increased mortality after elective and emergency AAA repair [2-4]. Vascular surgeons should aim for optimum preparation and technical skill to reduce ischaemic time and use endovascular techniques, where appropriate, to reduce tissue ischaemia. The use of cell salvage and mannitol may help to reduce the damage caused by IRI. Anticipation for the development of abdominal compartment syndrome in patients undergoing major aortic surgery, particularly in the emergency setting, should allow for proactive intra-abdominal pressure measurement and prophylactic manoeuvres.

Acute compartment syndrome in a limb is a surgical emergency and clinical assessment remains the cornerstone of diagnosis [51]. A high index of suspicion should be maintained especially in patients presenting with prolonged acute ischaemia before intervention. A low threshold for prevention of compartment syndrome by prophylactic fasciotomy undoubtedly saves legs in these high-risk patients, and may save lives.

Key points

♦ Ischaemia reperfusion injury and multi-organ failure significantly increase operative morbidity and mortality, as well as increasing hospital stay and ITU requirements.

♦ A well-briefed and rehearsed operating team with optimum preparation can improve time efficiency during aortic cross-clamping.

♦ Surgical skill and economy of motion may translate to improved outcomes in all aspects of operative surgery, not just reduced clamp times.

♦ Endovascular techniques, where appropriate, decrease lower torso ischaemia.

♦ Remote ischaemic preconditioning and mannitol may help to ameliorate IRI.

♦ A high index of suspicion is needed for a compartment syndrome in all patients who have revascularisation of prolonged or profound limb ischaemia, or those undergoing emergency aortic surgery.

♦ Minimising hypotension, hypothermia and acidosis, and reducing bank blood transfusion with cell salvage techniques reduce the risk of systemic inflammatory response syndrome.

References

1. Blankensteijn JD, Lindenbourg FP, Van der Graaf Y, Eikleboom BC. Influence of study design on reported mortality rates after abdominal aortic aneurysm repair. *Br J Surg* 1998; 85: 1624-30.

2. Sayers RD, Thompson MM, Nasim A, *et al*. Surgical management of 671 abdominal aortic aneurysms: a 13-year review from a single centre. *Eur J Vasc Endovasc Surg* 1995; 9: 239-43.

3. McLean RF, Tarshis J, Mazer CD, Szalai JP. Death in two Canadian intensive care units: institutional difference and change over time. *Crit Care Med* 2000; 28: 100-3.

4. Barratt J, Pararajasingam R, Sayers RD, Feehally J. Outcome of acute renal failure following surgical repair of ruptured abdominal aortic aneurysms. *Eur J Vasc Endovasc Surg* 2000; 20: 163-8.

5. American College of Chest Physcians/Society of Critical Care Medicine Consensus Conference: definitions for sepsis and organ failure and guidelines for the use of innovative therapies in sepsis. *Crit Care Med* 1992; 20: 864-74.

6. Moore FA, Moore EE. Evolving concepts in the pathogenesis of post injury multiple organ failure. *Surg Clin North Am* 1995; 75: 257-77.

7. Welbourn CRB, Goldman G, Paterson IS, *et al*. Pathophysiology of ischaemia-reperfusion injury: The central role of the neutrophils. *Br J Surg* 1991; 78: 651-5.

8. Oberholzer A, Oberholzer C, Moldawer LL. Cytokine signalling-regulation of the immune response in normal and critically ill states. *Crit Care Med* 2000; 28: N3-12.

9. Baigrie RJ, Lamont PM, Kwiatkowski D, *et al*. Systemic cytokine response after major surgery. *Br J Surg* 1992; 79: 757-60.

10. Davies MG, Hagen PO. Systemic inflammatory response syndrome. *Br J Surg* 1997; 84: 920-35.

11. Brown MJ, Nicholson ML, Bell MD, Sayers RD. The systemic inflammatory response syndrome, organ failure, and mortality after abdominal aortic aneurysm repair. *J Vasc Surg* 2003; 37: 600-6.

12. Norwood MGA, Bown MJ, Lloyd G, *et al*. The clinical value of the systemic inflammatory response syndrome (SIRS) in abdominal aortic aneurysm repair. *Eur J Vasc Endovasc* 2004; 27: 292-8.

13. Smail N, Messiah A, Edouard A, *et al*. Role of systemic inflammatory response syndrome and infection in the occurrence of early multiple organ dysfunction syndrome following severe trauma. *Intensive Care Med* 1995; 21: 813-6.

14. Salvo I, De Cian W, Musicco M, *et al*. The Italian sepsis study: preliminary results on the incidence and evolution of SIRS, sepsis, severe sepsis and septic shock. *Intensive Care Med* 1995; 21: S244-9.

15. Opal SM. The uncertain value of the definition for SIRS. Systemic inflammatory response syndrome. *Chest* 1998; 113: 1442-3.

16. Vincent JL. Dear SIRS I'm sorry to say that I don't like you. *Crit Care Med* 1997; 25: 372-4.

17. Carden DL, Granger DN. Pathophysiology of ischaemia-reperfusion injury. *J Pathol* 2000; 190: 255-66.

18. Kellog EW. Superoxide, hydrogen peroxide and siglet oxygen in lipid peroxidation by xanthine oxidase system. *J Biol Chem* 1975; 250: 8812-7.

19. Grace PA. Ischaemia-reperfusion injury. *Br J Surg* 1994; 81: 637-7.

20. Homer-Vanniasinkam S, Crinnon JN, Gough MJ. Post-ischaemic organ dysfunction: a review. *Eur J Vasc Endovasc Surg* 1997; 14: 195-203.

21. Shanley TP, Warner RL, Ward PA. The role of cytokines and adhesion molecules in the development of inflammatory injury. *Mol Med Today* 1995; 1: 405.

22. Lindsey TF, Luo XP, Lehotay DC, *et al.* Ruptured abdominal aortic aneurysm, a 'two-hit' ischaemia-reperfusion injury: evidence from an analysis of oxidative products. *J Vasc Surg* 1999; 30: 219-28.

23. Defraigne JO, Pincemail J. Local and systemic consequences of severe ischaemia and reperfusion of skeletal muscle. Physiopathology and prevention. *Acta Chir Belg* 1998; 98: 176-86.

24. Anner H, Kaufmann RP, Valeri CR, *et al.* Reperfusion of ischaemic lower limbs increases pulmonary microvascular permeability. *J Trauma* 1988; 28: 607-10.

25. Paterson IS, Klausner JM, Pugatch R, *et al.* Noncardiogenic pulmonary oedema after abdominal aortic aneurysm surgery. *Ann Surg* 1989; 209: 231-6.

26. Fantini GA, Conte MS. Pulmonary failure following lower torso ischaemia: clinical evidence for a remote effect of reperfusion injury. *Am Surg* 1995; 61: 316-9.

27. O'Donnell D, Clarke G, Hurst P. Acute renal failure following surgery for abdominal aortic aneurysm. *Aust NZ J Surg* 1989; 59: 405-8.

28. Gornick CC Jr, Kjellstrand CM. Acute renal failure complicating aortic aneurysm surgery. *Nephron* 1983; 35: 145-57.

29. Durrani NK, Trisal V, Mittal V, Hans SS. Gastrointestinal complications after ruptured aortic aneurysm repair. *Am Surg* 2003; 69: 330-3; discussion 333.

30. Yassin MM, Barros D'Sa AA, Parks TG, *et al.* Lower limb ischaemia-reperfusion injury alters gastrointestinal structure and function. *Br J Surg* 1997; 84: 1425-9.

31. Thompson MM, Nasim A, Sayers RD, *et al.* Oxygen free radical and cytokine generation during endovascular and conventional aneurysm repair. *Eur J Vasc Endovasc Surg* 1996; 12: 70-5.

32. Jacobs MJ, de Mol BA, Legemate DA, *et al.* Retrograde aortic and selective organ perfusion during thoracoabdominal aortic aneurysm repair. *Eur J Vasc Endovasc Surg* 1997; 14: 360-6.

33. Walsh SR, Tang TY, Sadat U, Gaunt M. Remote ischaemic preconditioning in major vascular surgery. *J Vasc Surg* 2008; 49: 240-3.

34. Reimer KA, Murray CE, Yamasawa I, Hill ML. Four brief periods of ischaemia have no cumulative ATP loss or necrosis. *Am J Physiol* 1986; 251: H1306-5.

35. Yellon DM, Alkhulaifi AM, Pugsley WB. Preconditioning the human myocardium. *Lancet* 1993; 342: 276-7.

36. Cheung MM, Kharbanda RK, Konstantinov IE, *et al.* Randomized controlled trial of the effects of remote ischaemic preconditioning on children undergoing cardiac surgery: first clinical application in humans. *J Am Coll Cardiol* 2006; 47: 2277-82.

37. Ali ZA, Callaghan CJ, Lim E, *et al.* Remote ischaemic preconditioning reduces myocardial and renal injury after elective abdominal aortic aneurysm repair: a randomized controlled trial. *Circulation* 2007; 116: 95-106.

38. Wijnen MHWA, Roumen RMH, Vader HL, Goris RJA. A multiantioxidant supplementation reduces damage from ischaemia reperfusion in patients after lower torso ischaemia. A randomized trial. *Eur J Endovasc Surg* 2002; 23: 486-90.

39. Weinbroum AA, Shapira I, Ben-Abraham R, Szold A. Mannitol dose-dependently attenuates lung reperfusion injury following liver ischemia reperfusion: a dose-response study in an isolated perfused double-organ model. *Lung* 2002; 180: 327-38.

40. Magovern GJ Jr, Bolling SF, Casale AS, *et al.* The mechanism of mannitol in reducing ischemic injury: hyperosmolarity or hydroxyl scavenger? *Circulation* 1984; 70(3 Pt 2): I91-5.

41. Nicholson ML, Baker DM, Hopkinson BR, Wenham PW. Randomized controlled trial of the effect of mannitol on renal reperfusion injury during aortic aneurysm surgery. *Br J Surg* 1996; 83: 1230-3.

42. Oredsson S, Plate G, Qvarfordt P. The effect of mannitol on reperfusion injury and postischaemic compartment pressure in skeletal muscle. *Eur J Vasc Surg* 1994; 8: 326-31.

43. Tavare AN, Parvizi N. Does use of intra-operative cell-salvage delay recovery in patients undergoing elective abdominal aortic surgery. *Interact Cardiovasc Thorac Surg* 2011; 12: 1028-32.

44. Wolowczyk L, Nevin M, Lamont P, *et al.* The effect of acute normovolaemic haemodilution on the inflammatory response and clinical outcome in abdominal aortic aneurysm repair - results of a pilot trial. *Eur J Endovasc Surg* 2005; 30: 12-9.

45. Mayer D, Rancic Z, Meier C, Pfammatter T, *et al.* Open abdomen treatment following endovascular repair of ruptured abdominal aortic aneurysms. *J Vasc Surg* 2009; 50: 1-7.

46. Cheatham ML, White MW, Sagraves SG, *et al.* Abdominal perfusion pressure: a superior parameter in the assessment of intra-abdominal hypertension. *J Trauma* 2000; 49: 621-6.

47. Wattel F, Mathieu D, Neviere R, Bocquillon N. Acute peripheral ischaemia and compartment syndromes: a role for hyperbaric oxygenation. *Anaesthesia* 198; 53: 63-5.

48. Kearns SR, Kelly CJ, Barry M, *et al.* Vitamin C reduces ischaemia-reperfusion induced acute lung injury. *Eur J Vasc Endovasc Surg* 1999; 17: 533-6.

49. Joyce M, Kelly CJ, Chen G, Bouchier-Hayes DJ. Pravastatin attenuates lower torso ischaemia-reperfusion induced lung injury by upregulating constitutive endothelial nitric oxide synthase. *Eur J Vasc Endovasc Surg* 2001; 21: 295-300.

50. Pararajasingam R, Weight SC, Bell PRF, *et al.* Endogenous renal nitric oxide metabolism following experimental infra-renal aortic cross-clamping induced ischaemia-reperfusion injury. *Br J Surg* 1999; 86: 795-9.

51. Shadgan B, Menon M, O'Brien PJ, Reid WD. Diagnostic techniques in acute compartment syndrome of the leg. *J Orthop Trauma* 2008; 22: 581-7.

Chapter 12

The aetiology and management of the failed vascular bypass

Kaji Sritharan MD FRCS, Specialist Registrar in Vascular Surgery
Alun H. Davies MA DM FRCS FHEA FEBVS FACPh, Professor of Vascular Surgery
Academic Department of Vascular Surgery, Imperial College London, London, UK

Introduction

Critical limb ischaemia (CLI) affects approximately 20,000 people per year in the UK, and its incidence is set to rise as the population ages. For patients with CLI due to lower limb infra-inguinal occlusive disease, or in patients with long segment occlusions or severe infrapopliteal disease, surgical revascularisation remains the most effective method of treatment, with reported limb salvage rates of 88% and acceptable peri-operative mortality rates of 2.7% [1]. Evidence also exists to suggest that successful revascularisation is more cost effective than primary amputation [2]. In recent years, endovascular therapies have emerged, and provide a valuable alternative therapeutic option in selected patients.

Factors associated with graft outcome

Over the past 20 years, the demographics of patients with CLI have changed considerably. Patients now tend to be older, there are more females and patients are more likely to have diabetes mellitus, chronic kidney disease, and previous coronary artery bypass grafting, thus limiting the availability of vein as a bypass conduit. In addition, patients more frequently present with tissue necrosis and more distal levels of athero-occlusive disease [2]. These factors impact on the technical complexity of any procedure.

The aetiology of the failed infra-inguinal bypass graft is multifactorial. Factors associated with poor outcome include those related to technical aspects of the surgery, such as vein diameter [3], conduit type [3], inflow and run-off status [4] and graft length, and those which are patient-related, such as comorbid factors and the mode of presentation [5]. Referral pathways, multidisciplinary approaches, and hospital revascularisation policies may also influence outcome.

Regardless of the success of a bypass procedure, irreversible tissue ischaemia or progressive infection may necessitate amputation [6].

Supra-inguinal bypass grafts

Aorto-iliac, aortobifemoral and axillofemoral bypass grafts

The long-term patency of supra-inguinal grafts depends largely on their location. Occlusive iliac disease is primarily treated using endovascular techniques, although when the disease is extensive, aortobifemoral grafting is a good alternative. The high flow rate in these bypasses results in excellent primary patency, with rates of 88.5% at 5 years [7] for aorto-iliac and 93% at 3 years for aortobifemoral grafts [8]. Nevertheless, graft limb occlusion occurs in 10-20% of all grafts, resulting in limb ischaemia and necessitating a femorofemoral bypass [9].

Axillobifemoral bypass grafts are associated with a higher risk of complication or occlusion, due to the general health of patients undergoing the procedure, and the length of bypass; the primary and secondary patency rates are 67.7% and 80.3% at 5 years, respectively (Figure 1) [7]. Although these patency rates are lower than for aortobifemoral grafts [7, 8], this can be a fair trade-off for a less complex procedure in a sick patient with a limited life expectancy, or where no other option exists.

Iliofemoral bypass grafts

Iliofemoral bypass grafts are rarely performed, but may be indicated where a femorofemoral crossover graft is not appropriate; for example, in a patient with a hostile groin from previous surgery. Five-year patency rates are between 61.3% and 76.6% [10], with secondary patency rates of 80.5% [10] to 95% [11].

Femorofemoral crossover grafts

Femorofemoral grafts are indicated in patients with either unilateral iliac disease in which the lesion is diffuse and long and therefore not suitable for angioplasty [12], or in patients who are unfit for open aortic procedures. In addition, some EVAR techniques

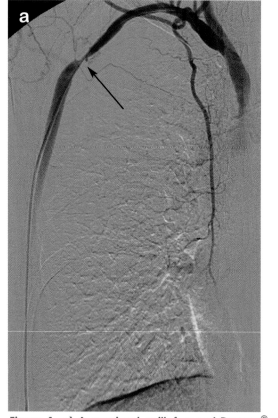 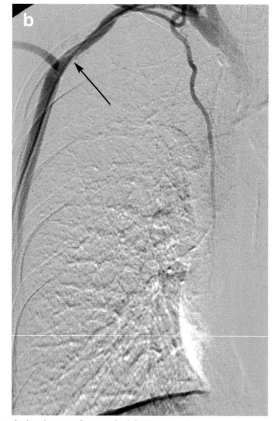

Figure 1. a) A proximal axillofemoral Dacron® graft stenosis is shown (arrow). b) The graft stenosis was successfully treated using balloon angioplasty (arrow).

utilize an aorto-uni-iliac prosthesis, necessitating femorofemoral bypass.

Five-year primary patency rates for femorofemoral bypasses range from 36% [13] to 62% [14], with limb salvage rates of 84%, reflecting the impact of a successful reoperation [9]. These patency rates are due to the use of prosthetic material, but when superficial femoral vein is used, 5-year primary and secondary patency rates of 76% and 90% can be achieved [15].

Occlusion of a femorofemoral bypass graft is associated with significant morbidity (amputation 20%) and mortality (20%) rates [16]. Graft surveillance can improve secondary patency rates, due to earlier detection and intervention of a failing bypass graft [14]; however, in many hospitals this is not done routinely.

Management of the failed supra-inguinal graft

Factors which influence graft failure include poor outflow, the presence of a synchronous infra-inguinal reconstruction [7], neotimal hyperplasia, femoral pseudoaneurysm formation and graft infection [17] (see Chapter 7).

Vascular graft infection has a reported incidence of 0.7-7% and most commonly affects the femoral site (13% incidence) [18]. In more than 50% of cases, *Staphylococcus aureus* is implicated as the causative organism. Excision of the infected graft and vascular reconstruction with an extra-anatomic bypass is the standard management. However, this approach is associated with mortality rates of between 10% and 30%, and amputation rates of 70% [18] (Figure 2).

Alternatives to graft excision include irrigation of the wound, radical debridement of unhealthy tissue with, or without local rotational muscle flap (Sartorius muscle) coverage of the exposed graft, vacuum-assisted wound closure or frequent dressing changes or skin grafting [18].

For an occluded aortofemoral bypass, extra-anatomic bypass options include axillosuperficial femoral and axillopopliteal bypasses. Primary patency rates of 75% at 1 year and 43% at 2 years have been reported with axillopopliteal bypass; acceptable secondary patency rates can be achieved by thrombectomy, revision and/or warfarin therapy [19]. Although subcutaneous extra-anatomic bypass is often favoured, the descending thoracic aorta can also be used for inflow, with primary graft patency rates of 98% and 70.4% at 1 and 5 years, respectively [20]. This approach can also be used in the management of the failed axillofemoral bypass. Marston *et al*, in their series of 28 patients, reported 2-year primary patency rates after secondary reconstructions to be significantly better than after thrombectomy alone (81% versus 10%), or graft revision (16%). More specifically, patients undergoing reconstruction with descending thoracic aorta to femoral artery bypass had an 89% primary patency rate at 24 months [21].

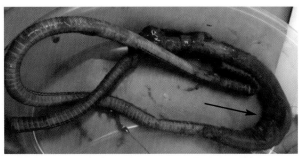

Figure 2. An excised infected axillofemoral bypass graft. A pseudo-membrane can be seen over the graft (arrow).

Other options for the management of infected aortofemoral, femorofemoral, and axillofemoral prosthetic grafts include obturator bypass, *in situ* replacement of the graft with a rifampin-soaked gelatin-impregnated polyester graft or reconstruction with autologous vein. In 2009, Ali *et al* reported a series of 187 patients who underwent successful excision of infected aortofemoral, aorto-iliac and axillofemoral grafts and replacement with large calibre superficial vein. Concomitant infra-inguinal bypass was necessary in 14% of patients and the cumulative 6-year primary and secondary patency rates were 81% and 91%, with limb salvage rates of 89% [22]. Similar primary patency rates of 87% (2 years) and 82% (5 years) were reported in a series of 240 patients by Beck *et al* [23].

Infra-inguinal bypass grafts

Conduit type

Autologous great saphenous vein is widely accepted as the conduit of choice for infra-inguinal bypass grafting, and in particular for bypass to the crural vessels [24]. Much debate has surrounded the virtues of its use *in situ* compared to reversed, with the former affording benefits of maintaining the integrity of the vasa vasorum, reducing myointimal hyperplasia and allowing for better vein to artery size matching at the proximal and distal anastomoses. Harris *et al*, in a randomised study, demonstrated that for veins >3.5mm in diameter, the *in situ* and reversed techniques for operation were equally effective [25]. However, for veins <3.5mm, there was a non-significant trend for improved patency with the *in situ* technique.

In a third of patients, ipsilateral saphenous vein is lacking or inadequate. For these patients, alternative conduits should be sought, and include the contralateral great saphenous vein (available in 38% of patients) [26], cephalic and/or basilic vein, or the deep veins [27]. Human umbilical vein (HUV) has fallen out of favour due to the long-term complications of graft dilatation and aneurysm formation [28].

Where an adequate length of single vein is lacking, two or more veins may be spliced. However, the PREVENT III trial database of 1404 patients with CLI undergoing infra-inguinal bypass reported a 2.1-fold increased risk of 30-day graft failure and reduced 1-year primary and secondary patency rates when non-single segment great saphenous vein conduits were used [3].

In the absence of any suitable vein, synthetic material such as Dacron® or polytetrafluoroethylene

(PTFE) may be used, but has been shown to be inferior to autologous vein as a bypass conduit [29]. Tilanus *et al* demonstrated patency rates of 37% and 70% for PTFE and saphenous vein, respectively, at 54 months for femoropopliteal bypass grafts [30]. Veith *et al*, in their randomised trial, demonstrated more subtle differences in graft patency; patency rates were comparable in the short term, but differed at 4 years for above-knee bypasses (68% vs. 47% for autologous saphenous vein and PTFE, respectively) [31]. For distal popliteal and tibioperoneal reconstruction, the superiority of autologous vein (including spliced arm vein) over PTFE is undisputed [29, 31]. PTFE should therefore only be used for below-knee bypasses if native vein is unavailable.

Cryopreserved allograft saphenous vein bypass grafts have been used as an alternative conduit. Although they have the benefit of being more resistant to infection than PTFE, results have been disappointing, with 1-year primary patency rates between 36.8% [32] and 56% [33].

Vein diameter, graft length and inflow and run-off status

The PREVENT III trial database revealed patency rates were negatively associated with a vein diameter <3.5mm, and graft lengths >50cm; a vein diameter of <3mm was linked to a 2.1-fold increased risk of 30-day graft failure [3]. A study by Ishii *et al* of 67 patients suggested that vein diameter may be more critical in femoropopliteal bypass grafts; in their series, all femoropopliteal bypass grafts were patent at 3 years if the vein was >3mm; for crural bypasses, primary patency rates were 66% versus 27% for vein diameters >3mm and <3mm, respectively [34].

The cause of bypass graft failure in approximately a third of all cases is inadequate inflow and/or run-off [35]. The latter in particular appears important for bypasses onto the tibial and peroneal vessels, where the presence of straight line flow to the foot and patent pedal vessels is critical.

Patient factors

Major amputation is often selected over infra-inguinal bypass in patients with significant comorbidities, on the assumption that it has lower peri-operative risks. Indeed, approximately 25% of patients with CLI undergo amputation without an attempt at revascularisation. In a recent retrospective study of high-risk patients, Barshes *et al* challenged this preconception, demonstrating bypass surgery to be associated with a lower 30-day postoperative mortality compared to amputation even in high-risk patients (6.54% vs. 9.97%) [36].

Predicting bypass graft failure

A number of scoring systems have been developed to try to identify grafts at high risk of failure. The Finnvasc and modified PREVENT III risk scoring methods are useful for predicting the long-term outcome of patients undergoing both surgical and endovascular infra-inguinal revascularisation for CLI. The Finnvasc score has also been shown to be useful in predicting immediate postoperative outcome [37].

Improving infra-inguinal graft patency

Vein cuffs

Strategies adopted to improve PTFE graft patency include the incorporation of a distal vein (Miller) cuff, St Mary's boot or Taylor patch. These aim to reduce the size mismatch between the graft and distal artery and reduce myointimal hyperplasia. One randomised controlled trial evaluated their efficacy, and showed that below the knee, PTFE with a vein cuff improved primary patency when compared to PTFE alone [29].

Graft surveillance

The incidence of vein graft stenosis is greatest in the first year following surgery and complicates up to 45% of infra-inguinal bypass grafts [38]. The potential merit of a graft surveillance programme following femoropopliteal and femorocrural vein bypass was addressed by the Vein Graft Surveillance Trial (VGST) [39], a multicentre, prospective, randomised, controlled trial of 594 patients. However, similar amputation and vascular mortality rates were observed, as well as primary patency, primary-assisted patency, and secondary patency rates in both groups over 18 months. This suggests that intensive surveillance with duplex scanning does not afford any additional benefit in terms of limb salvage rates for patients undergoing vein bypass surgery compared to clinical assessment [39]. Clinical deterioration or a drop in ABPI of >0.2 is reliable in detecting failing infra-inguinal vein bypasses.

Although the benefit of routine surveillance for all infra-inguinal bypass grafts remains unproven, there is an argument for surveying those at high risk of stenosis and subsequent failure (Figure 3). At risk grafts have been defined as those with a peak mean velocity (PMV) <45cm/s and an exit velocity/start velocity (V2/V1) of >2 at 6-week postoperative duplex [40, 41]. For prosthetic femorodistal bypass grafts, there is level 1b evidence to suggest that clinical review and ABPI measurements every 3 months is as effective as duplex imaging [42].

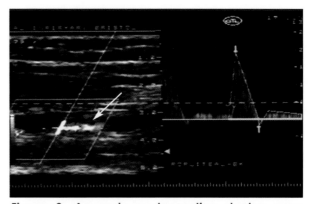

Figure 3. An early postoperative duplex scan demonstrating a technical error: intimal flap (arrow). This is likely to progress to myointimal hyperplasia later.

Aetiology of failed lower limb bypass graft

Re-operation after lower limb arterial bypass surgery is common, and infra-inguinal bypass graft failure can complicate up to 20% of bypasses at 1 month [35] and 50% at 5 years [43]. Early graft failure (<1 month) is largely attributed to operative technique or anatomical factors, and usually warrants early surgical exploration and surgical thrombectomy with correction of the underlying problem. In this cohort, short-term anticoagulation (1-4 weeks) may be considered; long-term anticoagulation with warfarin should be employed selectively, for example, in patients in whom no particular technical problem is identified [43]. By contrast, intermediate failure (within 1 year) is more likely to be due to intimal hyperplasia.

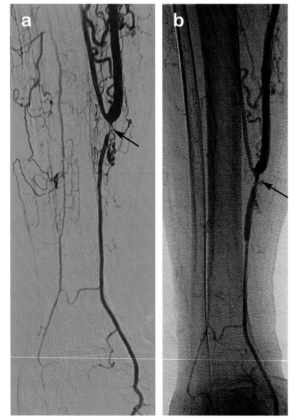

Figure 4. a) A digital subtraction angiogram showing a stenosis of a native posterior tibial artery (arrow) below a distal vein bypass. b) The stenosis was successfully treated with angioplasty (arrow).

Late graft failure is caused by progression of atherosclerotic disease within the inflow and outflow vessels (Figure 4).

Strategies for bypass graft salvage

Thrombosis of an infra-inguinal bypass graft can result in severe limb-threatening ischaemia, yet there is no clear consensus regarding its optimal management. This will be influenced by a number of factors including the time from bypass graft surgery to bypass graft failure, symptoms at presentation, patient comorbidities and functional status, and anatomical and practical considerations, such as the presence of additional autogenous vein for repeat bypass.

Graft thrombectomy

The therapeutic options for bypass graft salvage are diverse. They include graft thrombectomy alone, or combined with balloon angioplasty. The results of thrombectomy alone are poor with 5-year reported primary patency rates between 19% and 28% [44]. Longer patency is only achieved if the cause of graft failure is identified and treated.

Arterial reconstruction

Depending on the indication for the initial procedure and the patient's symptomatology, an aggressive approach to repeat arterial reconstruction following infra-inguinal bypass graft failure is generally advocated. Failure to re-intervene risks reduced limb salvage rates at 3 years of 51-70% [45]. Forty-four percent of patients in one series required further intervention in the form of graft revision/secondary revascularisation (Figure 5) or amputation following infra-inguinal bypass failure [45]. Results following subsequent vascular reconstruction are poor when compared to the index operation, with primary patency rates of 44-64% for redo vein bypass grafts at 5 years [45, 46].

Reasons for the lower primary patency rates observed after revisional surgery include inadequate inflow, less optimal target vessels with disease

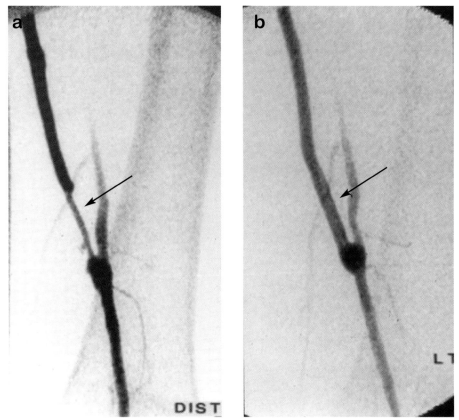

Figure 5. a) Digital subtraction angiogram demonstrating an in-graft stenosis (arrow). b) The stenosis is treated successfully with a short interposition vein graft (arrow).

progression, lack of adequate conduit and scarring within the reoperative field. Adequate planning prior to surgery is paramount and careful consideration should be given to the quality of the inflow and outflow vessels, and the availability of adequate calibre/length autogenous vein.

Graft failure is directly associated with limb loss, and a number of predictive factors have been identified in relation to redo infra-inguinal bypass surgery. These include reoperation for early primary graft failure (<3 months), distal outflow level [47], female gender, tissue loss and rest pain at the time of presentation [46], and the use of non-great saphenous vein as a bypass conduit [48]. Belkin *et al*, in a series of 300 consecutive reoperative bypass procedures, recorded 5-year primary patency rates and limb salvage rates to be superior when great saphenous vein was used compared to alternative autogenous

vein. In general, autogenous grafts outperformed prosthetic grafts with primary patency rates of 51.5% vs. 27.4% at 5 years [43].

Graft thrombolysis

Despite the obvious advantages of catheter-guided selective intra-arterial thrombolysis (Figure 6) over operative revascularisation (thrombectomy or bypass) for the treatment of occluded infra-inguinal vein bypass grafts, data regarding the long-term benefits of thrombolytic procedures are disappointing. In a recent cohort series by Bonhomme *et al*, although an initial success rate of 76% was reported, re-occlusion rates at 45 months were 58% [49]; similarly, other studies demonstrate patency rates of 23% at 5 years [50]. Thrombosed vein grafts, occlusions over 2 weeks old, poor run-off and

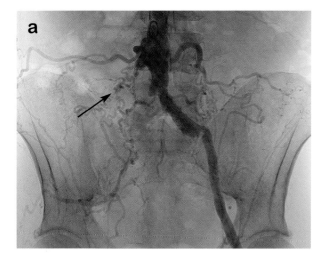
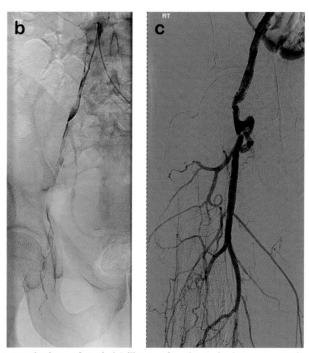

Figure 6. a) Digital subtraction angiogram demonstrating occlusion of a right ilio-profunda vein bypass graft (arrow). b) Catheter-directed thrombolysis into the bypass graft via a contralateral (left) groin approach. c) Check angiogram at day 1 following thrombolysis demonstrating successful salvage of the graft.

failure to identify or rectify an underlying causative stenosis have been identified as factors which influence long-term outcome following thrombolysis [49], and a judicious approach to its use is advocated.

Endovascular intervention

Endovascular techniques play a useful role in the threatened graft, where treatment of a flow-limiting stenosis may prevent graft thrombosis. Once a graft has failed, successful salvage strategies include subintimal, transluminal or cutting balloon angioplasty, and mechanical thrombectomy devices for PTFE graft thrombosis. Factors found to affect the success of angioplasty adversely include early graft stenosis (<3 months), and long (>2cm) or multiple stenoses. These lesions are best treated by surgical revision, if appropriate.

No randomised controlled trial exists to help establish the best management of the failed infra-

inguinal bypass. Endovascular options should therefore in general be reserved for patients with a reduced life expectancy, where suitable vein for bypass surgery is lacking or in patients with a high operative risk, or where there is less severe arterial occlusion.

Role of anticoagulants and antiplatelets

The Dutch Bypass Oral Anticoagulants or Aspirin Study is the largest study to evaluate the role of oral anticoagulants in patients undergoing infra-inguinal bypass grafting [51]. Comparing the use of warfarin versus 80mg aspirin alone, and using the primary outcome of graft occlusion, it demonstrated a benefit of warfarin in venous but not artificial grafts. A subsequent Cochrane review also reported in favour of oral anticoagulants for venous but not artificial grafts [52]. Two studies have compared the effect of warfarin with aspirin or aspirin/dipyridamole and have shown a positive effect of warfarin on the patency of venous but not on artificial grafts [52].

Most vascular surgeons do not use warfarin routinely but selectively in patients with grafts at risk of early thrombosis. These include redo bypass grafts, composite saphenous or alternative (arm or small saphenous) vein bypasses, grafts in which there is compromised distal outflow and prosthetic infrageniculate bypasses. The rationale in the latter group is that warfarin and aspirin compared to aspirin alone, reduces the severity of limb ischaemia if these grafts occlude [41].

Conclusions

Regardless of the intervention, 25% of patients with CLI die within a year and 50% within 5 years, and this is largely from myocardial infarction and stroke. The aim of treatment should therefore focus on a patient's quality of life, taking into account their comorbidity, functional status, and surgical risk, as well as factors affecting the long-term durability of the bypass employed.

Key points

- Thrombosis of an infra-inguinal bypass graft can result in severe limb-threatening ischaemia. There is no clear consensus regarding its optimal management.
- An active approach to arterial reconstruction, following infra-inguinal bypass graft failure, is generally advocated.
- Adequate planning prior to surgery is essential, with careful consideration of the quality of the inflow and outflow vessels, and the availability of adequate calibre and length of autogenous vein.
- Endovascular options for infra-inguinal graft salvage are useful in patients with a reduced life expectancy, where suitable vein for bypass surgery is lacking or in patients with a high operative risk.

References

1. Conte MS, Bandyk DF, Clowes AW, et al. Results of PREVENT III: a multicenter, randomized trial of edifoligide for the prevention of vein graft failure in lower extremity bypass surgery. J Vasc Surg 2006; 43: 742-51.

2. Conte MS, Belkin M, Upchurch GR, et al. Impact of increasing comorbidity on infrainguinal reconstruction: a 20-year perspective. Ann Surg 2001; 233: 445-52.

3. Schanzer A, Hevelone N, Owens CD, et al. Technical factors affecting autogenous vein graft failure: observations from a large multicenter trial. J Vasc Surg 2007; 46: 1180-90.

4. Alback A, Roth WD, Ihlberg L, et al. Preoperative angiographic score and intraoperative flow as predictors of the mid-term patency of infrapopliteal bypass grafts. Eur J Vasc Endovasc Surg 2000; 20: 447-53.

5. Nasr MK, McCarthy RJ, Budd JS, Horrocks M. Infrainguinal bypass graft patency and limb salvage rates in critical limb ischemia: influence of the mode of presentation. Ann Vasc Surg 2003; 17: 192-7.

6. Matzke S, Biancari F, Ihlberg L, et al. Increased preoperative c-reactive protein level as a prognostic factor for postoperative amputation after femoropopliteal bypass surgery for CLI. Ann Chir Gynaecol 2001; 90: 19-22.

7. Onohara T, Komori K, Kume M, et al. Multivariate analysis of long-term results after an axillobifemoral and aortobifemoral bypass in patients with aortoiliac occlusive disease. J Cardiovasc Surg (Torino) 2000; 41: 905-10.

8. Kashyap VS, Pavkov ML, Bena JF, et al. The management of severe aortoiliac occlusive disease: endovascular therapy rivals open reconstruction. J Vasc Surg 2008; 48: 1451-7, 1457 e1-3.

9. Nolan KD, Benjamin ME, Murphy TJ, et al. Femorofemoral bypass for aortofemoral graft limb occlusion: a ten-year experience. J Vasc Surg 1994; 19: 851-6.

10. Nazzal MM, Hoballah JJ, Jacobovicz C, et al. A comparative evaluation of femorofemoral crossover bypass and iliofemoral bypass for unilateral iliac artery occlusive disease. Angiology 1998; 49: 259-65.

11. Defraigne JO, Vazquez C, Limet R. Crossover iliofemoral bypass grafting for treatment of unilateral iliac atherosclerotic disease. J Vasc Surg 1999; 30: 693-700.

12. Norgren L, Hiatt WR, Harris KA, Lammer J. TASC II section F on revascularization in PAD. J Endovasc Ther 2007; 14: 743-4.

13. Piotrowski JJ, Pearce WH, Jones DN, et al. Aortobifemoral bypass: the operation of choice for unilateral iliac occlusion? J Vasc Surg 1988; 8: 211-8.

14. Stone PA, Armstrong PA, Bandyk DF, et al. Duplex ultrasound criteria for femorofemoral bypass revision. J Vasc Surg 2006; 44: 496-502.

15. D'Addio V, Ali A, Timaran C, et al. Femorofemoral bypass with femoral popliteal vein. J Vasc Surg 2005; 42: 35-9.

16. Hinchliffe RJ, Alric P, Wenham PW, Hopkinson BR. Durability of femorofemoral bypass grafting after aortouniiliac endovascular aneurysm repair. *J Vasc Surg* 2003; 38: 498-503.

17. Lau H, Cheng SW. Long-term outcome of aortofemoral bypass for aortoiliac occlusive disease. *Ann Acad Med Singapore* 2000; 29: 434-8.

18. Herrera FA, Kohanzadeh S, Nasseri Y, *et al.* Management of vascular graft infections with soft tissue flap coverage: improving limb salvage rates - a veterans affairs experience. *Am Surg* 2009; 75(10): 877-81.

19. McCarthy WJ, McGee GS, Lin WW, *et al.* Axillary-popliteal artery bypass provides successful limb salvage after removal of infected aortofemoral grafts. *Arch Surg* 1992; 127: 974-8.

20. Criado E, Johnson G, Jr., Burnham SJ, *et al.* Descending thoracic aorta-to-iliofemoral artery bypass as an alternative to aortoiliac reconstruction. *J Vasc Surg* 1992; 15: 550-7.

21. Marston WA, Risley GL, Criado E, *et al.* Management of failed and infected axillofemoral grafts. *J Vasc Surg* 1994; 20: 357-65; discussion 365-6.

22. Ali AT, Modrall JG, Hocking J, *et al.* Long-term results of the treatment of aortic graft infection by *in situ* replacement with femoral popliteal vein grafts. *J Vasc Surg* 2009; 50: 30-9.

23. Beck AW, Murphy EH, Hocking JA, *et al.* Aortic reconstruction with femoral-popliteal vein: graft stenosis incidence, risk and reintervention. *J Vasc Surg* 2008; 47: 36-43.

24. Brochado Neto FC, Cury MV, Costa VS, *et al.* Inframalleolar bypass grafts for limb salvage. *Eur J Vasc Endovasc Surg* 2010; 40: 747-53.

25. Harris PL, Veith FJ, Shanik GD, *et al.* Prospective randomized comparison of *in situ* and reversed infrapopliteal vein grafts. *Br J Surg* 1993; 80: 173-6.

26. Holzenbein TJ, Pomposelli FB, Jr., Miller A, *et al.* Results of a policy with arm veins used as the first alternative to an unavailable ipsilateral greater saphenous vein for infrainguinal bypass. *J Vasc Surg* 1996; 23: 130-40.

27. Kaczynski J, Gibbons CP. Experience with femoral vein grafts for infra-inguinal bypass. *Eur J Vasc Endovasc Surg* 2011; 41: 676-8.

28. Aalders GJ, van Vroonhoven TJ. Polytetrafluoroethylene versus human umbilical vein in above-knee femoropopliteal bypass: six-year results of a randomized clinical trial. *J Vasc Surg* 1992; 16: 816-23; discussion 823-4.

29. Twine CP, McLain AD. Graft type for femoro-popliteal bypass surgery. *Cochrane Database Syst Rev* 2010; 5: CD001487.

30. Tilanus HW, Obertop H, Van Urk H. Saphenous vein or PTFE for femoropopliteal bypass. A prospective randomized trial. *Ann Surg* 1985; 202: 780-2.

31. Veith FJ, Gupta SK, Ascer E, *et al.* Six-year prospective multicenter randomized comparison of autologous saphenous vein and expanded polytetrafluoroethylene grafts in infrainguinal arterial reconstructions. *J Vasc Surg* 1986; 3: 104-14.

32. Harris L, O'Brien-Irr M, Ricotta JJ. Long-term assessment of cryopreserved vein bypass grafting success. *J Vasc Surg* 2001; 33: 528-32.

33. Randon C, Jacobs B, De Ryck F, *et al.* Fifteen years of infrapopliteal arterial reconstructions with cryopreserved venous allografts for limb salvage. *J Vasc Surg* 2010; 51: 869-77.

34. Ishii Y, Gossage JA, Dourado R, *et al.* Minimum internal diameter of the greater saphenous vein is an important determinant of successful femorodistal bypass grafting that is independent of the quality of the runoff. *Vascular* 2004; 12: 225-32.

35. Alback A, Lepantalo M. Immediate occlusion of *in situ* saphenous vein bypass grafts: a survey of 329 reconstructions. *Eur J Surg* 1998; 164(10): 745-50.

36. Barshes NR, Menard MT, Nguyen LL, *et al.* Infrainguinal bypass is associated with lower perioperative mortality than major amputation in high-risk surgical candidates. *J Vasc Surg* 2011; 53: 1251-90.

37. Arvela E, Soderstrom M, Korhonen M, *et al.* Finnvasc score and modified Prevent III score predict long-term outcome after infrainguinal surgical and endovascular revascularization for critical limb ischemia. *J Vasc Surg* 2010; 52: 1218-25.

38. Wilson YG, Davies AH, Currie IC, *et al.* Vein graft stenosis: incidence and intervention. *Eur J Vasc Endovasc Surg* 1996; 11: 164-9.

39. Davies AH, Hawdon AJ, Sydes MR, Thompson SG. Is duplex surveillance of value after leg vein bypass grafting? Principal results of the Vein Graft Surveillance Randomised Trial (VGST). *Circulation* 2005; 112(13): 1985-91.

40. Tinder CN, Chavanpun JP, Bandyk DF, *et al.* Efficacy of duplex ultrasound surveillance after infrainguinal vein bypass may be enhanced by identification of characteristics predictive of graft stenosis development. *J Vasc Surg* 2008; 48: 613-8.

41. Brumberg RS, Back MR, Armstrong PA, *et al.* The relative importance of graft surveillance and warfarin therapy in infrainguinal prosthetic bypass failure. *J Vasc Surg* 2007; 46: 1160-6.

42. Carter A, Murphy MO, Halka AT, *et al.* The natural history of stenoses within lower limb arterial bypass grafts using a graft surveillance program. *Ann Vasc Surg* 2007; 21: 695-703.

43. Belkin M. Secondary bypass after infrainguinal bypass graft failure. *Semin Vasc Surg* 2009; 22: 234-9.

44. Li QL, Zhang XM, Shen CY. [Management of prosthetic graft occlusion after lower extremity bypasses]. *Zhonghua Yi Xue Za Zhi* 2010; 90(33): 2334-7.

45. Cheshire NJ, Noone MA, Wolfe JH. Re-intervention after vascular surgery for critical leg ischaemia. *Eur J Vasc Surg* 1992; 6: 545-50.

46. Henke PK, Proctor MC, Zajkowski PJ, *et al.* Tissue loss, early primary graft occlusion, female gender, and a prohibitive failure rate of secondary infrainguinal arterial reconstruction. *J Vasc Surg* 2002; 35: 902-9.

47. Nguyen LL, Conte MS, Menard MT, *et al.* Infrainguinal vein bypass graft revision: factors affecting long-term outcome. *J Vasc Surg* 2004; 40: 916-23.

48. Belkin M, Conte MS, Donaldson MC, *et al.* Preferred strategies for secondary infrainguinal bypass: lessons learned from 300 consecutive reoperations. *J Vasc Surg* 1995; 21: 282-93.

49. Bonhomme S, Trotteur G, Van Damme H, Defraigne JO. Thrombolysis of occluded infra-inguinal bypass grafts: is it worthwhile? *Acta Chir Belg* 2010; 110: 445-50.

50. Belkin M, Donaldson MC, Whittemore AD, *et al.* Observations on the use of thrombolytic agents for thrombotic occlusion of infrainguinal vein grafts. *J Vasc Surg* 1990; 11: 289-94.

51. Efficacy of oral anticoagulants compared with aspirin after infrainguinal bypass surgery (The Dutch Bypass Oral Anticoagulants or Aspirin Study): a randomised trial. *Lancet* 2000; 355(9201): 346-51.

52. Dorffler-Melly J, Buller HR, Koopman MM, Prins MH. Antithrombotic agents for preventing thrombosis after infrainguinal arterial bypass surgery. *Cochrane Database Syst Rev* 2003; 4: CD000536.

Case vignette   Difficult diagnosis of graft infection

Kaji Sritharan MD FRCS, Specialist Registrar in Vascular Surgery
Alun H. Davies MA DM FRCS FHEA FEBVS FACPh, Professor of Vascular Surgery
Academic Department of Vascular Surgery, Imperial College London, London, UK

A 76-year-old woman presented with acute onset right-sided short distance claudication, 10 years following bilateral axillo-unifemoral bypass grafts. Her inflammatory markers were elevated and a CT scan revealed a fluid collection around an occluded right-sided graft. Despite negative FDG-PET CT and technetium-99 labelled white cell scans, an infected right-sided graft (bathed in pus) was eventually excised. Her symptoms improved and no further revascularisation was required.

This case illustrates the difficulties that can be encountered in the diagnosis of graft infection. In the presence of new symptoms, graft occlusion, perigraft collection and raised inflammatory markers, infection is highly probable despite negative FDG-PET CT and technetium-99 labelled white cell scans.

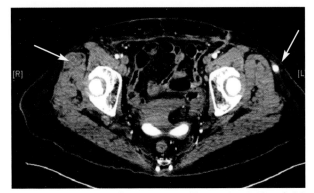

Figure 1. CT scan of the aorta with contrast. The right axillo-unifemoral graft is occluded, whilst the left remains patent (arrows). A perigraft collection is seen bilaterally but is more significant on the right.

Chapter 13

Complications after peripheral angiography, angioplasty and stenting

Jonathan Ghosh FRCS MD, Endovascular Fellow
Robert K. Fisher FRCS MD, Consultant Vascular & Endovascular Surgeon
Department of Vascular Surgery, Royal Liverpool University Hospital, Liverpool, UK

Introduction

Percutaneous transluminal angioplasty performed with stenting or in isolation has revolutionised the management of peripheral arterial disease. Innovations in technique and technology have broadened the scope for increasingly complex interventions and contributed towards a favourable safety profile. A large prospective audit of percutaneous peripheral inventions found major medical morbidity complicating 2.4% of procedures, emergency surgical intervention was required in 2.3%, and the overall amputation rate was 0.6% [1].

The true incidence of access site complications is unclear due to inconsistent reporting standards, although the rate of iatrogenic peripheral vascular injuries ranges from 1% after diagnostic angiography up to 9% following therapeutic intervention [2-4]. Furthermore, an inverse relationship between complication rates and number of procedures performed per annum has been described previously [5].

This chapter focuses on the recognition, prevention and management of the principal complications of percutaneous interventions, namely:

- haemorrhage;
- pseudoaneurysm;
- arteriovenous fistula;
- dissection;
- thrombo-embolism;
- contrast-induced renal injury.

Emphasis is given to the common femoral artery access site, though the principles are relevant to other anatomical regions.

Haemorrhage

Puncture site bleeding accounts for the majority of complications following arterial catheterisation. Whilst minor bruising occurs commonly, significant bleeding requiring resuscitation or reintervention is reported in fewer than 1% of procedures.

Two patterns of bleeding may be appreciated. The first is characterised by rapid onset of haematoma around the puncture site, which is associated with pain and bruising and is superficial and accessible. These haematomas are readily imaged by duplex ultrasonography and are amenable to surgical or non-surgical intervention. However, they may become complicated by pseudoaneurysm formation, nerve compression, deep venous thrombosis or compartment syndrome if unattended.

The second pattern refers to bleeding into the retroperitoneal space either from an inadvertent high groin puncture, tracking of blood along the femoral sheath (often related to posterior wall perforation), or perforation of the iliac system during the primary intervention. Retroperitoneal haemorrhage can potentially be devastating due to anatomical inaccessibility and lack of tamponade, which allows the haematoma to reach a considerable size before becoming clinically evident. In a review of iatrogenic retroperitoneal haematomas, the mean time to first clinical signs was 158 minutes: 42% of patients presented with abdominal pain, 46% groin discomfort, 23% back pain, 31% bradycardia, 58% sweating and 92% hypotension [6]. Femoral nerve compression and iliopsoas spasm can result in groin pain with radiation to the anterior thigh, flexion and external rotation of the hip, and paraesthesia in the anteromedial thigh. A low index of suspicion should be maintained in any patient presenting with post-procedural hypotension or the aforementioned symptoms.

Prevention

Puncture

Access site bleeding arises as a consequence of inadequate post-procedural haemostasis, which may be related to procedural or patient factors (Table 1). The common femoral artery is situated below the inguinal ligament midway between the anterior superior iliac spine and the pubic symphysis (mid-

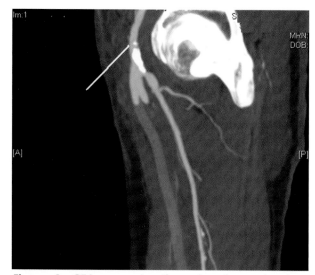

Figure 1. CTA reconstruction of a femoral artery overlying the femoral head. The white line indicates the optimum access point; cephalad risks retroperitoneal bleeding and caudal involves diseased vessel or a previous bypass graft. Such precision can only be gained through ultrasound-guided access.

inguinal point). Arterial puncture inadvertently cephalad to the inguinal ligament increases the risk of serious haematoma and retroperitoneal haemorrhage, whilst low puncture increases the risk of occlusion, dissection, arteriovenous fistula or pseudoaneurysm.

Radiologically, the common femoral artery is located over the medial half of the femoral head with puncture intended at the middle of the femoral head (Figure 1). Fluoroscopy can guide the puncture

Table 1. Risk factors for arterial puncture site complications.	
Procedure-related	**Patient-related**
Inadequate post-procedural compression	Glycoprotein IIB/IIIA inhibitor
Wide calibre access sheath (>7F)	Bleeding diathesis
Anticoagulation	Hypertension
Atherosclerotic access artery	Early mobilisation/patient non-compliance
Puncture site above inguinal ligament	Previous surgery/graft puncture

needle to the desired location in relation to the femoral head but cannot predict the subset of patients in whom the femoral bifurcation lies above this. Conversely, ultrasound-directed puncture has been shown to improve the accuracy of the arterial entry, speed of cannulation and risk of venepuncture relative to fluoroscopic-guided cannulation [7].

Haemostasis

Following catheter withdrawal, manual compression is directed to the site of access, noting that this will often be remote to the skin puncture site, dependent on the angle of needle puncture. The classic Seldinger method of manual compression required sustained pressure over the puncture site for at least 15-20 minutes followed by bed rest for an additional 6 hours, though in practice these intervals are often abridged. Ultrasound-directed pressure is of value in directing compression and will also inform when extravasation has stopped. Mechanical external compression devices such as the FemoStop™ (Radi Medical Systems) have also been demonstrated to augment haemostasis in patients undergoing coronary catheterisation [8].

Since the mid-1990s, a number of percutaneous closure devices have been developed that work either as passive sealants (e.g. Angio-Seal™, St Jude Medical) or by active wall apposition (e.g. Perclose™ and Starclose™, Abbott Laboratories) [9]. These aim to reduce the frequency of local complications and allow early mobilisation [10]. Overall, the success rate in achieving haemostasis is up to 98%, with low failure rates ranging from 1-3%. Anecdotal reports of infections, maldeployment, pseudoaneurysm, device embolism and limb ischaemia have been published, and there have been no largescale randomised clinical trials to demonstrate superiority of an individual device. Meta-analyses have failed to substantiate benefit over standard compression, although time to haemostasis is generally quicker [3, 11, 12]. One meta-analysis found closure devices to be associated with increased haematoma and pseudoaneurysm formation [3], although reviews suffer from underpowered and heterogenous source data. In view of their cost, application of these devices is generally restricted to those with risk factors for complications and people who cannot tolerate external compression

or who are immobile [13, 14]. Meta-analysis data would suggest that these adjuncts augment rather than replace external compression. The management of complications from closure devices is beyond the scope of this chapter but has been addressed elsewhere [9].

Management

During the procedure

Extravasation due to guide wire perforation noted at the time of injury can almost always be managed conservatively. This may be aided by low-pressure tamponade with an angioplasty balloon for up to 5 minutes. Extravasation during angioplasty is more treacherous as this implies a significant laceration to the artery that requires urgent and definitive treatment. Low-pressure inflation of an angioplasty balloon above the injury, ideally from the contralateral side, will allow proximal endoclamp control. With concurrent fluid resuscitation, the anatomy can then be reviewed to determine whether a stent graft can cover the injury or if surgical repair is required (Figure 2).

Post-procedural retroperitoneal bleeding

Clinical suspicion of retroperitoneal bleeding requires immediate pressure to be applied over the site of arterial puncture, patient resuscitation in the standard manner and assessment of distal perfusion. In the stable patient, additional imaging will localise the site of injury and allow planning of conservative, endovascular or surgical management. Duplex ultrasonography can visualise infra-inguinal vasculature clearly but pelvic views are limited by pain and the lack of a sonographic window. Accordingly, contrast-enhanced spiral CT allows optimal visualisation of the site and extent of the bleeding site (Figure 3) [15, 16].

In the presence of haemodynamic instability, urgent surgical exploration is mandated with sufficient proximal access to allow inflow control. A small-calibre single puncture may be repaired primarily, whereas a laceration requires vein patch repair. It is important to look for multiple sites of injury including the posterior arterial wall, and to check for coexisting dissection or thrombo-embolism. A single centre experience of surgical repairs found that

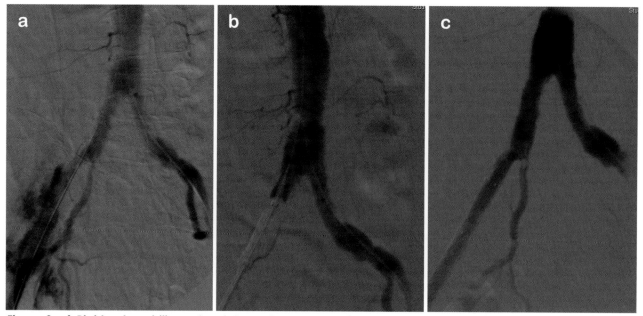

Figure 2. a) Right external iliac artery iatrogenic rupture with extravasation of contrast. Wire access has been maintained across the vessel during the completion angiogram, enabling subsequent control and salvage. b) Balloon tamponade gains temporary haemorrhage control. c) Deployment of two covered self-expanding stents achieves permanent haemostasis and preserves limb perfusion. *Images courtesy of Dr Richard McWilliams FRCR, Consultant Interventional Radiologist, Royal Liverpool University Hospital, UK.*

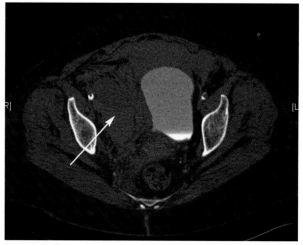

Figure 3. Unenhanced CT scan demonstrating a large right retroperitoneal haematoma (arrow) following a retrograde puncture of the common femoral artery and external iliac/common femoral artery angioplasty. Note the deviation of the bladder (filled with excreted contrast) indicating the significant size of the haematoma. Urgent surgery controlled the haemorrhage and identified an inadvertent high puncture.

approximately 20% of such injuries required a retroperitoneal exposure for proximal control [17]. Mortality in this series was 3.5% and, although there was no limb loss, morbidity was 25% due to subsequent myocardial infarction or wound complications.

Iliac injury is optimally managed by endovascular means using a covered stent, though care must be taken to ensure that this remains proximal to the hip joint. Though common femoral artery stenting has been reported, mechanical stresses predispose to device breakage, myointimal hyperplasia and occlusion [18]. As maximal conformational change of the external iliac artery during hip flexion is observed 35.1 +/- 30.1mm cranial to the inguinal ligament [19], injuries involving this region are best managed surgically.

Conservative management of retroperitoneal haematoma is reserved for patients that are haemodynamically stable and have no radiological evidence of active bleeding. Such patients require intensive monitoring in a high dependency environment, bed rest, normalisation of clotting, serial imaging and monitoring for compartment syndrome [16].

Pseudoaneurysm

A pseudoaneurysm arises when blood exits through a defect of the arterial wall to form a localized pocket of flow either within, or outside the adventitia. It shares the same risk factors and aetiologies as haemorrhage. These present as rapid onset of bruising, pain and swelling, and should be suspected in any patient with a pulsatile lump with an associated machinery murmur on auscultation at the site of cannulation, and is easily confirmed on duplex imaging (Figure 4). Necrosis of overlying skin is the most common complication, though rupture, compression neuropathy, deep venous thrombosis and infection may also occur. A small pseudoaneurysm may be indistinguishable from a haematoma, and any suspicion requires further imaging.

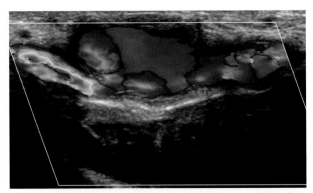

Figure 4. Pseudoaneurysm of radial artery following percutaneous coronary intervention.

Prevention

Accurate arterial puncture and effective haemostasis with consideration for patient risk factors will minimise the prospect of pseudoaneurysm formation; there is no convincing evidence that percutaneous closure devices reduce the risk.

Management

The goal of treatment is to exclude the pseudoaneurysm cavity from flow or to obliterate the lumen to convert it into a simple haematoma. Pseudoaneurysms with a small cavity (<6cm³ volume /1.8cm diameter) [20] or long necks (>9mm) [21] are associated with spontaneous thrombosis and may simply be monitored; larger or expanding cavities require intervention. There is no consensus as to which pseudoanerysms to treat conservatively, though it is reasonable to use 2cm as a size threshold, below which the lesion can be monitored and above which intervention considered.

Four treatment modalities are available: ultrasound-directed compression, thrombin injection, endovascular exclusion and surgical repair; they have been the subject of a Cochrane meta-analysis [22]. Ultrasound-guided compression, performed under analgesia or sedation, involves using the ultrasound probe to occlude the inflow to the aneurysm sac for 10-minute cycles. The force applied should cause cessation of colour flow within the aneurysm sac but not compromise the flow in the native artery. Inability to achieve this represents failure of the treatment. Using this technique, the aneurysm inflow may be thrombosed successfully in 63-88% of cases, although the Cochrane analysis found no advantage over blind Femostop compression [22].

Thrombin at a concentration of 1000U/ml may be injected slowly into the pseudoaneurysm under ultrasound visualisation, which causes rapid thrombosis after up to 98% of procedures. This approach is less labour intensive than compression but carries the risk of thrombin reflux into the true arterial lumen with the potential for thrombosis, embolisation and ischaemia. Delayed reperfusion of the aneurysm may occur in up to 6% of cases and there exists a concern over prion transmission with bovine-derived preparations. The UK National Institute for Health and Clinical Excellence has found evidence of sufficient advantage of thrombin over compression (success rates of 93-100% with thrombin vs. 65-93% compression) to support its use [23]. However, in the Cochrane analysis the advantage of thrombin over ultrasound-guided compression did not reach statistical significance. Peri-aneurysmal saline injection infiltration [24] and recombinant Factor VII injection [25] have also been described as percutaneous therapeutic options.

Endovascular management can either be by coil embolisation of the sac or intraluminal exclusion of the defect using a covered stent. Embolisation is disadvantaged by cost, prevention of sac shrinkage and sac pressurisation and rupture [26]. Sac exclusion using a covered stent is valuable when other methods have failed, but is contra-indicated at flexion points and should be used cautiously in young patients due to the risk of late thrombosis.

Surgical treatment, by oversewing the arterial defect neck, is reserved for those that have failed percutaneous treatments, have regional complications due to sac expansion or have sustained a rupture. The same operative principles for management of pseudoaneurysm apply as those highlighted above for haemorrhage control.

Arteriovenous fistula

Arteriovenous fistula is rare, and complicates up to 0.86% of femoral catheterisations with a statistically significant increase in incidence after interventional over diagnostic procedures [27]. Female sex, hypertension, anticoagulation and left groin puncture have been identified as independent risk factors. It has been hypothesised that the comparatively smaller luminal diameter in women increases the risk of technical error and that the left side preponderance may be related to positional issues, where an operator conventionally stands on the patient's right. Acutely, these rarely produce symptoms and diagnosis is often delayed by months or years [28]. The diagnosis may be made clinically by palpation of a thrill and auscultation of a bruit. In the long term a fistula may result in high-output cardiac failure, aneurysmal dilatation of the artery, and limb oedema.

Prevention

Arteriovenous fistula is an abnormal communication between artery and vein and arises following simultaneous arterial and venous puncture. Accordingly, the incidence can be reduced by accurate cannulation and avoidance of multiple passes; ultrasound-guided access is of value in this regard, particularly in scarred or deep groins [7]. Unlike the common femoral vessels that lie side-to-side, the superficial femoral vein is related deep to the artery and is thus more vulnerable to inadvertent puncture [29].

Puncture below the femoral bifurcation, particularly during antegrade cannulation therefore, should be undertaken with caution. In common with other puncture site complications, the importance of effective compression cannot be overstated.

Management

Clinical suspicion can be confirmed by colour Doppler ultrasonography (Figure 5), which can also identify the position and extent of the communication. Ultrasound compression is less successful than for pseudoaneurysm, with fewer than a third treated successfully, as the track is typically too short to be obliterated without occluding the adjacent vein [30, 31]. Prolonged bandaging (mean 15 days) was reported as a promising solution in one series of 12 patients, although skin breakdown and deep venous thrombosis were highlighted as potential complications [32].

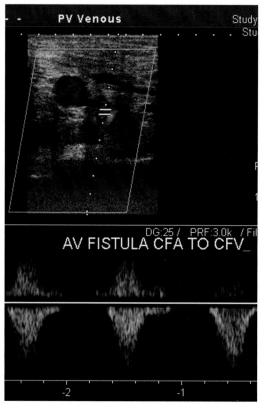

Figure 5. Arteriovenous fistula following arterial puncture. An arterialised waveform is demonstrated in the common femoral vein.

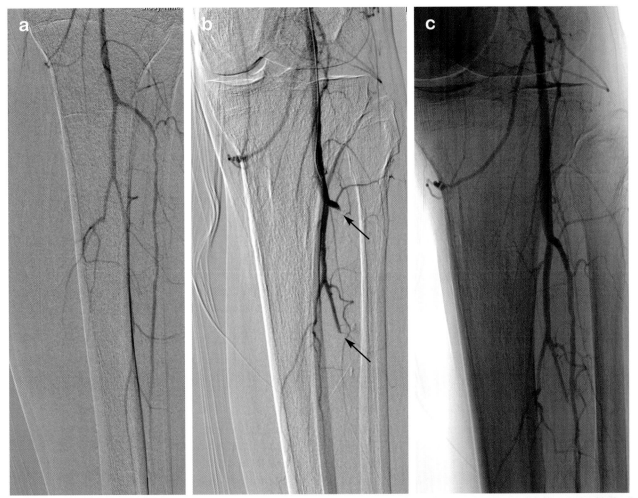

Figure 6. a) Peripheral digital subtraction angiogram prior to long superficial femoral artery subintimal angioplasty indicating patent anterior tibial and peroneal vessels. **b)** Post-angioplasty resulted in embolic occlusion of the anterior tibial and peroneal vessels (arrows). **c)** Thrombosuction recanalised the anterior tibial vessel whilst the peroneal remained occluded.

Endovascular exclusion of a fistula occurring distal to the femoral bifurcation has a high rate of technical success, a low complication profile and good short-term outcome [33, 34]. Technical considerations include the need to approach the lesion by crossing the aortic bifurcation from the contralateral side over a stiff guide wire, and accuracy in positioning and preservation of the profunda femoris. Fistulae that involve the common femoral artery are best managed surgically, although dissection of the arterialised venous system can risk haemorrhage.

Thrombo-embolism and dissection

Acute arterial occlusion may occur due to thrombo-embolism, dislodgement of plaque or dissection (Figure 6). Additionally, ischaemia following the use of a closure device should raise the suspicion of stenosis or embolisation. Macro-emboli present with the classical symptoms and signs of acute limb ischaemia, whereas micro-emboli occluding peripheral vessels manifest by trash foot, digital ischaemia and pain.

Dissection may occur either at the site of the puncture or the intervention. The latter may occur from subintimal passage of a guide wire, contrast injection or excessive dilatation during angioplasty. The resulting intimal injury and thrombosis may cause acute or delayed ischaemia.

Prevention

In general, the risk of peri-procedural arterial thrombosis may be diminished by adequate heparinisation (50-100u/kg plus 1000u/hour for prolonged procedures), hydration, low profile catheter systems and minimisation of procedural time. Intra-arterial use of heparin during radiological intervention is commonplace, although this is intuitive rather than evidence-based and represents off-label use of the drug.

Puncture

Risk of access site dissection can be minimised by avoiding calcified plaques or multiple punctures. Contrast injection through the puncture needle can confirm entry into the lumen and guide wire transit should never be forced; if resistance or bowing is encountered then the wire should be withdrawn and fluoroscopy performed. Passage of hydrophilic wires through puncture needles is contra-indicated as stripping of the coating can cause wire fracture and distal embolisation.

Crossing the lesion

For conventional or subintimal angioplasty, the guiding wire must be intraluminal either side of the target lesion. Low profile balloons are helpful for crossing tight lesions, and exchanging a floppy for a stiff wire may support a catheter in tracking along a heavily diseased artery. Excessive attempts to cross a lesion will increase the risk of micro-emboli and dissection and, in such circumstances, consideration should be given to abandoning the procedure.

Occasionally pre-dilatation of complex disease is required to allow the angioplasty system access to the target lesion, though caution must be taken not to embolise plaque during this manoeuvre. Additionally,

when managing complex disease, consideration should be given to placement of accessory guide wires in adjacent vessels. This is particularly applicable to the tibial vessels which may become occluded from thrombus or plaque embolising over the trifurcation during angioplasty of an adjacent artery. Pre-established access facilitates recanalisation of the vessel through techniques such as thrombosuction or angioplasty.

Dilation

Balloon over-dilatation is the main cause of dissection and rupture, and treating only clinically relevant lesions can reduce complications. Balloon diameter and length should be based on measured angiography images of the target vessel rather than estimation. Non-compliant-type balloons are generally preferable as expansion is limited to a predetermined nominal maximum diameter and enlarges very little thereafter despite inflation pressure increases. These balloon catheters can be inflated to high pressures in a controlled manner and the force focused on the stenosing plaque. It is advisable to perform dilatation in a step-wise manner, starting with small diameter balloons if the appropriate balloon size to select is not clear from the imaging, and escalating according to angiographic appearance. Similarly, balloon length should be determined on the basis of angiography, so that exposure to undiseased artery is minimised.

Management

During the procedure

Acute thrombo-embolism or dissection can often be recognised from the completion angiogram. If embolisation has been diagnosed during the procedure, an angiogram of run-off vessels should be obtained and thrombosuction or mechanical thrombectomy performed. Fresh thrombus may be treated by catheter-directed thrombolysis, though dislodgment of plaque will require surgical embolectomy. Intraprocedural dissection is significant if there is disturbance of distal flow. These can be tamponaded by low-pressure inflation of an angioplasty balloon for up to 5 minutes, with the aim of holding the flap against the vessel wall. Stenting across the dissection may be also considered, if anatomically suitable. If the lesion remains, then strong consideration must be given to urgent surgical thrombectomy and reconstruction.

Post-procedure

Clinical suspicion of acute limb ischaemia following completion of the procedure requires careful assessment to determine limb viability [35]: severe ischaemia with a neurosensory deficit is a requirement for urgent revascularisation.

Arterial imaging by duplex or CT/MR angiography determines the site and differentiates between dissection and thrombo-embolism. Flow-limiting macro-emboli are treated by surgical thrombectomy, though catheter-directed thrombolysis or mechanical thrombectomy remain options if there is no motor or sensory deficit. Symptomatic micro-emboli may be treated by thrombolysis, or conservatively with antiplatelet agents if symptoms are minor. An occluding dissection requires surgery, whereas a non-occluding lesion may be managed conservatively or by stenting depending on the severity of symptoms and anatomy. Although surgery allows rapid, definitive management, the process presents a significant physiological stress in the elderly comorbid patient; mortality and amputation rates for these patients are not insignificant.

Contrast-induced renal injury

Renal function may deteriorate after the administration of iodine contrast media. A commonly accepted definition of acute kidney injury (AKI) is a >25% increase from baseline of serum creatinine and/or an absolute elevation of 0.5mg/dL [36], although it is notable that over two dozen other definitions exist. Although it remains unclear whether contrast-induced AKI results from renal vasoconstriction and haemodynamic disturbance or tubular toxicity of the contrast material, the phenomenon has been associated with several risk factors, including: pre-existing renal insufficiency, diabetes mellitus, dehydration, cardiovascular disease and the use of diuretics, age over 70 years, myeloma, hypertension, and hyperuricaemia [37]. Of these, pre-existing renal insufficiency and diabetes mellitus appear to pose greatest risk.

Contrast-induced AKI is generally limited to a transient decline of renal function that is typically associated with a rise in serum creatinine within 24 hours following administration of intravenous contrast and peaking within 96 hours. Return of renal function to baseline is usually seen within 7-10 days, although chronic impairment may occur in those with multiple risk factors.

Prevention

Whilst the risk of developing contrast-induced AKI is a relative, rather than absolute contra-indication to the use of iodinated contrast media, the clinical need and patient risk factors should be assessed individually, with preventative strategies planned in advance (see also Chapter 3).

Hydration

Adequate hydration is the simplest and most effective way of maintaining renal function [38]. In patients with dehydration or those with risk factors, intravenous fluids should be commenced 6-12 hours before, and considered for up to 24 hours after the radiographic examination. Hydration with 0.9% saline has been found to reduce contrast-induced AKI risk more than 0.45% saline. Whilst some evidence has arisen that hydration with sodium bicarbonate may further reduce contrast-induced AKI, this benefit has been challenged [39].

Contrast

Renal excretion of contrast may take up to 24 hours. Accordingly, multiple contrast examinations within a short interval should be avoided as these may have a cumulative effect. Consideration should, in such circumstances, be given to the use of non-iodinated agents, particularly in the presence of severe chronic renal impairment. Carbon dioxide angiography is useful in this context as it is not allergenic or nephrotoxic and may be employed for diagnostic and therapeutic procedures [40].

Contrast-induced AKI can follow the use of high-, low- or iso-osmolar contrast agents. A meta-analysis of the literature concerning the relative nephrotoxity of high-osmolality contrast media versus low-osmolality contrast found that the latter reduced contrast-induced AKI in patients with pre-existing renal impairment but conferred no advantage in patients with normal renal function [41]. Similarly, iso-osmolality contrast has been found to confer no significant protection over low-osmolality agents [42].

Pharmacotherapy

The most commonly used prophylaxis for contrast-induced AKI is N-acetylcysteine, 600mg twice daily on the day before and on the day of exposure to iodinated contrast media. N-acetylcysteine is advantageous in being inexpensive and safe although there are conflicting published data on its efficacy [43]. Therefore, the role of N-acetylcysteine to prevent acute renal failure remains unclear. There is no evidence to support the use of mannitol or furosemide in this context [44].

Contrast-induced AKI is largely preventable, and institutions should ensure that pathways exist to identify patients at risk with poor renal function, and to ensure that they receive adequate hydration and monitoring. This applies to both diagnostic and therapeutic procedures in the angiography suite, but it should not be forgotten when intravenous contrast is employed during CT investigations.

Conclusions

Radiological intervention for vascular disease has revolutionised the treatment of patients but brings with it unique complications. Basic principles may reduce the frequency of such events, including careful case selection and planning, meticulous technique with regard to access, wire manipulation and angioplasty, and successful haemostasis. Awareness of the potential complications will facilitate their avoidance and reduce their implications when they (inevitably) occur.

Key points

- Ultrasound-directed puncture provides safest access.
- Accurate puncture and effective haemostasis will avoid most complications.
- Closure devices allow faster haemostasis but have a failure/complication profile.
- Have a low threshold for suspecting retroperitoneal bleeding – signs may be masked or delayed.
- Pseudoaneurysm can be avoided by effective post-procedural haemostasis.
- Small (<2cm) and narrow-necked pseudoaneurysms may be observed.
- Compression and thrombin treatments are both effective for pseudoaneurysms.
- Surgery for pseudoaneurysms is reserved for failed percutaneous treatments, regional effects of sac expansion or rupture.
- Arteriovenous fistulae may be avoided by accurate cannulation above the femoral bifurcation (US directed) and the avoidance of multiple passes.
- Ultrasound compression for arteriovenous fistulae is less effective than for pseudoaneurysm.
- Stent graft coverage away from flexion points is effective for arteriovenous fistulae.
- Surgery is required if arteriovenous fistulae are anatomically unsuitable for a stent.
- The risk of thrombo-embolism and dissection can be reduced with anticoagulation, accurate cannulation, careful lesion passage and balloon catheter selection.
- Pre-existing renal impairment and diabetes mellitus are leading risk factors for contrast-induced AKI.
- Pre-hydration with 0.9% saline and contrast reduction are principal methods of renal protection.
- Low and iso-osmolar contrast agents should be used if there is pre-existing renal impairment.
- There are conflicting data regarding the use of N-acetylcysteine in preventing contrast-induced AKI.

References

1. Axisal B, Fishwick G, Bolia A, *et al*. Complications following peripheral angioplasty. *Ann R Coll Surg Engl* 2002; 84: 39-42.

2. Eternad-Rezai R, Peck DJ. Ultrasound-guided thrombin injection of femoral artery pseudoaneurysms. *Can Assoc Radiol J* 2003; 54: 118-12.

3. Koreny M, Riedmüller E, Nikfardjam M, *et al*. Arterial puncture closing devices compared with standard manual compression after cardiac catheterization. *JAMA* 2004; 291: 350-7.

4. Omoigui NA, Califf RM, Pieper K, *et al*. Peripheral vascular complications in the Coronary Angioplasty versus Excisional Atherectomy Trial (CAVEAT-I). *J Am Coll Cardiology* 1995; 26: 922-30.

5. Hessel SJ, Adams DF, Abrams HL. Complications of angiography. *Radiology* 1981; 138: 273-81.

6. Farouque HM, Tremmel JA, Raissi Shabari F, *et al*. Risk factors for the development of retroperitoneal hematoma after percutaneous coronary intervention in the era of glycoprotein IIb/IIIa inhibitors and vascular closure devices. *J Am Coll Cardiol* 2005; 45: 363-8.

7. Seto AH, Abu-Fadel MS, Sparling JM, *et al*. Real-time ultrasound guidance facilitates femoral arterial access and reduces vascular complications: FAUST (Femoral Arterial Access With Ultrasound Trial). *JACC Cardiovasc Interv* 2010; 3: 751-8.

8. Jaspers L, Benit E. Immediate sheath removal after PCI using a Femostop is feasible and safe. Results of a registry. *Acta Cardiol* 2003; 58: 535-7.

9. Bechara CF, Annambhotla S, Lin PH. Access site management with vascular closure devices for percutaneous transarterial procedures. *J Vasc Surg* 2010; 52: 1682-96.

10. Wilde NT, Bungay P, Johnson L, *et al*. Outpatient angioplasty and stenting facilitated by percutaneous arterial suture closure devices. *Clin Radiol* 2006; 61: 1035-40.

11. Vaitkus PT. A meta-analysis of percutaneous vascular closure devices after diagnostic catheterization and percutaneous coronary intervention. *J Invasive Cardiol* 2004; 16: 243-6.

12. Nikolsky E, Mehran R, Halkin A, *et al*. Vascular complications associated with arteriotomy closure devices in patients undergoing percutaneous coronary procedures: a meta-analysis. *J Am Coll Cardiol* 2004; 44: 1200-29.

13. Resnic FS, Blake GJ, Ohno-Machado L, *et al*. Vascular closure devices and the risk of vascular complications after percutaneous coronary intervention in patients receiving glycoprotein IIb-IIIa inhibitors. *Am J Cardiol* 2001; 88: 493-6.

14. Patel MR, Jneid H, Derdeyn CP, *et al*. Arteriotomy closure devices for cardiovascular procedures: a scientific statement from the American Heart Association. *Circulation* 2010; 122: 1882-93.

15. Scialpi M, Scaglione M, Angelelli G, *et al*. Emergencies in the retroperitoneum: assessment of spread of disease by helical CT. *Eur J Radiol* 2004; 50: 74-83.

16. Chan YC, Morales JP, Reidy JF, *et al*. Management of spontaneous and iatrogenic retroperitoneal haemorrhage: conservative management, endovascular intervention or open surgery? *Int J Clin Pract* 2008; 62: 1604-13.

17. Franco CD, Goldsmith J, Veith FJ, *et al*. Management of arterial injuries produced by percutaneous femoral procedures. *Surgery* 1993; 113: 419-25.

18. Stricker H, Jacomella, V. Stent-assisted angioplasty at the level of the common femoral artery bifurcation: midterm outcomes. *J Endovasc Ther* 2004; 11: 281-6.

19. Park SI, Won JH, Kim BM, *et al*. Femoral artery pseudoaneurysm: Doppler sonographic features predictive for spontaneous thrombosis. *Cardiovasc Intervent Radiol* 2005; 28: 173-7.

20. O'Sullivan GJ, Ray SA, Lewis JS, *et al*. A review of alternative approaches in the management of iatrogenic femoral pseudoaneurysms. *Ann R Coll Surg Engl* 1999; 81: 226-34.

21. Samuels D, Orron DE, Kessler A, *et al*. Femoral artery pseudoaneurysm: Doppler sonographic features predictive for spontaneous thrombosis. *J Clin Ultrasound* 1997; 25: 497-500.

22. Tisi PV, Callam, M.J. Treatment for femoral pseudoaneurysms. *Cochrane Database Syst Rev* 2009; 15(2): CD004981.

23. National Institute for Health and Clinical Excellence. Thrombin injections for pseudoaneurysms: guidance (IPG60), 2004. http://guidance.nice.org.uk/IPG60/Guidance/pdf/English (accessed March 2011).

24. Finkelstein A, Bazan S, Halkin A, *et al*. Treatment of post-catheterization femoral artery pseudo-aneurysm with para-aneurysmal saline injection. *Am J Cardiol* 2008; 101: 1418-22.

25. Liem AK, Biesma DH, Ernst SM, *et al*. Recombinant activated Factor VII for false aneurysms in patients with normal haemostatic mechanisms. *Thromb Haemost* 1999; 82: 150-1.

26. Morgan R, Belli AM. Current treatment methods for postcatheterization pseudoaneurysms. *J Vasc Interv Radiol* 2003; 14: 697-710.

27. Perings SM, Kelm M, Jax T, *et al*. A prospective study on incidence and risk factors of arteriovenous fistulae following transfemoral cardiac catheterization. *Int J Cardiol* 2003; 88: 223-8.

28. Marsan RE, McDonald V, Ramamurthy S. Iatrogenic femoral arteriovenous fistula. *Cardiovasc Intervent Radiol* 1990; 13: 314-6.

29. Sidawy AN, Neville RF, Adib H, *et al*. Femoral arteriovenous fistula following cardiac catheterization: an anatomic explanation. *Cardiovasc Surg* 1993; 1: 134-7.

30. Paulson EK, Kliewer MA, Hertzberg BS, *et al*. Ultrasonographically guided manual compression of femoral artery injuries. *J Ultrasound Med* 1995; 14: 653-9.

31. Schaub F, Theiss W, Heinz M, *et al*. New aspects in ultrasound-guided compression repair of postcatheterization femoral artery injuries. *Circulation* 1994; 90: 1861-5.

32. Zhou T, Liu ZJ, Zhou SH, *et al*. Treatment of postcatheterization femoral arteriovenous fistulas with simple prolonged bandaging. *Chin Med J (Engl)* 2007; 120: 952-5.

33. Baltacioglu F, Cimsit NC, Cil B, *et al*. Endovascular stent-graft applications in iatrogenic vascular injuries. *Cardiovasc Intervent Radiol* 2003; 26: 434-9.

34. Onal B, Ilgit ET, Kosar S, *et al*. Endovascular treatment of peripheral vascular lesions with stent-grafts. *Diagn Interv Radiol* 2005; 11: 170-4.

35. Rutherford RB, Baker JD, Ernst C, *et al.* Recommended standards for reports dealing with lower extremity ischemia: revised version. *J Vasc Surg* 1997; 26: 517-38.

36. Barrett BJ, Parfrey PS. Preventing nephropathy induced by contrast medium. *N Engl J Med* 2006; 354: 379-86.

37. Gleeson TG, Bulugahapitiya S. Contrast-induced nephropathy. *Am J Roentgenol* 2004; 183: 673-89.

38. Eisenberg RL, Bank WO, Hedgock MW. Renal failure after major angiography can be avoided with hydration. *Am J Roentgenol* 1985; 136: 859-63.

39. Brar SS, Shen AY, Jorgensen MB, *et al.* Sodium bicarbonate vs. sodium chloride for the prevention of contrast medium-induced nephropathy in patients undergoing coronary angiography: a randomized trial. *JAMA* 2008; 300: 1038-46.

40. Shaw DR, Kessel DO. The current status of the use of carbon dioxide in diagnostic and interventional angiographic procedures. *Cardiovasc Intervent Radiol* 2006; 29: 323-31.

41. Barrett BJ, Carlisle EJ. Meta-analysis of the relative nephrotoxicity of high- and low-osmolality iodinated contrast media. *Radiology* 1993; 188: 171-8.

42. Heinrich MC, Haberle L, Muller V, *et al.* Nephrotoxicity of iso-osmolar iodixanol compared with nonionic low-osmolar contrast media: meta-analysis of randomized controlled trials. *Radiology* 2009; 250: 68-86.

43. Hoffmann U, Fischereder M, Krüger B, *et al.* The value of N-acetylcysteine in the prevention of radiocontrast agent-induced nephropathy seems questionable. *J Am Soc Nephrol* 2004; 15: 407-10.

44. Solomon R, Werner C, Mann D, *et al.* Effects of saline, mannitol, and furosemide to prevent acute decreases in renal function induced by radiocontrast agents. *N Engl J Med* 1994; 331: 1416-20.

Case vignette   Distal embolisation of an Angio-Seal vascular closure device

Alex Torrie MRCS, Orthopaedic Specialist Registrar
Jonathan J. Earnshaw DM FRCS, Consultant Surgeon
Gloucestershire Royal Hospital, Gloucester, UK

Vascular closure devices are increasingly used after percutaneous endovascular procedures as an alternative to sustained mechanical compression of the puncture site. This reduces the delay before mobilisation and thus increases the rate of same day discharge. Angio-Seal™ is a vascular closure device that uses an absorbable collagen anchor on the intraluminal side of the artery and a collagen plug on the outside, connected by a suture (Figure 1) [1].

A 37-year-old man developed intermittent claudication in his right calf immediately after recovering from cardio-ablative treatment for atrial flutter. The procedure was conducted via the ipsilateral common femoral artery, and the arteriotomy was closed using an Angio-Seal™ device. Arterial duplex imaging identified an occlusion at the level of the tibioperoneal trunk, reducing flow in the posterior tibial and peroneal arteries (Figure 2).

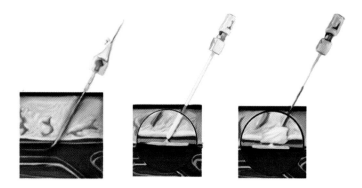

Figure 1. Diagram of the Angio-Seal™ vascular closure device. a) The guide wire is inserted intra-arterially through the Angio-Seal™ insertion sheath. b) The Angio-Seal™ collagen anchor is deployed on the luminal surface of the artery. c) Withdrawal of the insertion sheath secures the intra-arterial anchor by deploying collagen extra-luminally, sealing the arterial puncture site.

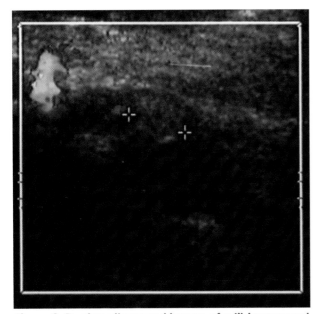

Figure 2. Duplex ultrasound image of a tibioperoneal artery occlusion due to a collagen anchor. The thrombus in the tibioperoneal trunk is located between the two markers.

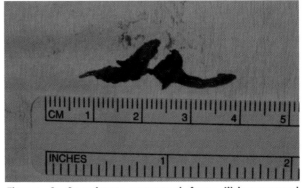

Figure 3. Specimen removed from tibioperoneal artery, consisting of the collagen anchor at the centre of an organising thrombus.

At operation, the collagen anchor from the Angio-Seal device was found surrounded by organising secondary thrombus occluding the tibioperoneal trunk (Figure 3). It was removed through a longitudinal arteriotomy that was repaired with a vein patch. Postoperatively, the patient made an uneventful recovery with resolution of his claudication symptoms and restoration of foot pulses.

Angio-Seal™ is a biodegradable plug-type vascular closure device that can achieve arterial haemostasis quickly and safely when used after interventional procedures. The collagen anchor is thought to resorb within 60-90 days. There have been a number of reports of arterial occlusion following their use.

Previous reports of complications with Angio-Seal™ usually describe occlusion of the common or superficial femoral arteries [2]. This case is unusual because the collagen anchor embolised beyond the popliteal artery, into the tibioperoneal trunk. Vascular specialists should be aware of this possible complication after use of a vascular closure device, even if the occlusion is distal to the popliteal artery [3]. The collagen anchor may dissolve more slowly than originally thought, possibly due to the influence of surrounding secondary thrombus.

References

1. Aker UT, Kensey KR, Heuser RR, *et al*. Immediate arterial haemostasis after cardiac catheterisation: initial experience with a new puncture closure device. *Cathet Cardiovasc Diagn* 1994; 31: 228-32.
2. Wille J, de Vries J-P. Acute leg ischaemia: the dark side of a percutaneous femoral artery closure device. *Ann Vasc Surg* 2006; 20: 278-81.
3. Shaw JA, Gravereaux EC, Winters GL, *et al*. An unusual case of claudication. *Cathet Cardiovasc Interv* 2003; 60: 562-5.

Chapter 14

Complications specific to peripheral intravascular stents

James McCaslin MBBS MRCS MD, Specialist Registrar in Vascular Surgery

Sumaira Macdonald MBChB (Comm.) FRCR FRCP PhD, Consultant Interventional Radiologist

Freeman Hospital, Newcastle upon Tyne, UK

Introduction

The origins of endovascular stenting can be traced to experimental work on canine popliteal arteries by Dotter in 1969 [1]; however, the routine use of stents has only been seen over the past two decades [2]. Stent technology continues to advance, allowing the deployment of devices in an increasing variety of locations, and a widening number of applications. From the original Palmaz stainless steel closed cell design, which conferred excellent radial force with limited flexibility, to the latest nitinol, self-expanding, tapered, hybrid and membrane mesh carotid stents, there is a huge range of stents to select from. Stents can be classified by their construction material (stainless steel, cobalt-chromium or nitinol), their structural design (open or closed cell), their deployment method (self-expanding or balloon mounted), whether or not they are covered (stent grafts) or finally, whether they are constructed specifically for the arterial territory in question. Most stents are available in a range of diameters and lengths to suit their purpose and the patient's anatomy.

For the majority, stenting is used as an adjunct to angioplasty in two main settings: first, when the result from angioplasty alone is suboptimal (e.g. elastic recoil of a vessel) and second, as a bail-out from complications related to angioplasty (e.g. flow-limiting dissection). Occasionally circumstances dictate that a stent should be used primarily to give a superior result, e.g. renal ostial stenoses or long occlusions of the superficial femoral artery (SFA) [3, 4]. This chapter examines the evidence for stenting, reviews the complications generic to all endovascular stents, and highlights the specific complications in certain arterial territories.

The evidence for vascular stenting

Iliac artery lesions

Meta-analysis of the results of stenting the aorto-iliac segment versus angioplasty alone in 2116 patients revealed higher technical success rates and no difference in 30-day complication rates [5]. Four-year stent patency rates were 77% for stenoses and 61% for occlusions, with a reduction in long-term failure of 39% after stent placement compared with angioplasty alone. Two trials have examined primary versus selective stenting in iliac lesions [6, 7]. The Dutch Iliac Stent Trial Study Group found equivocal results [7], although more recently it has been shown that in TASC C and D lesions, primary stenting was beneficial [6]. The choice of stent did not appear to have a major impact on outcome [8]. The STAG trial also reported equivalent outcomes between stenting and angioplasty at 2 years, but a higher primary success rate and lower complication rate (mainly from distal emboli) in stenting occlusive iliac disease [9]. It can be argued that stenting iliac lesions, particularly occlusions, should be performed routinely.

Femoropopliteal lesions

Endovascular treatment of infra-inguinal disease is well established in patients with intermittent claudication; however, the evidence for stenting here is less robust. Pooled results from open studies show equivocal 3-year patency rates in stenoses (61% angioplasty versus 66% stent), although encouraging results in occlusive disease (48% angioplasty versus 64% stent) [10]. A Cochrane review of SFA stenting showed a small but significant radiological benefit at 6 months, but not beyond this. Clinical outcomes followed a similar pattern with ankle brachial pressure index (ABPI) improved only initially, although treadmill walking distance remained significantly improved for 12 months [11]. It is important to note, however, that the Cochrane review included studies using stents primarily designed for use in the iliac arteries. The Vienna Absolute trial was the only trial included which used a flexible stent more suited to use in the SFA which had much more favourable results [12]. Other reviews have come to similar conclusions, but again concede that the early trials used stents that would now be considered obsolete [13]. Modern stent design, with increased flexibility and reduced vessel trauma seems to be improving the outcome of SFA stenting, with results from recent trials such as Resilient and Durability-1 suggesting ongoing improvement [4, 14-16].

Current trials such as VIBRANT will provide more information on the use of covered stents for long SFA lesions; they have the potential to improve patency by reducing neointimal hyperplasia associated with bare metal stenting.

Infrapopliteal lesions

Endovascular procedures below the popliteal artery are used almost exclusively for limb salvage; because of the high rate of complications, there is no current evidence base for this treatment in patients with claudication. In most cases, infrapopliteal angioplasty is combined with more proximal treatment [17, 18]. Stenting of the tibial arteries is usually reserved as a bailout procedure in the case of flow-limiting dissection, residual stenosis >30%, or elastic recoil, and experience is growing rapidly [19]. Driven by the success of drug-eluting stents in the coronary vessels, sirolimus-eluting stents in tibial vessels have shown promising results, with significantly better 3-year patency and lower reintervention rates than with bare metal stents [20]. With bio-absorbable stents in development and under trial, and dedicated tibial stents with thin struts that do not encroach on the small lumen inherent to tibial vessels new to the market, there may be an increased role for stenting in tibial vessels for limb salvage in the future. Whilst the cost-benefit of these products will need to be examined given the poor prognosis of patients with critical limb ischaemia, quality of life and cost-effectiveness analyses tend to favour limb-salvage strategies in this group [21, 22].

Carotid artery stenting

This is a specialised area with specific demands to include high-level technical expertise, an in-depth understanding of the indications for carotid intervention and of periprocedural haemodynamics, an understanding of specialised equipment used rarely outside of this vascular territory (to include a wide range of embolic protection devices) and complications specific to this procedure [23]. This is covered in more detail in Chapter 19.

Renal artery stenting

Renal artery stenosis (RAS) frequently represents an extension of aortic atheroma into the renal artery ostium and is therefore often stented primarily rather than relying on angioplasty alone. This is due to the elastic recoil seen particularly with lesions of the renal artery ostium. Stenting of RAS may be beneficial in the treatment of hypertension (particularly hypertension refractory to pharmacological control or malignant hypertension); a recent meta-analysis described a small but significant benefit [24]. It is also used in the treatment of renal insufficiency, although at present the evidence is mixed and probably only supports treatment in rapidly progressing renal failure or flash pulmonary oedema [25]. The results of the CORAL trial are expected in 2012, and are expected to guide the role of stenting for RAS.

Generic complications of vascular stenting

The generic complications of stent placement should include all the potential complications of angiography and angioplasty such as access problems, contrast reactions and toxicity, arterial dissection and distal embolisation (see Chapter 13).

Complications of stent deployment

During the deployment of a stent (Figures 1 and 2), three main problems can occur. First, the stent can either fail to deploy, or deploy in a faulty manner. This is especially true of balloon-mounted stents, where the stent can become dislodged from the balloon if sufficient care is not taken during its delivery to the area of deployment. This can largely be avoided by using a sheath to access the necessary area, and not passing the balloon-mounted stent 'bareback' through the arteries. If a stent does slip from a balloon, it is often possible to retrieve it provided the guide wire is still in place through the stent, using the partially inflated balloon to grip the stent and reposition it. If repositioning of the stent is not possible, then deploying the stent in a 'safe' location is often the best solution. If the stent is not retrievable using the balloon, then it is often possible to try to withdraw it back into the sheath followed by removal of the sheath and the stent.

The second major problem is maldeployment of the stent in the wrong position (Figure 3). The stent may cover the ostium of another vessel, or simply not adequately treat the target stenosis. Familiarity with the stent markers and the behaviour of the stent during its deployment (some stents advance or

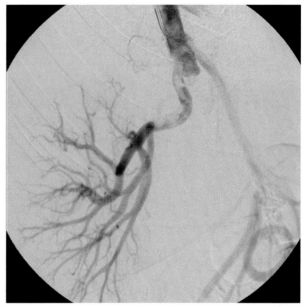

Figure 1. A heavily diseased left renal artery prior to treatment. Note that the aorta is occluded below the renal arteries.

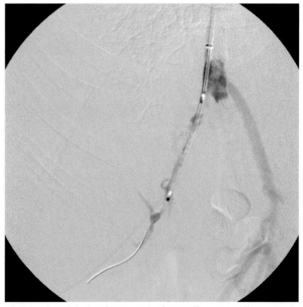

Figure 2. Mid-deployment of a self-expanding stent. Note the position markers just proximal to the first branch.

retreat fractionally), along with adequate angiography should avoid this complication. Certain self-expanding stents can be resheathed and moved following deployment, but on the whole, prevention is better than cure in this situation, and good planning is essential.

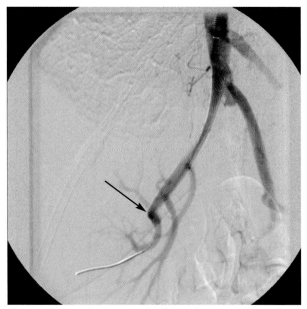

Figure 3. Maldeployment of a self-expanding stent. The stent has ridden forwards on deployment, ending up in a renal artery branch.

Third, the vessel can rupture during deployment of a stent. The external iliac artery is particularly prone to rupture, although any vessel can be affected in theory. Vessel wall calcification and steroid medication put the patient at increased risk [26, 27]. Care should be taken to observe the patient during balloon insufflation for pain. Pain that increases on balloon deflation, or that does not resolve, should raise concern, and the patient should be monitored for hypotension/tachycardia. Treatment of a rupture starts with early recognition, and there should be no delay in reacting to the situation. Care should be taken following iliac stent deployment and post-stenting balloon dilatation to maintain the balloon on the wire outside of the sheath during post-procedure angiography. In this way, rapid reinsertion of the balloon and its inflation across a rupture is straightforward and can be life-saving. No-one wants to be fumbling about for a balloon to tamponade the rupture. If balloon tamponade is insufficient to gain

control of the situation (demonstrated by continued extravasation despite 5 minutes or more of low-pressure inflation – 4 to 6 atmospheres is usually adequate) revealed by angiography via the opposite common femoral artery, a covered stent can rapidly be prepared, and after inevitable upsizing of the vascular sheath, deployed across the rupture [26]. Many experienced operators only perform iliac interventions with bilateral common femoral artery access, mindful of the potential for arterial rupture, but also to obtain accurate intra-arterial pressure measurements [28]. No iliac intervention should be commenced without prior placement of an intravenous cannula of 19 gauge or larger. Care should be taken to ensure that the patient's blood pressure is well controlled before the procedure (iliac artery rupture can rapidly be fatal and due care is warranted) [29]. Furthermore, experienced units advocate the use of bowel peristaltic agents such as buscopan or glucagon intravenously in order to ensure optimal angiographic images and thus minimise the chances of overlooking rupture due to degradation of the image by bowel gas movement.

Post-procedural complications

The long-term patency of stents varies according to location, but may be as high as 80-90% at 5 years in iliac stenoses [5]. Stent thrombosis, either primarily or secondary to stent fracture is the main mid- to long-term complication of stenting (Figures 4 and 5). Treatment of stent occlusion can be difficult, particularly radiologically. In the acute setting, a recently thrombosed stent can be recanalised by a combination of thrombolysis and restenting, but often this is not the favourable option, with patients either better managed conservatively, depending on clinical need, or with surgical revascularisation if necessary.

Restenosis within a stent can be a significant long-term problem. Restenting within the previous stent is the first-line treatment, although further restenosis can still occur (Figures 6 and 7). Drug-eluting stents, cryoplasty and brachytherapy are alternatives, but none of these has yet been shown definitively to prevent further restenosis of stented vessels [30-32].

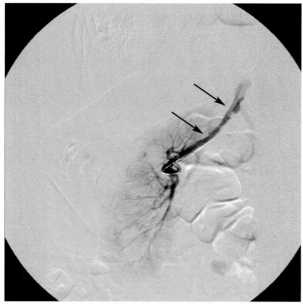

Figure 4. In-stent restenosis.

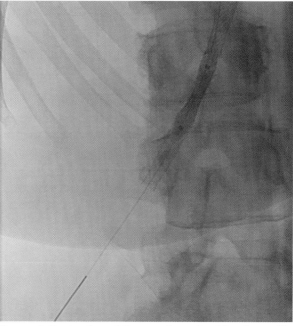

Figure 6. Restenting of the previous stent fracture with a covered stent.

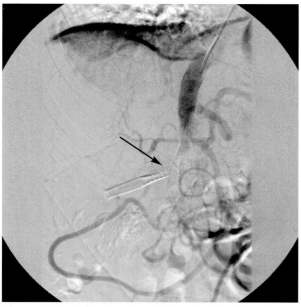

Figure 5. Stent fracture.

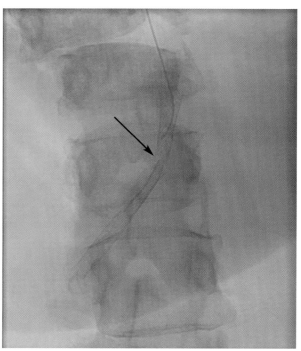

Figure 7. Re-fracture of the stent despite a second (covered) stent _in situ_.

Complications in specific stent locations

Renal artery

The renal artery is particularly prone to elastic recoil, and is often stented primarily for this reason. When stenting the renal arteries, close attention should be given to contrast volume, as renal toxicity is more of a problem here. It is also important to be especially careful with wire manipulations, as the renal parenchyma is particularly sensitive to cholesterol embolism.

Upper limb arteries

During endovascular treatment of the upper limb vessels, consideration should be given to the increased risk of stroke caused by embolisation of cholesterol fragments to either the carotid or vertebral arteries.

Tibial arteries

Due to their size and their relatively thin intimal lining, these vessels are prone to spasm and rupture. Spasm may be controlled by the local intra-arterial administration of antispasmodics such as papaverine and isosorbide dinitrate. Guide wire perforation is seldom associated with clinical sequelae but often means that the procedure has to be abandoned, though it may be rescheduled.

Conclusions

Endovascular stenting has a wide ranging set of applications, which are likely to expand in the future. Complications are relatively rare, and on the whole have endovascular solutions. Many complications can be avoided by planning and care during the procedure, and by following established guidelines. Rarely, stent complications necessitate surgical treatment, and an awareness of the problems encountered is important to the modern vascular surgeon.

Key points

- Endovascular stenting continues to develop as a technique and is likely to become more frequent with time.
- Stenting is used both primarily (e.g. iliac occlusions) and as a bailout option following angioplasty.
- Procedural complications are uncommon, and can largely be avoided with good planning and technique.
- Complications often have endovascular solutions, although surgery is occasionally necessary.
- Long-term patency of stents is reasonable, and is likely to improve with further stent development.

References

1. Dotter CT. Transluminally-placed coilspring endarterial tube grafts. Long-term patency in the canine popliteal artery. *Investigative Radiology* 1969; 4: 329-32.
2. Rosch J, Keller FS, Kaufman JA. The birth, early years, and future of interventional radiology. *J Vasc Interv Radiol* 2003; 14: 841-53.
3. van de Ven PJ, Kaatee R, Beutler JJ, *et al.* Arterial stenting and balloon angioplasty in ostial atherosclerotic renovascular disease: a randomised trial. *Lancet* 1999; 353: 282-6.
4. Sabeti S, Czerwenka-Wenkstetten A, Dick P, *et al.* Quality of life after balloon angioplasty versus stent implantation in the superficial femoral artery: findings from a randomized controlled trial. *J Endovasc Ther* 2007; 14: 431-7.
5. Bosch JL, Hunink MG. Meta-analysis of the results of percutaneous transluminal angioplasty and stent placement for aortoiliac occlusive disease. *Radiology* 1997; 204: 87-96.
6. AbuRahma AF, Hayes JD, Flaherty SK, Peery W. Primary iliac stenting versus transluminal angioplasty with selective stenting. *J Vasc Surg* 2007;46: 965-70; e962.
7. Tetteroo E, Van Der Graaf Y, Bosch JL, *et al.* Randomised comparison of primary stent placement versus primary angioplasty followed by selective stent placement in patients with iliac-artery occlusive disease. *Lancet* 1997; 351: 1153-9.

8. Ponec D, Jaff MR, Swischuk J, *et al*. The nitinol SMART stent vs. wallstent for suboptimal iliac artery angioplasty: CRISP-US trial results. *J Vasc Interv Radiol* 2004; 15: 911-8.

9. Goode SD, Hersey N, Cleveland TJ, Gaines P. STAG trial: A multicentre randomised clinical trial comparing angioplasty and stenting for the treatment of iliac occlusion. *Cardiovasc Interv Radiol* 2010; 33: 174-5.

10. Norgren L, Hiatt WR, Dormandy JA, *et al*. Inter-Society Consensus for the Management of Peripheral Arterial Disease (TASC II). *J Vasc Surg* 2007; 45: S5-67.

11. Twine CP, Coulston J, Shandall A, McLain AD. Angioplasty versus stenting for superficial femoral artery lesions. *Cochrane Database Syst Rev* 2009: CD006767.

12. Schillinger M, Sabeti S, Loewe C, *et al*. Balloon angioplasty versus implantation of nitinol stents in the superficial femoral artery. *N Engl J Med* 2006; 354: 1879-88.

13. Perrio S, Holt PJE, Patterson BO, *et al*. Role of superficial femoral artery stents in the management of arterial occlusive disease: review of current evidence. *Vascular* 2010; 18: 82-92.

14. Laird JR, Katzen BT, Scheinert D, *et al*. Nitinol stent implantation versus balloon angioplasty for lesions in the superficial femoral artery and proximal popliteal artery: twelve-month results from the RESILIENT randomized trial. *Circulation: Cardiovascular Interventions* 2010; 3: 267-76.

15. Schillinger M, Minar E. Past, present and future of femoropopliteal stenting. *J Endovasc Ther* 2009; 16: 147-52.

16. Bosiers M, Torsello G, Gissler H-M, *et al*. Nitinol stent implantation in long superficial femoral artery lesions: 12-month results of the DURABILITY I study. *J Endovasc Ther* 2009; 16: 261-9.

17. Rastogi S, Stavropoulos SW. Infrapopliteal angioplasty. *Tech Vasc Interv Radiol* 2004; 7: 33-9.

18. Bosiers M, Hart JP, Deloose K, *et al*. Endovascular therapy as the primary approach for limb salvage in patients with critical limb ischemia: experience with 443 infrapopliteal procedures. *Vascular* 2006; 14: 63-9.

19. Karnabatidis D, Katsanos K, Siablis D. Infrapopliteal stents: overview and unresolved issues. *J Endovasc Ther* 2009; 16: 153-62.

20. Siablis D, Karnabatidis D, Katsanos K, *et al*. Infrapopliteal application of sirolimus-eluting versus bare metal stents for critical limb ischemia: analysis of long-term angiographic and clinical outcome. *J Vasc Interv Radiol* 2009; 20: 1141-50.

21. Rogers LC, Lavery LA, Armstrong DG. The right to bear legs - an amendment to healthcare: how preventing amputations can save billions for the US Health-care System. *J Am Podiatr Med Ass* 2008; 98: 166-8.

22. Boutoille D, Raille A, Maulaz D, Krempf M. Quality of life with diabetes-associated foot complications: comparison between lower-limb amputation and chronic foot ulceration. *Foot Ankle Int* 2008; 29: 1074-8.

23. Macdonald S, Stansby G, Eds. *Practical Carotid Artery Stenting*, 1st ed. Springer, UK, 2009.

24. Symonides B, Gaciong Z. The effect of percutaneous revascularisation of atherosclerotic renal artery stenosis on blood pressure. Meta-analysis of randomised trials. *J Hypertens* 2010; 28: e510.

25. Steichen O, Amar L, Plouin PF. Primary stenting for atherosclerotic renal artery stenosis. *J Vasc Surg* 2010; 51: 1574-80.

26. Allaire E, Melliere D, Poussier B, *et al*. Iliac artery rupture during balloon dilatation: what treatment? *Ann Vasc Surg* 2003; 17: 306-14.

27. Lois JF, Takiff H, Schechter MS. Vessel rupture by balloon catheters complicating chronic steroid therapy. *Am J Roentgenol* 1985; 144: 1073-4.

28. McWilliams RG, Robertson I, Smye SW, *et al*. Sources of error in intra-arterial pressure measurements across a stenosis. *Eur J Vasc Endovasc Surg* 1998; 15: 535-40.

29. NCEPOD. Interventional Vascular Radiology and Interventional Neurovascular Radiology, 2000: http://www.ncepod.org.uk/pdf/2000/ir/Radiofull.pdf.

30. Duda SH, Pusich B, Richter G, *et al*. Sirolimus-eluting stents for the treatment of obstructive superficial femoral artery disease: six-month results. *Circulation* 2002; 106: 1505-9.

31. Hansrani M, Overbeck K, Smout J, Stansby G. Intravascular brachytherapy for peripheral vascular disease. *Cochrane Database Syst Rev* 2002; 4: CD003504.

32. McCaslin JE, Macdonald S, Stansby G. Cryoplasty for peripheral vascular disease. *Cochrane Database Syst Rev* 2007; 4: CD005507.

Chapter 15 Vascular complications in patients belonging to other specialties

Robin Windhaber MD FRCS, Specialist Registrar in Vascular Surgery
Simon Parvin MD FRCS, Consultant Vascular Surgeon
Royal Bournemouth Hospital, Bournemouth, UK

Introduction

Although vascular surgeons can cause inadvertent injuries to adjacent vessels during vascular reconstruction, it is not uncommon for vascular injuries to be caused by surgeons from other specialties. The commonest complications encountered arise as a result of puncture-site complications from coronary and peripheral angiography, and these are covered in the preceding chapters. Vascular complications can arise in an almost infinite and surprising number of ways; however, a number of specialties have earned the reputation of frequent flyers with repeatable patterns of injury. In this chapter we aim to describe the injuries that may reasonably be encountered along with suggestions for potential management strategies that may be followed. Rather than describe these complications by specialty they have been described anatomically, although it must be recognised that orthopaedics, general surgery, and gynaecology provide the majority of cases.

Vascular injuries

Types of vascular injury

Arterial injuries fall into one of five broad groups:

- vascular compression leading to distal ischaemia;
- intimal tear leading to occlusion and distal ischaemia;
- laceration leading to haemorrhage, arteriovenous fistula or false aneurysm formation;
- transection leading to both haemorrhage and distal ischaemia;
- embolisation.

Any of these mechanisms may be followed by a compartment syndrome after revascularisation. A rapid revascularisation is essential when dealing with loss of distal circulation and should take precedence over any other manoeuvre or procedure which may also be required.

Causes of vascular injury

The aetiology of an iatrogenic vascular injury is primarily due to one of three main causes:

- direct damage;
- external compression;
- tumour invasion.

Direct damage to a blood vessel with a surgical instrument is common. Examples include inadvertent scalpel or scissor injuries and trocar injuries, and no matter how careful the surgeon is, such injuries will happen from time to time. Surgical trauma may result from swelling in a confined space. Examples of this type of injury include ischaemic tissue damage following the prolonged application of a tourniquet to a leg during elective orthopaedic surgery or from haemorrhage following long bone fracture. Local invasion by tumour is an unusual problem, and can lead to either occlusion of, or haemorrhage from a blood vessel. In the past, dealing with such injuries was fraught with difficulty, but the ready availability of interventional radiological techniques has significantly improved the management of these patients.

Repair techniques

Repair techniques include:

- simple ligation with, or without bypass;
- simple suture;
- vein patching;
- vessel replacement;
- endovascular interventions including embolisation or stenting.

Treating a vascular complication follows the well-established routine of controlling the haemorrhage, debriding damaged tissue, and restoring the circulation with a bypass or endovascular procedure or by direct repair of the damaged blood vessel.

Vascular complications by anatomical region

Arterial injuries involving the upper limb

Injuries around the clavicle and axilla

The subclavian artery and vein may be damaged as a result of a clavicular fracture or more rarely following internal fixation of a fracture. Common injury patterns include an intimal flap resulting in occlusion, pseudoaneurysm formation or vessel transection.

Following occlusion, if the patient has a good collateral supply, is asymptomatic, and particularly when the non-dominant hand is involved, treatment may be conservative. For patients with subclavian artery occlusion where the limb is threatened, or when the patient may place significant demands upon the limb (dominant limb or active lifestyle), a more invasive approach may be adopted. Standard surgical bypass often requires wide exposure and dissection in traumatised tissues with significant associated morbidity. Radiological intervention, often with the deployment of an endovascular stent graft is an effective alternative technique which has been shown to be associated with a shorter procedure time and reduced blood loss compared to standard surgical techniques [1] (Figure 1).

False aneurysms of the subclavian or axillary artery have been described following clavicular fracture and fixation, anterior shoulder dislocation, shoulder surgery, and proximal humeral fractures. Conservative treatment with ultrasound-guided compression is a safe and effective treatment, provided that the site of injury can be accessed and compressed externally [2]. Alternative radiological treatments are ultrasound-guided injection of thrombin and the placement of an endovascular covered stent [3, 4]. Modern stents are flexible with a low fracture potential and have the major advantage of avoiding the acute area of injury when compared with traditional surgical approaches [5]. Surgery is usually reserved for situations when radiological support is not available. The standard surgical approach involves primary suture repair with or

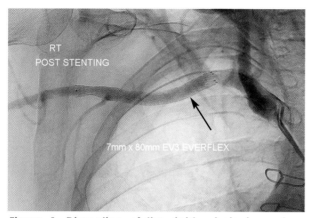

Figure 1. Dissection of the right subclavian artery caused by a fractured clavicle treated with an endovascular stent (arrow).

without the use of a vein patch. Occasionally, if the injury is extensive, formal ligation may be undertaken followed by bypass if necessary.

Arterial transection is best treated by open surgical repair in order to arrest bleeding and restore circulation to the arm. Re-anastomosis following mobilisation, interposition grafting (with either vein or prosthetic material) and ligation with bypass have all been described as effective treatments [6, 7]. The choice of technique is largely dependent on anatomical considerations and the surgeon's preference. If the injury is closed, and the transection is either incomplete or the vessel ends are in close apposition, endovascular insertion of a covered stent may be an effective strategy [8].

Injuries around the elbow

Brachial artery entrapment or occlusion following a supracondylar humeral fracture of the elbow is a common pattern of injury in children, occurring in up to 14% of cases [9]. Studies have shown that early recognition of the injury along with prompt surgical exploration improves outcome compared with the traditional approach of watch and wait if pulses are not restored following closed reduction [10, 11]. In one recent series, failure to restore brachial artery patency following supracondylar fracture was associated with the development of ischaemic contracture of the forearm in almost every case (23 of 26 total cases). In only four of the injuries was the brachial artery

explored surgically, three being performed successfully and in one case unsuccessfully (at 48 hours); this patient went on to develop an ischaemic contracture [12].

Injures of the vessels in the forearm and at the wrist

A number of mechanisms have been described in which the blood vessels may be injured below the elbow, commonly involving trauma at a fracture site, traction during dislocation, direct injury during internal fracture fixation or following radial artery puncture (increasingly common as cardiologists use this route as access to coronary angiography). In individuals with normal anatomy, an occlusion of either the radial or ulnar arteries is unlikely to cause significant symptoms and frequently requires no treatment. When either the radial or ulnar artery is transected, they may be ligated with impunity, providing that the integrity of the collateral circulation is confirmed. Primary repair is possible in experienced hands, but is usually unnecessary.

False aneurysm formation following vessel trauma in the forearm is usually seen after radial artery puncture during cardiac catheterisation or line insertion, but may also occur following forearm fracture or following internal fixation [13, 14]. Timely operative intervention is indicated in these patients if false aneurysm rupture is to be avoided [15]. Thrombin injection or the use of a covered stent is rarely indicated in the forearm or elbow.

Complications involving the neck vessels

Carotid artery injuries

Sharp injuries to the carotid artery may occur during central venous catheterisation and neck surgery. In addition, accidental catheterisation of the carotid artery during central venous cannulation can occur and is associated with obesity, emergency puncture and lack of ultrasound guidance. If an arterial injury has been identified, and it is not safe just to remove the catheter, consideration should be given to leaving it in place, and seeking advice about possible surgical or radiological intervention [16].

Whilst ultrasound guidance has certainly made the procedure safer, it has not eliminated the risk of arterial injury completely. The carotid artery is at risk during most surgical procedures involving the anterior or posterior triangles of the neck. It has been well described following ENT, maxillofacial, orthopaedic and general surgical procedures. The approach to treatment depends on surgical access and the site and extent of the vessel injury. Traditional open surgical procedures have more recently been replaced by endovascular interventions.

Blunt injuries affecting the carotid artery have been described as a result of a diverse array of mechanisms including rugby tackles [17], cervical spine fractures [18] and even following love bites [19]. The symptomatology may be inconspicuous, and the presentation is frequently delayed. The mechanism is carotid dissection due to hyperextension of the neck with rotation, basal skull (K) fracture or direct blunt trauma. The diagnosis can be confirmed by CT angiography or MRI, although selective angiography and duplex imaging may play a role. In major injuries, the management requires a multidisciplinary approach, addressing airway issues, management of cervical spine and neurological injuries, alongside control of bleeding or maintenance of cerebrovascular blood supply. Treatment of the carotid injury depends on the location of the damage within the artery. Prognosis is good in most patients with carotid dissection due to blunt trauma, and in most cases no intervention is required, other than a consideration about whether anticoagulation might prevent secondary thrombosis.

Complications involving the neck veins

Direct injury to the internal and external jugular veins can occur during surgery, following direct penetrating trauma or after venous cannulation. Small defects can be controlled adequately with direct pressure; however, significant injuries usually require open surgical repair or ligation which can usually be carried out with impunity.

Occlusion of the neck veins may occur due to compression from tumour, haematoma or from thrombosis (usually surrounding a catheter). The mainstay of treatment is medical, although on rare occasions endovascular stenting may be indicated for symptom control in patients with superior vena caval syndrome.

Vascular injuries involving the thorax and abdomen

Aortic injuries

Spinal fractures and surgery place not only the thoracic and abdominal aorta at risk, but also the iliac vessels. Injuries are rare but potentially lethal. Aortic and iliac injuries may occur following instrumentation of the disc space [20] or following placement of pedicle screws [21]. During the posterior spinal approach, prone positioning and the need to prevent contamination of exposed bone and metalwork poses additional problems to the vascular surgeon attempting management of a major vessel injury. In a stable patient where the expertise is available, endovascular repair has been used to treat aortic injuries [22]; however, in the event of acute life-threatening bleeding it may be necessary to adopt a standard open approach with either repair or replacement of the affected segment.

There have been a number of great vessel injuries described as a result of laparoscopic procedures. The incidence of major vessel injury during the establishment of laparoscopic access is low (approximately 0.05%) for closed entry using a Verres needle, but is reduced to almost zero by the use of an open access technique [23]. When major vessel injury occurs, immediate conversion to laparotomy is usually required to control bleeding. Simple closure or patch repair is often possible, with graft repair reserved for the most serious of injuries.

Injuries to the epigastric and visceral arteries

More commonly, an epigastric or pre-peritoneal vessel can be injured leading to bleeding or false aneurysm formation. The treatment options are suture ligation or radiological intervention by means of embolisation. Figure 2 shows an injury to a branch of the inferior epigastric artery, which occurred during gynaecological laparoscopy. This was successfully treated with coil embolisation (Figure 3) and the patient made a full recovery.

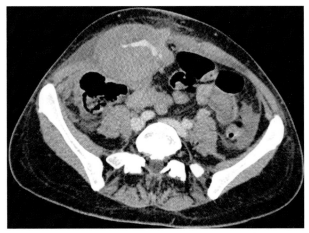

Figure 2. A large rectus sheath haematoma following a trocar injury.

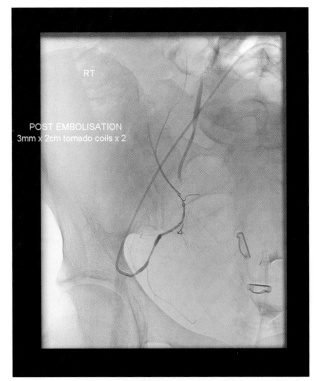

RT

POST EMBOLISATION
3mm x 2cm tornado coils x 2

Figure 3. Coil embolisation of the injured inferior epigastric artery.

Rarely, intestinal surgery may lead to delayed arteriovenous fistula formation, usually as a consequence of joint ligation of an artery and a vein. This has been seen in the ileocolic artery following appendicectomy [24]. Modern treatment would be by embolisation of the fistula where previously, right hemicolectomy would have been indicated. False aneurysms of the ileocolic artery, following laparoscopic right hemicolectomy for Crohn's disease, have been successfully treated endovascularly [25].

Injuries to the great veins

Venous injuries may occur in a similar way during spinal surgery and are often concomitant with arterial injury, particularly in the common iliac region where the veins lie posterior and adjacent to the arteries. Usually these venous injuries can be repaired primarily; however, if the damage is extensive, primary repair may not be possible and ligation of the iliac veins or inferior vena cava (IVC) may be required. Long-term sequelae are rare, and even ligation of the suprarenal IVC is possible in a damage control situation [26]. General surgical and vascular procedures are occasionally associated with venous injury and frequently affect the pelvic veins during the mobilisation of pelvic organs or arteries. Immediate surgical repair is the rule, as access is already in place. Simple suture of the vein is facilitated by proximal and distal control.

Lower limb vascular injuries

Injuries to the iliac and femoral arteries

Arterial injury is a rare complication of hip arthroplasty, occurring in fewer than 0.2% of cases. The commonest sites for injury (in decreasing frequency) are the external iliac and common femoral arteries followed by the internal iliac and then the profunda femoris artery [27]. Most are direct vessel injuries [28] although ruptured false aneurysm following revision of an infected prosthesis has been well described [29]. The management of non-infected arterial injuries is dependent on the vessel involved, the extent of the injury and available expertise.

Injuries to the external iliac artery can be treated safely by primary repair with, or without vein patch, excision and interposition grafting, ligation and bypass or insertion of an endovascular covered stent. Injuries to the internal iliac artery or its branches can often be treated by radiological embolisation; if this technique is not available, surgical ligation may be possible. Providing that the contralateral internal iliac artery is patent, significant sequelae from embolisation are rare [30].

Injuries to the common femoral artery are preferably treated by primary open surgical repair and a vein patch. Occasionally it may be necessary to excise the damaged artery and use an interposition graft; prosthetic material such as Dacron® or PTFE is adequate unless there is a risk of local sepsis when long saphenous vein is the conduit of choice.

Injuries involving the profunda femoris artery usually involve its branches rather than the main trunk and these can safely be ligated or embolised, with little risk to the limb.

A rare complication of varicose vein surgery is damage to the femoral artery bifurcation. Rarer still is inadvertent stripping of the femoral artery instead of the long saphenous vein. When this happens the long saphenous vein may be suitable for restoring the arterial circulation (Figure 4).

Injures around the knee

Popliteal arterial injury following total knee replacement is a rare but limb-threatening injury with an incidence of approximately 0.2%. Injury patterns include intra-operative haemorrhage, thrombosis, false

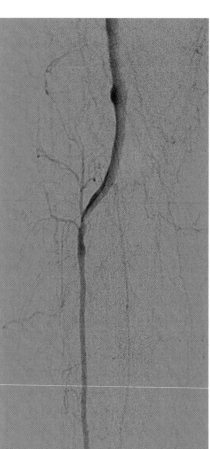

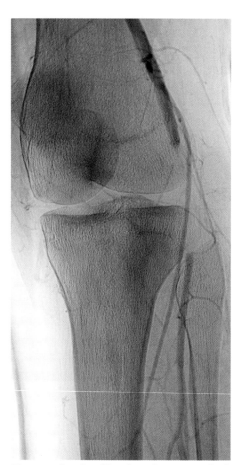

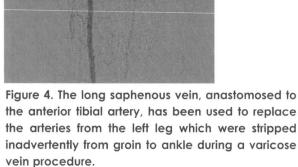

Figure 4. The long saphenous vein, anastomosed to the anterior tibial artery, has been used to replace the arteries from the left leg which were stripped inadvertently from groin to ankle during a varicose vein procedure.

Figure 5. Popliteal artery occlusion following traumatic dislocation of the knee.

aneurysm and arteriovenous fistula formation. Early recognition of the injury and prompt intervention are vital if limb loss is to be prevented. Definitive treatment of the arterial injury can be by open primary repair, interposition grafting, bypass grafting or endovascular stenting [31]. The application of a tourniquet in the presence of peripheral vascular disease has been implicated in the increased incidence of arterial complications during total knee arthroplasty [32]. At present, there are little hard data to show at what level of ischaemia the use of a tourniquet becomes unsafe.

Failure to recognise popliteal artery damage following dislocation of the knee can lead to amputation, and a high index of suspicion is important following this uncommon injury (Figure 5). Regular examination of the circulation to the leg is an important component of care after joint replacement, particularly in a high-risk patient.

Miscellaneous vascular injuries

An embarrassing injury can occur during a midline laparotomy incision when a femorofemoral graft is divided. Once bleeding is controlled, however, the graft can usually be re-anastomosed, providing that there is no contamination from the abdominal contents.

Conclusions

Iatrogenic vascular injury is thankfully uncommon. If unrecognised, it can have very important long-term consequences for the patient and frequently leads to litigation. The advent of endovascular techniques has led to a dramatic reduction in the need for surgical intervention and most false aneurysms can now be treated radiologically. The pattern of these iatrogenic injuries has changed over the years as surgical techniques evolve. The rise of laparoscopic surgery, while reducing the incidence of some injuries, has led to an increase in others.

There will always be vascular injuries caused by other specialties, but in the future most will be dealt with by interventional radiological techniques. Iatrogenic vascular injuries are very distressing for the responsible clinician and in the acute situation it can be impossible for that individual to retrieve the situation. The experienced vascular surgeon or interventional radiologist should always be called in to help. They should remain calm and follow the basic principles of emergency surgery, namely to control the haemorrhage and to then maintain or restore the circulation.

Key points

- Vascular surgeons are frequently required to assist in the management of vascular complications occurring in patients belonging to non-vascular specialties.
- Most of these injuries can be managed using a combination of interventional radiology and open surgical techniques.
- Rapid revascularisation is essential when dealing with injuries which involve loss of circulation to the extremities and vital organs.
- Valuable time can often be bought with the judicious use of both arterial and venous temporary shunts.
- Injury to the major veins can be life-threatening and ligation is often required, with little subsequent morbidity.
- Compartment syndrome following major flow disruption to the extremities must be considered and fasciotomy performed at an early stage.
- Endovascular techniques are continuing to develop and it is essential that these are always available for the treatment of patients who develop vascular complications.

References

1. Castelli P, Caronno R, Piffaretti G, *et al*. Endovascular repair of traumatic injuries of the subclavian and axillary arteries. *Injury* 2005; 36: 778-82.

2. Szendro G, Golcman L, Klimov A, *et al*. Successful non-surgical management of traumatic pseudoaneurysm of the axillary artery by duplex-guided compression obliteration. *Eur J Vasc Endovasc Surg* 1997; 13: 513-4.

3. Kumar RM, Reddy SS, Sharma R, *et al*. Endovascular repair of a traumatic axillary artery pseudoaneurysm. *Cardiovasc Intervent Radiol* 2009; 32: 598-600.

4. Schonholz CJ, Uflacker R, De Gregorio MA, *et al*. Stent-graft treatment of trauma to the supra-aortic arteries. A review. *J Cardiovasc Surg* (Torino) 2007; 48: 537-49.

5. Michaluk BT, Deutsch E, Moufid R, *et al*. Endovascular repair of an axillary artery pseudoaneurysm attributed to hyperextension injury. *Ann Vasc Surg* 2009; 23: 412: e5-9.

6. Sriussadaporn S. Vascular injuries of the upper arm. *J Med Assoc Thai* 1997; 80: 160-8.

7. Pillai L, Luchette FA, Romano KS, *et al*. Upper-extremity arterial injury. *Am Surg* 1997; 63: 224-7.

8. Danetz JS, Cassano AD, Stoner MC, *et al*. Feasibility of endovascular repair in penetrating axillosubclavian injuries: a retrospective review. *J Vasc Surg* 2005; 4: 246-54.

9. Louahem DM, Nebunescu A, Canavese F, *et al*. Neurovascular complications and severe displacement in supracondylar humerus fractures in children: defensive or offensive strategy? *J Pediatr Orthop B* 2006; 15: 51-7.

10. Korompilias AV, Lykissas MG, Mitsionis GI, *et al*. Treatment of pink pulseless hand following supracondylar fractures of the humerus in children. *Int Orthop* 2009; 33: 237-41.

11. Mangat KS, Martin AG, Bache CE. The 'pulseless pink' hand after supracondylar fracture of the humerus in children: the predictive value of nerve palsy. *J Bone Joint Surg Br* 2009; 91: 1521-5.

12. Blakey CM, Biant LC, Birch R. Ischaemia and the pink, pulseless hand complicating supracondylar fractures of the humerus in childhood: long-term follow-up. *J Bone Joint Surg Br* 2009; 91: 1487-92.

13. Amrani A, Dandane M, El Alami Z, *et al*. False aneurysm of the radial artery: unusual complication of both-bone forearm fracture in children: a case report. *Cases J* 2008; 1: 170.

14. Dao KD, Venn-Watson E, Shin AY. Radial artery pseudoaneurysm complication from use of AO/ASIF volar distal radius plate: a case report. *J Hand Surg Am* 2001; 26: 448-53.

15. Erdoes LS, Brown WC. Ruptured ulnar artery pseudoaneurysm. *Ann Vasc Surg* 1995; 9: 394-6.

16. Pikwer A, Acosta S, Kolbel T, *et al*. Management of inadvertent arterial catheterisation associated with central venous access procedures. *Eur J Vasc Endovasc Surg* 2009; 38: 707-14.

17. Thakore N, Abbas S, Vanniasingham P. Delayed rupture of common carotid artery following rugby tackle injury: a case report. *World J Emerg Surg* 2008; 3: 14.

18. Leach JC, Malham GM. Complete recovery following atlantoaxial fracture-dislocation with bilateral carotid and vertebral artery injury. *Br J Neurosurg* 2009; 23: 92-4.

19. Wu TY, Hsiao J, Wong EH. Love bites: an unusual cause of blunt internal carotid artery injury. *NZ Med J* 2010; 123(1326): 112-5.

20. Smythe WR, Carpenter JP. Upper abdominal aortic injury during spinal surgery. *J Vasc Surg* 1997; 25: 774-7.

21. Kakkos SK, Shepard AD. Delayed presentation of aortic injury by pedicle screws: report of two cases and review of the literature. *J Vasc Surg* 2008; 47: 1074-82.

22. Minor ME, Morrissey NJ, Peress R, *et al*. Endovascular treatment of an iatrogenic thoracic aortic injury after spinal instrumentation: case report. *J Vasc Surg* 2004; 39: 893-6.

23. Larobina M, Nottle P. Complete evidence regarding major vascular injuries during laparoscopic access. *Surg Laparosc Endosc Percutan Tech* 2005; 15: 119-23.

24. De Gregorio MA, Gimeno MJ, Medrano J, *et al*. Ileocolic arteriovenous fistula with superior mesenteric vein aneurysm: endovascular treatment. *Cardiovasc Intervent Radiol* 2004; 27: 556-9.

25. Edden Y, Shussman N, Cohen MJ, *et al*. Endovascular treatment of ileocolic pseudoaneurysm after a laparoscopic-assisted bowel resection for Crohn disease. *Vasc Endovascular Surg* 2008; 42: 173-5.

26. Sullivan PS, Dente CJ, Patel S, *et al*. Outcome of ligation of the inferior vena cava in the modern era. *Am J Surg* 2010; 199: 500-6.

27. Leiva L, Arroyo A, Gil J, Rodriguez AI, *et al*. Arterial trauma in hip arthroplasty. *Cir Esp* 2008; 83: 125-8.

28. Parvizi J, Pulido L, Slenker N, *et al*. Vascular injuries after total joint arthroplasty. *J Arthroplasty* 2008; 23: 1115-21.

29. Wera GD, Ting NT, Della Valle CJ, *et al*. External iliac artery injury complicating prosthetic hip resection for infection. *J Arthroplasty* 2010; 25: 660 e1-4.

30. Travis T, Monsky WL, London J, *et al*. Evaluation of short-term and long-term complications after emergent internal iliac artery embolization in patients with pelvic trauma. *J Vasc Interv Radiol* 2008; 19: 840-7.

31. Pal A, Clarke JM, Cameron AE. Case series and literature review: popliteal artery injury following total knee replacement. *Int J Surg* 2010; 8: 430-5.

32. Smith DE, McGraw RW, Taylor DC, *et al*. Arterial complications and total knee arthroplasty. *J Am Acad Orthop Surg* 2001; 9: 253-7.

Case vignette   Ruptured axillary artery

Robin Windhaber MD FRCS, Specialist Registrar in Vascular Surgery
Simon Parvin MD FRCS, Consultant Vascular Surgeon
Royal Bournemouth Hospital, Bournemouth, UK

A 64-year-old gentleman was referred to the vascular team with complications arising from axillary metastases, having originally presented 4 years previously with squamous cell carcinoma of the thumb. Despite radiotherapy the axillary mass caused axillary vein thrombosis and invaded the axillary artery with eventual rupture and bleeding. Figure 1 shows disruption of the right axillary artery and the feeding vessels of the tumour mass; there was no active extravasation at this point. Bleeding was arrested and the blood supply restored to the arm by insertion of a covered stent (Figure 2).

The symptoms were relieved for 4 months, but unfortunately the disease progressed leading to further erosion of the axillary artery and subsequent rebleeding. After careful discussion, a repeat angiogram was performed (Figure 3) showing vessel

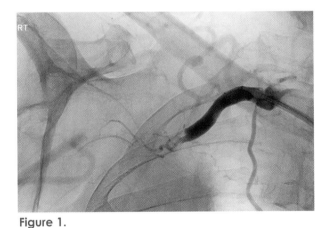

Figure 1.

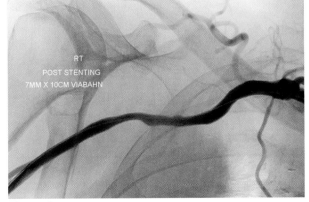

Figure 2.

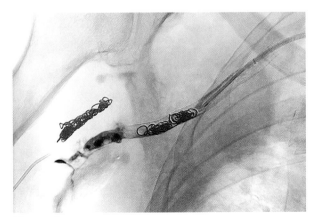

Figure 3.

Figure 4.

rupture at the distal end of the covered stent. Embolisation of the distal axillary and proximal brachial arteries was performed and the bleeding controlled (Figure 4). Whilst the arm suffered an initial degree of ischaemia, his symptoms were much improved and the axillary wound became manageable allowing him to go home. Figure 5 shows the axilla and highlights the difficulties that would have been encountered if an open surgical approach had been adopted.

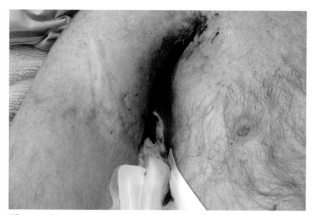

Figure 5.

Case vignette Radiation arteritis

Frank C. T. Smith BSc MD FRCS FRCSEd, Reader & Honorary Consultant Vascular Surgeon
University of Bristol & Bristol Royal Infirmary, Bristol, UK

A 72-year-old right-handed man presented with debilitating right arm claudication. Some years earlier he had undergone axillary radiotherapy for squamous cell carcinoma. Wrist pulses were diminished, and post-radiation telangiectasia was apparent in the axilla and upper arm (Figure 1). Duplex ultrasonography confirmed reduced brachial artery blood flow and arteriography demonstrated focal stenotic disease in the distal brachial artery, above the elbow (Figure 2). The artery was explored under general anaesthesia, confirming peri-adventitial inflammation and fibrosis. A reversed saphenous vein interposition graft was employed to bypass the diseased segment, with good restoration of blood flow to the forearm and hand (Figure 3).

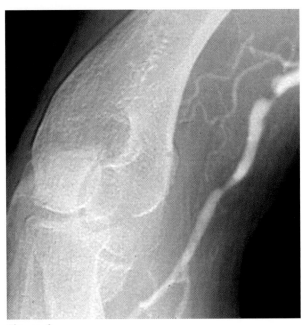

Figure 2.

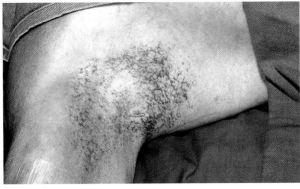

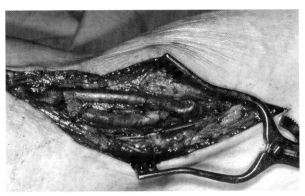

Figure 1.

Note that bypass for focal radiation-induced strictures is often successful, whereas surgery carries a poor prognosis for the diffuse disease of giant cell arteritis; administration of steroids may be the treatment of choice for arteritis.

Figure 3.

Part 2

Complications related to specific vascular and endovascular procedures

Chapter 16 Abdominal aortic aneurysm

Peng Foo Wong MB ChB MD FRCS (Gen Surg), Specialist Registrar in Vascular Surgery
Michael G. Wyatt MSc MD FRCS, Consultant Vascular Surgeon and Honorary Reader
Freeman Hospital, Newcastle upon Tyne, UK

Introduction

An aneurysm is defined as localised dilatation of all three layers of a blood vessel, resulting in an increased vessel diameter of more than 50% compared to the adjacent normal vessel. Most authorities use an aortic diameter of 3cm or more to define an abdominal aortic aneurysm (AAA). The prevalence of AAA increases with age; it occurs in up to 4% in men aged between 65 and 74 years old.

The main risk of an untreated AAA is progressive expansion leading to rupture, exsanguination and death; the overall mortality rate from rupture is about 85%. Less commonly, an AAA can undergo thrombosis or embolise distally to the legs. The risk of AAA rupture is related to its size. Most asymptomatic AAA which are less than 5.5cm can be managed by ultrasound surveillance, since the risk of rupture is low, as shown by the UK Small Aneurysm Trial (UKSAT) [1] and the Veterans Administration Aneurysm Detection and Management (ADAM) Trial [2]. Urgent surgical intervention is justified in ruptured and symptomatic AAA, regardless of size, provided there is no terminal pre-morbid diagnosis. Some have suggested that an AAA expansion rate of more than 0.5cm in 6 months in an AAA <5.5cm warrants surgical intervention, but there is scant evidence.

The main aim of treating asymptomatic large AAA is prevention of rupture with its inherent high mortality rate. The decision to perform an elective intervention involves weighing the risk of aneurysm rupture against the risk of complications or death. To understand the risk: benefit ratio of elective asymptomatic AAA repair, it is important to know the annual rupture rate of an AAA in relation to its diameter (Table 1). The peri-operative mortality after elective open and endovascular AAA repair (EVAR) is between 5-10% and 2-5%, respectively, and varies with the workload (volume) of a particular unit or surgeon. The mortality rate after open repair of a ruptured AAA is

Table 1. Annual rupture rate for AAA [3].

AAA diameter (cm)	Rupture risk (%/year)
<4	<0.5
4.1 - 4.9	0.5 - 5
5.0 - 5.9	3 - 15
6.0 - 6.9	10 - 20
7.0 - 7.9	20 - 40
>8.0	30 - 50

considerably higher, and ranges between 40% and 50%.

Open abdominal aortic aneurysm repair

Pre-operative knowledge of the anatomy of the AAA is crucial for planning an appropriate operative approach and anticipating potential problems. All patients undergo pre-operative CT. An aneurysm that extends to, or above the level of the renal arteries will probably need suprarenal clamping. An aneurysmal iliac artery of more than 3cm will require simultaneous repair.

Haemorrhage

Major haemorrhage during open AAA surgery can require massive blood transfusion that has serious postoperative consequences: cardiorespiratory, metabolic and haematological complications. Intra-operative haemorrhage is self-perpetuating, since hypothermia, metabolic acidosis and coagulopathy further inhibit clot formation. All possible avenues to limit the amount of blood loss should be considered.

Control of arteries

Rapid proximal aortic control of a ruptured AAA is fundamental; intraperitoneal rupture often results in unsalvageable catastrophic exsanguination; however, many people who survive to reach the operating theatre have a contained retroperitoneal leak. At operation, haemodynamic decompensation can occur immediately on induction of anaesthesia, once muscular tamponade of the haematoma is lost. Therefore, abdominal incision must commence as soon as anaesthetic induction is achieved; this means the operative site should be prepared and draped with the patient awake. Rapid proximal aortic control is often facilitated by manual compression of the supracoeliac aorta or applying a vertical aortic clamp at the level of the diaphragmatic crura. The clamp can be moved below the renal arteries after exposing the neck of the aneurysm. Other options for proximal control include an intra-aortic balloon catheter

introduced directly through the aneurysm or via a transfemoral or left brachial approach. Similarly, distal control can be achieved in difficult situations with balloon embolectomy catheters. A Foley catheter can be used for proximal control if an aortic balloon is not available.

Graft anastomosis

In a heavily diseased and friable aneurysm neck, suture lines can be reinforced with Dacron strips or pledgets. The use of glue has been discussed in a previous chapter (Chapter 6). A slackened suture can be tightened using a nerve hook; an additional suture is then inserted through the slack segment and tied to a buttress suture. Proximal anastomotic suture hole bleeding can be controlled with pressure or by repeat flushing of the graft with aspirated extruded blood. An alternative is to use a piece of muscle harvested from the rectus abdominis sutured as a buttress over the defect.

Lower limb ischaemia

The risk of distal embolisation to the lower limbs and viscera is minimised by the use of intravenous heparin and limiting direct manipulation of the AAA. Clamping the distal arteries before cross-clamping the aorta may reduce embolisation of mural thrombus. Before lower extremity blood flow is restored, the graft and outflow vessels should be allowed to back bleed and then irrigated with heparin-saline solution and any thrombus removed.

An absent femoral pulse following declamping needs further exploration. This may require a femoral embolectomy, either directly through the graft or by performing a separate incision in the groin. If the flow is still inadequate, revision of the graft is required and could involve an aortofemoral or femorofemoral bypass.

The lack of an audible Doppler signal in the popliteal artery after AAA repair is suspicious of embolisation; thrombo-embolectomy should be performed with a balloon catheter. Loss of ankle pulses can be ignored if perfusion of the foot is satisfactory. Ischaemic feet with palpable ankle pulses (trash foot) should be treated conservatively as the occlusions cannot be cleared by balloon catheters. Heparin or low-molecular-weight heparin should be used to prevent further clot propagation.

Colonic ischaemia

Colonic ischaemia is rare after elective open AAA repair (<1%), but occurs after 15-20% of operations for ruptured AAA. A number of methods have been used to try and detect colonic ischaemia intra-operatively: measurement of inferior mesenteric artery (IMA) stump pressure, Doppler, laser Doppler and pulse oximetry. The problem is that colonic ischaemia generally develops postoperatively and not whilst the patient is fully oxygenated under general anaesthetic. The classical early postoperative signs of bloody diarrhoea with signs of peritonitis are non-specific and unreliable, being absent in at least one third of patients. Plasma lactate elevated above 2.5mmol/L is sensitive for detecting colonic ischaemia, but not specific. Shock, major blood loss and loss of blood flow to the internal iliac arteries are all known risk factors.

When colonic ischaemia is predicted, some surgeons reimplant the inferior mesenteric artery (IMA) at the time of AAA repair. However, this is usually unnecessary due to collateralisation from the coeliac and superior mesenteric arteries (SMA). Reimplantation should be considered if there is evidence of stenosis to both the SMA and coeliac arteries, occlusion of both internal iliac arteries and/or the sigmoid colon remains dusky after perfusion of the viscera and lower limbs. The IMA may be reimplanted directly into the aortic graft or the left limb of a bifurcated graft. The Carrel patch technique is often useful here, although the cuff of native aorta around the origin of the IMA should be kept small to prevent subsequent aneurysm formation.

There should be a high index of suspicion of colonic ischaemia postoperatively in patients who do not seem to be progressing as expected in the presence of leukocytosis, and elevated lactate and D-dimer levels. Early sigmoidoscopy has been advocated, but this can be challenging in the unprepared bowel in a very ill patient. An urgent CT scan, or even exploratory laparotomy will often be more useful; if confirmed, segmental colonic resection with colostomy formation is the treatment of choice.

Graft infection

Graft infection following open AAA repair has been reported to occur in 2-3% of patients. The main organisms implicated are *Staphylococcus epidermidis*, *Staphylococcus aureus* and *Streptococcus faecalis*. More recently, methicillin-resistant *Staphylococcus aureus* (MRSA) has emerged as a major pathogen in graft infection. Early infection is often due to seeding of the organisms (which are more virulent) at the time of surgery. Late infections often involve less virulent bacteria such as *Staphylococcus epidermidis*, which may have been implanted at the time of surgery, or arrived by haematogenous or lymphatic seeding. Apart from the classical systemic features of sepsis, aortic graft infections can present with anaemia, a purulent wound discharge, local or gastrointestinal haemorrhage, false aneurysm formation and septic emboli. The investigation and management of aortic graft infection is similar to that for graft-enteric or aorto-enteric fistulae and is described below. It is essential that empirical broad-spectrum antibiotics should by prescribed for all patients.

Aorto-enteric fistula

Aorto-enteric fistula (AEF) is rare and can be classified as primary or secondary. An AEF is defined as a communication between the native aorta and the gastrointestinal (GI) tract. Primary AEF is excessively rare. Secondary AEF usually develops following open AAA repair with an incidence of 0.6-4% of aortic procedures. They often present months and even years following aortic surgery. Secondary AEF are subdivided into two types: Type 1, termed a true AEF, develops between the proximal aortic suture and bowel wall and usually presents with a massive haematemesis, although there may have been a number of previous smaller herald bleeds; Type 2, or para-prosthetic-enteric fistula, do not develop a communication between bowel and graft. Bleeding from the GI tract is caused by erosion of the bowel wall by mechanical pulsation of the aortic graft and may present with melaena. Sepsis is more frequently associated with Type 2 AEF. In order to prevent AEF, after AAA repair, the aortic sac and the retroperitoneum should be closed over the graft in layers. If the aneurysm sac and retroperitoneum cannot be used to cover the graft completely, a pedicle of omentum should be mobilised with its arterial supply. The omentum is drawn through an opening in the transverse mesocolon and secured over the prosthetic graft, to prevent its contact with bowel.

The clinical manifestation of AEF is always gastrointestinal bleeding. There should be a high index of suspicion in any patient with haematemesis or melaena and a past history of aortic surgery. Due to their anatomical proximity, the majority of cases involve the duodenum and the proximal suture line of an aortic graft. The diagnosis is confirmed on CT (Figure 1) or by the use of selective mesenteric angiography. Upper GI endoscopy may be helpful to exclude other causes of bleeding, and the diagnosis is strongly implicated in the absence of alternative pathology.

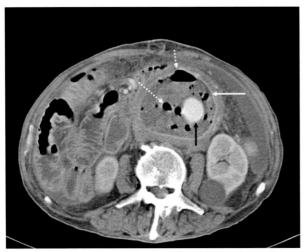

Figure 1. CT scan showing extensive peri-graft gas (dotted white arrow) as a result of graft (black arrow) infection. There is also ring enhancement of the old aneurysm sac (solid white arrow) further suggesting infection.

Prompt diagnosis and surgical intervention are crucial in managing AEF, since the reported mortality rates for all forms of treatment are high (50-60%). Standard treatment is graft excision with extra-

anatomic bypass; *in situ* replacement with antibiotic-bonded graft or autogenous femoral vein are alternatives. In order to achieve adequate aortic control, supracoeliac clamping is often required. This is followed by distal control and graft excision. If an extra-anatomic graft is used, the aortic stump is oversewn after debridement of all necrotic tissue to reduce the risk of further infection and aortic stump blow-out. Removal of all necrotic aorta, so that healthy aorta is sutured to close the aortic stump is the best way to prevent this complication. A flap of pre-vertebral fascia or pledgets from the rectus sheath may be used to buttress the stump closure, followed by omentoplasty to limit reinfection. The duodenal defect is debrided to healthy edges and closed in two layers. Modern *in situ* grafting involves the use of harvested superficial femoral veins from both legs. These can be fashioned into a tube or bifurcated aortic graft and used to replace the infected prosthetic aortic graft. An end-to-end anastomosis of the vein to the aorta is performed with 'downsizing' of the aorta using two or three separate through-and-through sutures. The second vein graft is anastomosed to the first vein 5cm below this proximal anastomosis. Alternative configurations involve making a bifurcate graft or a unilateral aorto-iliac/femoral bypass with a femorofemoral extension. Harvesting superficial femoral vein is contra-indicated in patients with previous deep venous thrombosis. It is also a more time-consuming and demanding procedure and may not be suitable for many patients with AEF who are often extremely ill. Furthermore, this procedure carries a risk of venous hypertension and lower limb compartment syndrome. Despite a higher risk of mortality than standard treatment, infection is usually eliminated in survivors, which makes it the procedure of choice for selected patients [4].

A possible endovascular approach to AEF, particularly in unfit or unstable patients is to place a covered stent across the aortic anastomotic defect. This is described as a useful bridging technique to gain time before planning a definitive procedure

Sexual dysfunction

The autonomic nerve plexus lies anterior and to the left of the aorta, encircling the origin of the inferior mesenteric artery and crosses the left common iliac artery. Injury to the plexus can result in impotence and retrograde ejaculation in as many as 80% of men. Prinssen and colleagues, however, reported that the incidence of sexual dysfunction is high in patients with AAA, even before treatment [5]. In order to avoid these complications, the peritoneum and aneurysm sac should be opened along the right anterolateral aspect onto the right common iliac artery, thus avoiding the inferior mesenteric plexus. Dissection of the left common iliac artery is performed at its bifurcation. The approach is lateral, rather than anterior, to the sigmoid mesocolon.

Additionally, at least one internal iliac artery should be preserved during open aorto-iliac aneurysm surgery to maintain pelvic blood supply. Retrospective studies have shown that EVAR carries a lower risk of sexual dysfunction than open AAA surgery, as long as at least one internal iliac artery is preserved. In one study, both open AAA repair and EVAR had an impact on sexual function, but after EVAR, recovery to pre-operative levels was faster. At 3 months, sexual function was similar in both groups [5].

Compartment syndrome

Abdominal compartment syndrome is defined as a sustained intra-abdominal pressure of more than 20mmHg (with or without abdominal perfusion pressure <60mmHg) combined with new organ dysfunction/failure and is primarily associated with open repair of ruptured AAA. Compartment syndrome is prevented by leaving the abdominal cavity open after AAA repair, when closure would cause high intra-abdominal pressure. The resulting wound can be treated open, using negative pressure therapy and temporary mesh approximation of abdominal fascia. This may require repeated changing of the abdominal dressing in theatre under general anaesthesia until the fascia is sufficiently lax for abdominal closure. (See also Chapter 11.)

Visceral injury

Supracoelic aortic dissection is often required to achieve supracoeliac clamping and can occasionally result in inadvertent iatrogenic oesophageal injury. In order to minimise this risk, a large-bore nasogastric tube should be inserted to help locate the oesophagus.

Strategies to avoid renal failure have been discussed in detail in Chapter 3. Intra-operative ischaemia associated with extended suprarenal clamping can become consequential after 20 minutes, and becomes likely if cross-clamping exceeds 40 minutes. The ischaemic tolerance of kidneys can by increased by perfusing them with 4°C heparinised saline.

Other anatomical considerations

Inflammatory AAA with its classical triad of thickened aortic wall, marked peri-aneurysmal/retroperitoneal fibrosis and dense neighbouring adhesions accounts for 3-10% of all AAA. They are often associated with ureteric obstruction, requiring ureteric stenting prior to AAA repair in order to minimise the risk of postoperative renal failure, and to aid identification of the ureter during dissection. Exposure of the neck of the aneurysm is often hampered by inflammatory fibrosis involving the duodenum. This often necessitates supracoeliac control of the aorta, minimal dissection of the duodenum and balloon occlusion of iliac arteries. For these reasons, both morbidity and mortality are higher after open repair of an inflammatory AAA.

Endovascular abdominal aortic aneurysm repair

EVAR is increasingly used for AAA repair since its introduction in the early 1990s. Randomised trials have suggested that the peri-operative mortality rate is half that of open repair, with shorter operating time, reduced in-hospital stay, and less blood loss and transfusion requirement [6, 7]. However, there are concerns regarding the high reintervention rates during follow-up, and its long-term durability due to late endograft rupture. The early benefits of EVAR with regards to all-cause and aneurysm-related mortality dissipate beyond 2 years [8]. Reintervention rates as high as 30% are recorded 8 years after EVAR (although most reinterventions are also endovascular), and there are concerns about substantial aneurysm-related mortality beyond 4 years [8, 9]. All patients will require routine follow-up after EVAR for life, with either regular CT or ultrasound imaging, and plain abdominal X-ray.

Endoleak

An endoleak is defined as persistent blood flow outside the lumen of the stent graft, but within the aneurysm sac or the adjacent vascular segment. Endoleaks are associated with the potential for continued aneurysm expansion and rupture. Endoleaks are classified according to the source of blood flow within the aneurysm sac (Table 2). Untreated Type I and III endoleaks are associated with a high risk of rupture (3.4% per year).

The prevention of endoleak begins with careful patient selection. The following morphology suggests anatomical suitability for EVAR:

- infrarenal aortic neck length – at least 10-15mm, depending on neck angulation;

- limited neck angulation. New devices such as Endurant® and Aorfix® are now licensed in angulated necks up to 60° and 90°, respectively. Most devices are suitable up to angulation of 60°;
- neck diameter – no more than 32mm;
- neck morphology – conical neck (contour change >10%), mural thrombus (>90°) and extensively calcified neck all increase risk of stent graft migration and are therefore relative contra-indications for EVAR;
- iliac artery diameter – at least 7mm, to facilitate passage of delivery system. If the diameter of the common iliac artery (CIA) is too large, the stent graft can be extended into the external iliac artery (EIA) with embolisation of the internal iliac artery. Alternatively, an aneurysmal aorto-iliac segment could be repaired using a Zenith® Iliac Branched Device (in conjunction with standard Zenith components), extending the landing zone to the EIA without occluding the internal iliac artery (IIA), thus avoiding ischaemic complications in the pelvis;
- length of distal sealing zone – at least 10-15mm (see above point);
- iliac artery tortuosity – small, calcified and tortuous iliac arteries make passage of the

Table 2. Classification of endoleak.

Type of endoleak	Subclassification	Source of persistent leak
I	a: proximal b: distal c: iliac occluder (in the case of iliac occluder in aorto-uni-iliac stent)	Graft attachment site
II	a: simple (single vessel) b: complex (>2 vessels)	Collateral vessel (lumbar or IMA)
III	a: junctional leak b: fabric tear	Graft failure
IV		Fabric porosity
V		Endotension (no visible aberrant blood flow seen)

delivery system difficult. In these situations, the use of an extra-stiff wire or a double wire will help to straighten the iliac artery. Alternatively, access to the CIA can be obtained directly using an iliac conduit, fashioned through an incision in the iliac fossa. Endovascular recanalisation may help traverse calcified or stenosed iliac arteries. Low-profile devices (Zenith® Low Profile and Ovation®) are now available and are designed for patients with difficult access.

Type I endoleak

Type I endoleak is caused by failure of sealing at the proximal (Type Ia) or distal (Type Ib) fixation points. This may be due to primary failure at initial deployment or late failure due to graft migration. Type I endoleak always needs treatment as the aneurysm sac is still under systemic pressure (Figure 2).

The majority of Type I endoleaks will seal after the use of a compliant moulding balloon (Figure 3) which improves apposition between the endoluminal surface of the vessel and the external aspect of the stent. Caution is needed to avoid ballooning above the main body of the covered stent especially in the presence of supra-renal fixation devices, as this can potentially result in aortic rupture. A giant Palmaz stent can be used to prevent recoil and encourage stent apposition if balloon moulding fails. In the event that stent migration results in a late proximal Type I endoleak, the stent graft can be extended proximally to increase the length of neck contact; a proximal aortic cuff (or graft limb distally) is employed and is generally oversized by 10-20%.

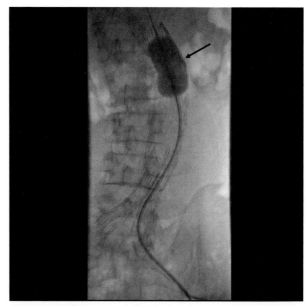

Figure 3. Balloon moulding to treat a Type Ia endoleak.

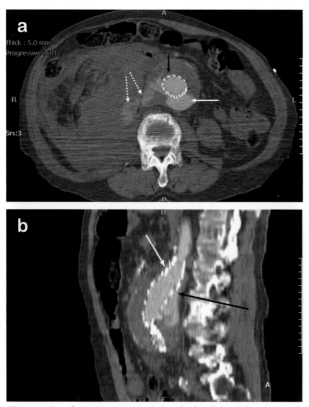

Figure 2. a) Type Ia endoleak (solid white arrow) resulting in rupture (dotted white arrows showing contrast leaking from the aneurysm sac; solid black arrow depicting the stent graft). b) Sagittal view showing the stent graft (white arrow) with a posterior Type I endoleak (black arrow).

Persistent Type I endoleak, despite the above technique, will require conversion to open repair or peri-aortic banding. For banding, following dissection of the aortic neck, nylon tapes are snugged down onto the aortic neck until the pulsatile motion of the aneurysm is diminished, without opening the aneurysm sac. This can be facilitated by inserting a Palmaz stent at the proximal anastomosis prior to aortic banding, to prevent overtightening, aortic stenosis or occlusion. Open repair may yet be difficult, as conventional cross-clamping may cause occlusion of the stent graft. Supracoeliac clamping or

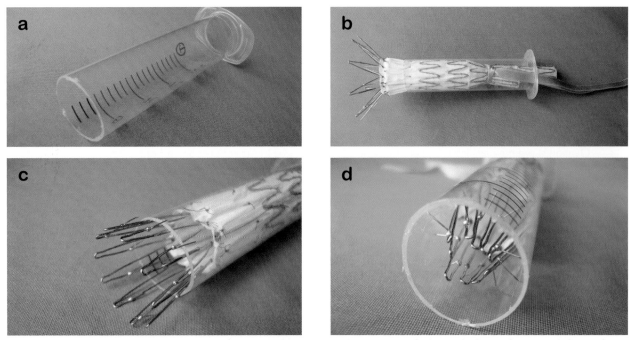

Figure 4. a) Modified syringe. b) Nylon tape used to retract the stent graft through the syringe and the syringe is advanced cranially. c) Top stent collapsed into device. d) Suprarenal fixation hooks retracted from the wall of the aorta into the device.

the use of an intra-aortic occlusion balloon supported by a sheath may be valuable techniques. The sheath prevents distal migration of the occlusion balloon.

If it is decided to convert to open aneurysm repair, the stent graft can be removed easily unless it has suprarenal fixation hooks and barbs. When these are present, the infrarenal component can be separated using wire cutters, leaving the suprarenal component *in situ*; open repair is then performed in the conventional manner. Stent grafts with suprarenal fixation can often be removed intact using a 20ml syringe (Figure 4a). First, the syringe plunger is removed. The end involving the needle hub is removed with a sharp knife, exposing the barrel of the syringe. The caudal end of the graft is grasped with forceps or with a nylon encircling tape. These are passed through the modified syringe with the cut hub end directed cranially (Figure 4b). The main body of the graft is resheathed by advancing the cylinder cranially while keeping the graft in a stable position (Figure 4c). In this way, the graft collapses and the hooks are withdrawn without tearing the wall of the aorta [10] (Figure 4d). Occasional cranial pressure is required to disengage the barbs safely from the aortic wall.

Type II endoleak

Type II endoleaks are the most common and occur after up to 43% of EVARs. They carry only a small risk of subsequent AAA rupture (0.52%); the majority seal spontaneously without the need for intervention. They often communicate with sac vessels such as the IMA (Figure 5), lumbar or internal iliac arteries. Treatment

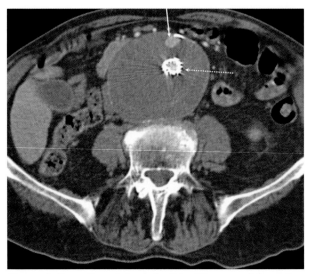

Figure 5. Type II endoleak (solid white arrow) from the IMA. The stent graft is depicted by a dotted white arrow.

is only required for endoleaks which persist for more than a year, or are associated with increasing aneurysm diameter.

Type II endoleaks associated with continued AAA expansion are usually treated with percutaneous embolisation either via a transarterial or translumbar route. Transarterial embolisation involves a femoral puncture and super-selective catheterisation of the SMA or the internal iliac artery to access the IMA via the marginal artery or the iliolumbar collaterals, respectively (Figure 6). The translumbar technique involves direct puncture of the aneurysm sac under CT or ultrasound guidance to enable embolisation of both the inflow and outflow vessels, and the endoleak cavity within the aneurysm sac. Various materials have been used, often combining coil and liquid embolic agents (such as Onyx® and cyan acrylic glue). Laparoscopic ligation of the IMA to treat a Type II endoleak has also been described.

Type III endoleak

Type III endoleak is associated with a significant risk of rupture due to the continued pressurisation of the aneurysm sac. It is often a result of structural

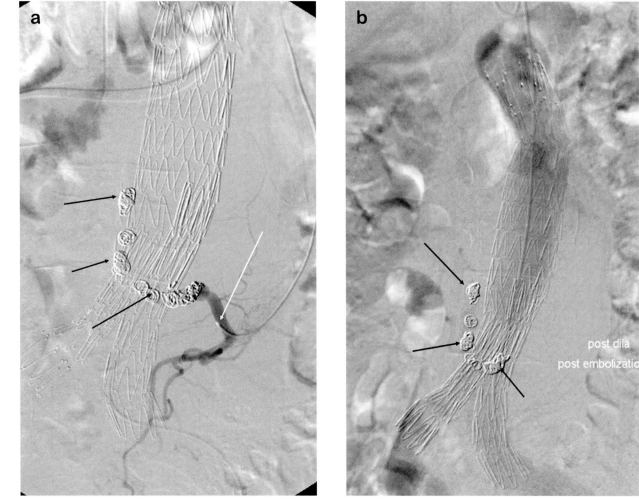

Figure 6. a) Coil (black arrows) embolisation of a Type II endoleak from the IMA, with super-selective mesenteric catheterisation (white arrow). b) Completion angiogram after coil embolisation with no visible endoleak.

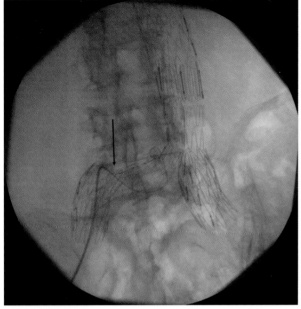

Figure 7. Stent dislocation (black arrow) resulting in a Type III endoleak.

failure of the stent, either due to separation of modular components (IIIa) (Figure 7) or fabric tear (IIIb). Primary Type IIIa endoleak can be identified intra-operatively and is treated with balloon moulding of the stent junctions; a stent extension may be required if there is insufficient overlap of the components. Type IIIb endoleak is rare with the new generation of stent grafts and is often a diagnosis of exclusion. It may require restenting across the torn segment, or even conversion from a bifurcated to an aorto-uni-iliac system.

Delayed Type III endoleak is often a consequence of aneurysm sac remodelling leading to separation of graft components, or mechanical stress causing stent and fabric failure. The treatment is the same as primary Type III endoleak, but often with a significant risk of conversion to open operation.

Type IV endoleak

Type IV endoleak is as a result of graft porosity and is rare with the new generation of stent grafts. It is recognised on completion angiography as an early diffuse blush of the aneurysm sac and resolves within hours of implantation and with reversal of heparin. As a consequence it is almost never associated with sac expansion or rupture.

Type V endoleak

Type V endoleak is defined as continuous aneurysm sac enlargement without signs of endoleak. In this phenomenon, the aneurysm is pressurised from an unapparent endoleak and this has been termed endotension. Contrast-enhanced ultrasound, CT and/or conventional angiography is required to rule out a true endoleak before making the diagnosis. Possible sources of endotension include pressure transmission through thrombus-lined areas of poor apposition at the proximal and distal sealing zones of the stent graft, or exudation through the graft. Untreated Type V endoleaks may lead to continuous sac enlargement and rupture. Treatment options include re-lining with a second device or open conversion. Open operation is complicated by probable supracoeliac clamping as discussed above. The sac may be opened to rule out a small undetected endoleak (which should be transfixed), and the aneurysm neck banded with nylon tape. Alternative open methods include wrapping of the endograft in a tube of Dacron® and closing the sac firmly over the endograft/wrap combination. There is insufficient evidence to compare the efficacy of these various treatments.

Late rupture

Late rupture of an EVAR-treated AAA occurs at a rate of up to 1.5% per year. The treatment of late rupture is dependent on local expertise and may involve both open or endovascular approaches.

Graft failure

Early EVAR stent grafts were associated with high rates of graft failure due to metallic stent fracture or fabric tear. Most of these patients have since undergone graft explantation or restenting with new generation, more durable stents.

Graft kinking and occlusion

The older generations of unsupported endovascular stents were prone to thrombosis due to kinking or twisting of the graft limbs within the native aorta. Stent kinking and twisting can also be caused by a change in the morphology of the treated AAA (sac remodelling), both in length and diameter (Figure 8). Postoperative graft kinking has been reported after up to 3.7% of procedures. Left untreated, this can lead to flow reduction, and eventually thrombosis. Treatment for this depends on the severity of the deformity and may include thrombectomy and restenting of the kinked limb. An alternative open approach is to construct a femorofemoral cross-over bypass, but this is usually only required following graft limb occlusion.

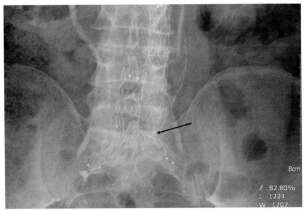

Figure 8. Kinking in the left limb of the graft (black arrow).

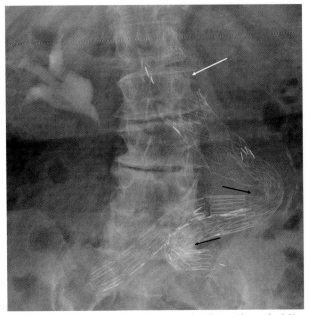

Figure 9. Stent migration and disruption (white arrow). The graft is also kinked (black arrows).

Graft migration and dislocation

Graft migration and disruption can be caused by a combination of sac remodelling and device failure (Figure 9), especially at the attachment sites. Significant stent migration at the sealing zones can lead to a Type I endoleak, whereas excess movement of the modular components can result in a dislocation and, eventually, a Type III endoleak. The newer generation of stent grafts have a better fixation mechanism and columnar strength, all of which reduces the risk of Type I endoleak. Treatment in suitable anatomy may involve restenting for limb dislocation, or aortic cuff placement for proximal migration.

Conclusions

Both open repair and EVAR have their unique benefit and risk profiles. Despite the initial advantages of EVAR, recent long-term trials show that they dissipate after 2 years. The results from the randomised trials should be interpreted with caution, as most were initiated over 10 years ago and involved earlier devices. Endovascular stent graft design has improved significantly and in conjunction with the enhanced experience of surgeons, better patient selection and the improved treatment of graft complications, the current outcomes following EVAR may be better than those from the previous randomised trials.

For patients with an AAA, the treatment decision should be individualised. Treatment options have to consider both aneurysm morphology and the risk benefit balance to the patient. For example, in patients with indolent malignancy, AAA repair is usually only considered if the patient has a minimum life expectancy of 2 years. Younger patients (under 60 years) who are generally in good health may benefit from the durability of open repair. Nevertheless, careful selection of patients for EVAR, adequate follow-up and the continuing development of new devices should reduce the incidence of complications associated with this procedure. All patients must be given full information regarding the risks and benefits of both open repair and EVAR. They should be involved in the choice of procedure, knowing that although EVAR is a lesser procedure with a significantly lower short-term mortality risk, it is associated with the need for lifelong follow-up, and with a significant late reintervention rate. Open repair, although a major procedure with a higher peri-operative mortality, is associated with improved durability and long-term follow-up is not required.

Key points

- Management of AAA will need to take into consideration the risk:benefit ratio and the patient's life expectancy.
- Both open and EVAR have their unique complications.
- Open AAA repair carries a higher risk of 30-day mortality compared to EVAR. EVAR requires long-term surveillance with an annual reintervention rate of 10%.
- Type I and III endoleaks are associated with a higher incidence of aneurysm sac expansion and rupture, and require further treatment.
- New evidence suggests that initial benefits of EVAR dissipate after 2 years.
- Newer generations of stent grafts have better durability and this has to be taken into consideration when interpreting trial results.

References

1. The UK Small Aneurysm Trial Participants. Mortality results for randomised controlled trial of early elective surgery or ultrasonographic surveillance for small abdominal aortic aneurysms. *Lancet* 1998; 352: 1649-55.
2. Lederle FA, Johnson GR, Wilson SE, *et al.* Prevalence and associations of abdominal aortic aneurysm detected through screening. Aneurysm Detection and Management (ADAM) Veterans Affairs Cooperative Study Group. *Ann Intern Med* 1997; 126: 441-9.
3. Brewster DC, Cronenwett JL, Hallett JW Jr, *et al*, Joint Council of the American Association for Vascular Surgery and Society for Vascular Surgery. Guidelines for the treatment of abdominal aortic aneurysms. Report of a subcommittee of the Joint Council of the American Association for Vascular Surgery and Society for Vascular Surgery. *J Vasc Surg* 2003; 37: 1106-17.
4. Daenens K, Fourneau I, Nevelsteen A. Ten-year experience in autogenous reconstruction with the femoral vein in the treatment of aortofemoral prosthetic infection. *Eur J Vasc Endovasc Surg* 2003; 25: 240-5.
5. Prinssen M, Buskens E, Nolthenius RP, *et al.* Sexual dysfunction after conventional and endovascular AAA repair: results of the DREAM trial. *J Endovasc Ther* 2004; 11: 613-20.
6. The EVAR Trial Participants. Endovascular aneurysm repair versus open repair in patients with abdominal aortic aneurysm (EVAR Trial 1): randomised controlled trial. *Lancet* 2005; 365 (9478): 2179-86.
7. Prinssen M, Verhoeven EL, Buth J, *et al*; Dutch Randomized Endovascular Aneurysm Management (DREAM)Trial Group. A randomized trial comparing conventional and endovascular repair of abdominal aortic aneurysms. *N Engl J Med* 2004; 351(16): 1607-18.
8. United Kingdom EVAR Trial Investigators, Greenhalgh RM, Brown LC, Powell JT, *et al.* Endovascular versus open repair of abdominal aortic aneurysm. *N Engl J Med* 2010; 362(20): 1863-71.
9. De Bruin JL, Baas AF, Buth J, *et al*; DREAM Study Group. Long-term outcome of open or endovascular repair of abdominal aortic aneurysm. *N Engl J Med* 2010; 362(20): 1881-9.
10. Koning OH, Hinnen JW, van Baalen JM. Technique for safe removal of an aortic endograft with suprarenal fixation. *J Vasc Surg* 2006; 43: 855-7.

Case vignette Aortic stent graft infection

Peng Foo Wong MB ChB MD FRCS (Gen Surg), Specialist Registrar in Vascular Surgery
Michael G. Wyatt MSc MD FRCS, Consultant Vascular Surgeon and Honorary Reader
Freeman Hospital, Newcastle upon Tyne, UK

A 67-year-old man who had an aorto-uni-iliac stent and femorofemoro crossover graft 8 months previously presented with general malaise, rigors, vague left-sided abdominal pain and an abscess in the left groin. Postoperatively, following his initial aortic stent, he had developed bilateral groin infection which necessitated femorofemoral graft excision and replacement with superficial femoral vein.

CT on this admission showed extensive peri-aortic stent graft gas (Figure 1) with a left common iliac

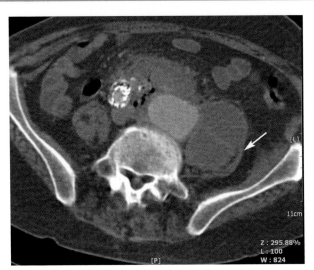

Figure 2.

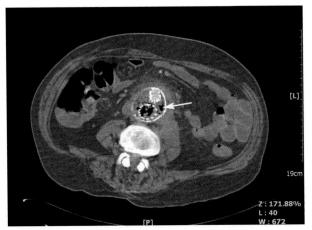

Figure 1.

pseudoaneurysm and psoas abscess tracking down to the left groin (Figure 2). He required explantation of the aortic stent graft with right axillofemoral bypass. Intra-operatively, his large bowel was noted to be ischaemic, requiring sub-total colectomy. He developed multi-organ failure and did not recover from his operation.

Chapter 17 Arch and thoracic aortic aneurysms

Peter L. Harris MD FRCS, Head of Multidisciplinary Endovascular Team
Jason Constantinou MD MRCS, Specialist Registrar in Vascular Surgery
Multidisciplinary Endovascular Team, University College London and University College London Hospital, London, UK

Introduction

Aneurysms involving the aorta within the chest represent both the most simple and the most complex challenges to the cardiothoracic and endovascular surgeon. In the absence of confounding comorbidities, a localised aneurysm in the mid-descending thoracic aorta is a straightforward matter for either open or endovascular repair. The latter is now preferred in most circumstances, and the results are impressive enough to render a randomised trial difficult to justify in modern clinical practice. In contrast, aneurysms located within the arch and thoraco-abdominal aorta represent some of the most interesting challenges to surgical and endovascular ingenuity. The high mortality rate in the early days of attempted surgical repair of the aortic arch led one of the great pioneers, Denton Cooley, to conclude, somewhat tongue-in-cheek, that "the arch is the seat of the soul". Results have improved dramatically since those days, but complication rates associated with treatment of arch and thoraco-abdominal aortic aneurysms remain relatively high. The brain and spinal cord are particularly at risk and much energy continues to be expended in devising techniques of cerebral and spinal protection. Other vital organs are similarly subject to potential ischaemic injury and, in the endovascular era, contrast-induced acute kidney injury has become a significant factor. In this chapter we will describe measures designed to ameliorate the risks associated with these procedures.

Aortic arch aneurysms

The aortic arch has been described as the final frontier of both conventional open and endovascular surgery. In both cases the challenge is to protect the brain from ischaemic injury, global hypoperfusion or embolic cerebrovascular occlusion.

Open surgery

Open surgery for total graft replacement of the aortic arch lies within the province of the cardiothoracic rather than the vascular surgeon. Nevertheless, although endovascular surgeons are encroaching increasingly upon this territory with hybrid, and now total endovascular, alternative options, they do need to be aware of what has been achieved with traditional approaches. Of necessity, open arch replacement requires temporary interruption of aortic blood flow and perfusion of all its supra-aortic branches. Techniques developed to protect the brain from ischaemic injury during interruption of normal cerebral blood flow include profound hypothermic circulatory arrest (PHCA) or moderate hypothermic circulatory arrest (MHCA) with, or without retrograde cerebral perfusion (RCP) or selective antegrade cerebral perfusion (SACP). Several experimental and clinical studies indicate that SACP presents significant advantages compared with PHCA with, or without RCP. Antegrade SCP can extend the safe duration of circulatory arrest by up to 90 minutes [1], allowing meticulous aortic arch repair. It is more effective in supplying oxygenated blood to the brain, thus ensuring a more physiological brain metabolism. It also obviates the need for deep hypothermia, thereby reducing pump time and the risk of hypothermia-related complications such as pulmonary insufficiency and coagulopathy. Cannulation of the right axillary artery via a Dacron® conduit has been found to be associated with a lower risk of cerebral emboli than conventional femoral cannulation [2]. Another recent advance is the use of trifurcated grafts with separate branches for the supra-aortic arteries in preference to implantation of a patch of aorta bearing the origins of these vessels. Selective cerebral perfusion has considerably prolonged the safe time of circulatory arrest, thereby allowing more complex and time-consuming aortic arch reconstructions and is considered to be the most reliable method of preventing ischaemic injury to the brain. In a series of 150 patients having total arch replacement over 16 years, the overall combined death and permanent stroke rate was 14%; 16% in those who had HCA alone or HCA plus SCP, but reducing to 8% in those having HCA plus SCP via axillary cannulation and arch replacement with a trifurcated graft [3].

One of the major challenges associated with open surgery in this area is how to address pathology that extends beyond the arch. This is a situation which occurs commonly following Type A aortic dissection and in Marfan's syndrome. The descending thoracic aorta is not surgically accessible from a median sternotomy, through which the ascending aorta and arch must be approached. The solution is a two-stage elephant trunk procedure, first described in 1983 by Borst [4]. The ascending aorta and arch are repaired using the techniques for cerebral protection described above and a tube of Dacron® graft is extended from the distal arch anastomosis and left floating-free within the descending thoracic aorta. The second stage involves a left thoracotomy, through which the distal aortic reconstruction is completed including a graft-to-graft anastomosis to the free end of the elephant trunk. Svensson reported a low 30-day mortality of 2.1% and permanent stroke rate of 5.3% after the first stage of this procedure [5]; however, only 50% of the patients underwent the second procedure with 13% suffering fatal rupture in the interim. The others did not proceed for a variety of reasons with an overall mortality rate of 56% at 5 years. These results signal the need for a better surgical approach and one recent significant development is known as the frozen elephant trunk procedure. This is a one-stage hybrid technique with incorporation of a stent into the distal end of the elephant trunk and the retrograde placement of a conventional stent graft within it to complete the repair (vide infra) [6].

Hybrid procedures

The frozen elephant trunk procedure is an example of how patients may benefit from image-guided wire and catheter techniques applied in combination with conventional open vascular surgery. In a contemporary series of 156 patients treated with a frozen elephant trunk, the in-hospital mortality and permanent stroke rates were 3.2% and 2.6%, respectively [7]. These results compare favourably with those of wholly open surgery with avoidance of the notable drawbacks associated with a two-stage procedure. This is, however, a relatively unusual hybrid operation and more commonly a hybrid arch repair is performed in which open surgery plays an adjuvant or permissive role to support endovascular reconstruction of the thoracic aorta.

Total debranching of the arch requires a sternotomy, but when the disease is confined to the distal arch with sufficient sealing zone beyond the origin of the innominate artery, the open surgical component can be confined to an extra-anatomic, carotid/carotid/subclavian bypass in the neck. In either circumstance, requirements for cardiopulmonary bypass, hypothermic circulatory arrest and retrograde or antegrade cerebral perfusion are obviated and the risk of complications is lower than that of conventional open surgery.

Technical tips to minimise risk include the following:

♦ to avoid phrenic nerve injury and diaphragmatic palsy when exposing the subclavian artery in the neck, visualise the nerve on the anterior surface of scalenus anterior muscle and divide the tendinous part of the muscle as close as possible to its insertion into the scalene tubercle on the upper surface of the first rib;

♦ to avoid incision, contamination or infection of the cross-neck bypass, in the event of subsequent tracheostomy, use a retro-oesophageal route. However, if transoesophageal echo (TOE) is being used to guide deployment of the stent graft, take care that it does not compress the bypass;

♦ the author's preference is for a right common carotid to left subclavian artery bypass with end-to-side anastomosis, followed by end-to-side anastomosis of the transected left common carotid artery onto the top of the graft, the proximal stump being oversewn;

♦ access to the left subclavian artery proximal to the vertebral artery origin can be difficult. There is also a case for retaining access to the arch via this route until completion of the procedure.

For these reasons occlusion of the left subclavian origin with coils following deployment of the aortic stent graft is preferred to surgical ligation or oversewing for prevention of Type 2 endoleak;

♦ in the case of total debranching via sternotomy, preformed trifurcated grafts are available commercially. However, it is a simple matter to stitch a side arm to one limb of a standard presealed bifurcated vascular graft. For women 12 x 6mm and for men 14 x 7mm grafts are usually appropriate;

♦ if access of the endograft into the arch is difficult from the groin (e.g. when the descending thoracic aorta is tortuous), an additional side arm sutured to the body of the graft will accommodate a through-and-through stiff guide wire from the groin and allow the endograft to be pulled rather than pushed into position (Figure 1);

♦ to avoid compression or kinking of the graft on closure of the sternotomy, it is essential that the body of the graft is not anastomosed to the front or anterior surface of the ascending aorta. The graft will lie comfortably without kinking if anastomosed to the right outer curve of the aorta;

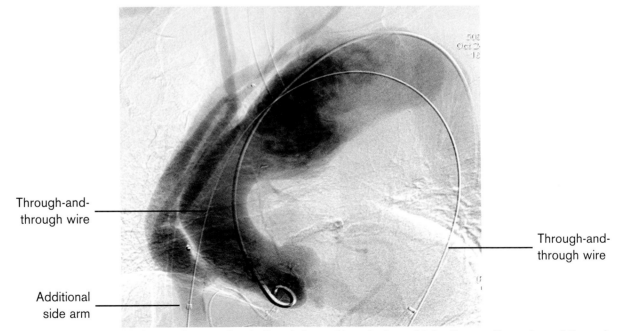

Through-and-through wire

Through-and-through wire

Additional side arm

Figure 1. A separate limb is anastomosed onto the debranching device which allows a through-and-through wire to be passed from the groin allowing the endograft to be pulled into position.

- to preserve an optimum length of sealing zone, this anastomosis must be placed as proximally as possible on the ascending aorta without the risk of clamp encroachment on, or flow restriction to the right coronary artery;
- to avoid slippage of the aortic side clamp, reduce the systolic blood pressure to less than 60mmHg before application. It is advisable to keep a second clamp close to hand, just in case!;
- to avoid anastomotic dehiscence or leak, the aortic anastomosis should always be buttressed with polytetrafluoroethylene (PTFE) felt pads;
- mark the distal edge of the aortic anastomosis with an easily identified radio-opaque marker. A large surgical clip or the thread from a surgical swab, securely sutured in place are both effective for this purpose;
- to minimise the risk of iatrogenic dissection of supra-aortic target arteries, it is the author's preference to construct the distal anastomosis obliquely end to end. The proximal stumps are then doubly oversewn;
- the required properties of an endograft for arch replacement are:
  - stability during deployment to enable accurate positioning; and
  - ability to conform to the curvature of the arch.

The Zenith TX2® Pro-Form™ device (Cook Medical Inc.) meets these requirements. A trigger wire constrains the proximal end of the endograft to allow blood to flow past it until deployment is complete. This, together with a through-and-through wire makes for a very stable and accurate deployment. However, to ensure that there is no loss of position, with compromise of seal at the last second, one option is to suspend cardiac output temporarily by ventricular overpacing;

- to ensure that the endograft conforms well to the curve of the arch and the aortic knuckle, it is important to push the device forward gently as the stents are deployed. Failure to do this results in the device taking a 'racing line' across the arch and risks malalignment of the sealing stent (Figure 2).

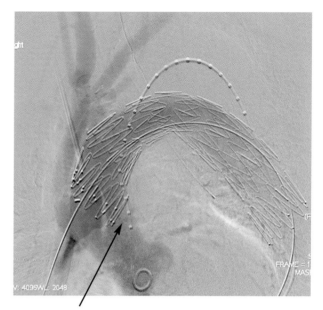

Malaligned stent

Figure 2. Failure to push the device as the stent is deployed may result in the device taking a racing line across the arch leading to malalignment of the sealing stent (arrow).

A recent meta-analysis of 463 hybrid arch reconstructions revealed a 30-day mortality rate of 8.3% and a stroke rate of 4.4% [8]. There was also a paraplegia rate of 3.9%, presumably as a consequence of extension of the reconstruction distally in a large proportion of the cases. The endoleak rate overall was 9.2%.

Wholly endovascular procedures

Three different techniques have been attempted so far to overcome the challenges associated with repair of the aortic arch by endovascular means alone with varying degrees of success:

- chimney endografts;
- *in situ* fenestration; and
- branched arch devices.

Of these, the latest iterations of branched devices hold the greatest promise of displacing open surgery and hybrid procedures as the method of choice. The other two will be discussed only briefly.

Chimney endograft technique

This involves placement of a stent, open or covered, proximally from a target supra-aortic artery that has been covered by an aortic arch endograft [9]. The chimney stent lies outside the endograft and projects proximally beyond its proximal edge to maintain perfusion of the vessel. The problem with this technique is that either the chimney stent or the aortic stent graft becomes compressed and gutters are created alongside the chimney stent, which are a potential and frequent source of Type 1 endoleaks. Therefore, safe use of this technique demands that there must be an adequate sealing zone distal to the target vessel. In other words it can optimise but not extend a short but adequate seal zone. The chimney stent technique can be a very valuable bail-out option in the event of inadvertent over-stenting of a critical supra-aortic branch, but it cannot be recommended as an elective procedure.

In situ fenestration

First described in 2003 [10] this technique involves perforation of the aortic arch stent graft *in situ* from the target vessel followed by insertion of a stent to maintain patency and the position of the fenestration that has been created. It has been applied clinically, with success, to preserve the patency of the over-stented left subclavian artery [11]. There is one report of its application for total reconstruction of the arch with *in situ* fenestration of the left carotid and innominate arteries [12]. In this case, an extracorporeal circuit with a pump was used to maintain cerebral perfusion during the time taken to re-establish flow from the aorta via the *in situ* created fenestrations. While it may have a place for maintenance of perfusion of an over-stented left subclavian artery, this technique has obvious limitations with respect to more extensive arch reconstructions.

There is concern also about the durability of a fenestration created by cutting a hole in the fabric of an endograft, especially within the very hostile haemodynamic environment of the aortic arch. Further developments in graft technology may overcome some of these concerns, but, for the present, *in situ* fenestration cannot be recommended for routine use.

Branched arch devices

The first branched arch device to be applied clinically was inserted into the aorta via the right common carotid artery [13]. It was bifurcated with a smaller diameter limb engaging in the innominate artery and a larger diameter limb extending distally into the arch to be accessed by a second endograft inserted from the groin to complete the repair. An extra-anatomic carotid/carotid/subclavian bypass was necessary to safeguard cerebral perfusion. A large sheath had to be introduced into the right common carotid artery following this adjuvant procedure with potential to compromise blood flow to both sides of the brain. Although there were a number of successes, a third of the patients suffered strokes and this type of device has been abandoned in favour of the next generation of branched arch devices.

The current design of branched arch device is delivered by the transfemoral route. The only commercially available graft is manufactured by Cook Medical Inc., as a customised version of their Zenith TX2® Pro-Form™ thoracic endograft. It incorporates two internalised sleeves for the left common carotid and innominate arteries with wide funnel-shaped openings to facilitate retrograde cannulation.

The endograft is mounted on a precurved cannula (Figure 3) within a precurved sheath and is prevented

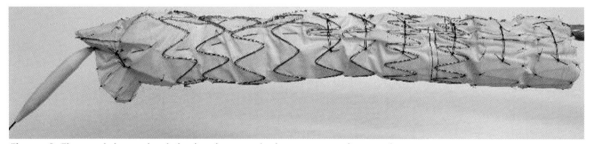

Figure 3. The arch branched device is mounted on a curved cannula.

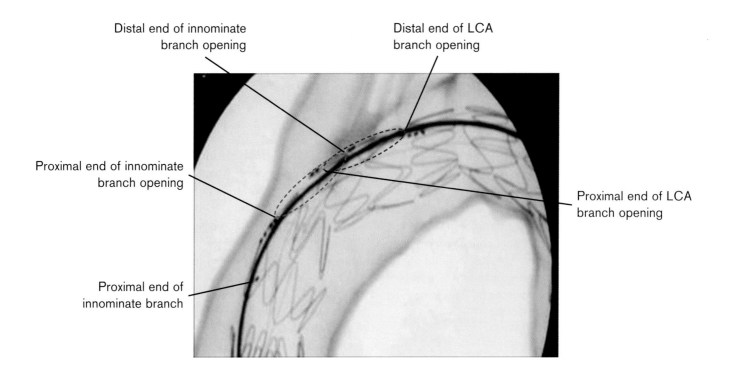

Distal end of innominate branch opening

Distal end of LCA branch opening

Proximal end of innominate branch opening

Proximal end of LCA branch opening

Proximal end of innominate branch

Figure 4. Radio-opaque markers on the endograft assist in the alignment of the funnels with the orifices of the target vessels.

from rotating during insertion by a spiral trigger wire that fixes it to the central cannula. By this means the endograft reliably orientates itself within the arch with the funnels on the outer curve. A system of radio-opaque markers assists longitudinal alignment of the funnels with the orifices of the target vessels (Figure 4). Withdrawal of trigger wires deploys the first two sealing stents, while the diameter of the funnel-bearing portion of the stent graft remains restricted by a diameter-reducing wire. This allows continued perfusion of the supra-aortic branches via the funnels.

Prior to insertion of the stent graft, a surgical conduit is placed onto the right subclavian artery and a left carotid to subclavian bypass is performed. A sheath with a radio-opaque tip is inserted to mark the orifice of the innominate artery.

The device is unsheathed under rapid pacing to ensure accurate positioning. The funnels, identified by their markers, are positioned slightly proximal to the orifices of the target vessels to facilitate cannulation. Bridging stents inserted retrograde via the funnels engage with the internal sleeves to complete the repair.

Fewer than ten of these procedures have been undertaken worldwide and each device has had some unique feature. Therefore, it is impossible to say whether or not this is the future of arch replacement but the anecdotal evidence is promising (see case vignette). An alternative is transapical access via a mini-thoracotomy to permit antegrade cannulation and stenting of the supra-aortic branches thereby avoiding the necessity for surgical exposure and manipulation of the neck vessels.

Aneurysms of the descending thoracic aorta

Spinal cord ischaemia

The most feared complication associated with both open replacement and endovascular repair of the descending thoracic aorta is paraplegia. For focal aneurysms, localised to the mid-descending aorta, the risk is minimal. However, the incidence of paraplegia increases with the length of aorta replaced and is in the order of 10% for extensive Type II thoraco-abdominal aneurysms. The majority of patients who develop dense paraplegia do not survive for long, but for those who do, the disability and distress caused are severe.

At open surgery, intercostal arteries that may give rise to spinal arteries can be preserved by reimplanting them into the graft. This is, however, not possible with an endograft as these intercostal arteries are too small to accommodate stents. However, there are various methods that can be employed to protect the spinal cord, some of which are of proven value, and one of which is not (at least not yet).

Left subclavian, lumbar and internal iliac arteries

Many aneurysms affecting the descending thoracic aorta arise at, or close to the origin of the left subclavian artery such that there is no safe seal zone distal to this vessel. Under these circumstances, the left subclavian artery must be over-stented. Initially it was considered that this manoeuvre could be undertaken with impunity and that revascularisation was unnecessary, except on the rare occasions when the patient developed troublesome claudication in the arm. This practice was challenged in 2007 when data from the EUROSTAR registry provided conclusive statistical evidence that over-stenting of the left subclavian artery without prophylactic revascularisation was associated with an increased risk of paraplegia [14]. Therefore, it follows that this artery must always be revascularised under these circumstances. Options include carotid subclavian bypass or subclavian transposition, chimney endograft and *in situ* fenestration.

Patency of the subclavian artery preserves flow into the vertebral artery and intercostal collaterals. Other important sources of collateral circulation to the spinal cord are the lumbar and internal iliac arteries. The risk of paraplegia is increased by concomitant thoracic and abdominal aortic aneurysm repair, which should be avoided. Every effort should be made to preserve patency of at least one if not both internal iliac arteries.

Spinal fluid and systemic blood pressures

Since spinal cord perfusion depends upon systemic blood pressure which is the perfusion force and spinal fluid pressure which resists it, it follows that manipulation of these two pressures relative to each other might be beneficial. Clinical benefit associated with withdrawal of spinal fluid to reduce pressure in the spinal canal was first demonstrated in respect of open surgical repair of thoraco-abdominal aortic aneurysms [15]. This technique is, however, equally effective in preventing or reversing spinal cord ischaemia associated with endovascular repair.

Prophylactic insertion of a spinal drain is recommended for all open and endovascular thoraco-abdominal procedures. It should also be performed for any thoracic aneurysm repair that involves exclusion of large intercostal arteries, particularly those at the T8 to T12 level from which the artery of Adamkiewicz often arises. In the absence of neurological symptoms, the spinal fluid pressure is maintained at 13cm H_2O by setting the manometer at this level and withdrawing 10ml of fluid per hour. In the event of neurological symptoms developing, the manometer is set to 10cm H_2O and up to 20ml per hour is withdrawn. Maintaining a systolic blood pressure above 140mmHg and a mean arterial pressure (MAP) above 80mmHg is equally important. The systolic pressure should be increased to 160 or even 180mmHg and the MAP over 100mmHg if the patient develops weakness in his legs.

Spinal drains are not without risk. Cerebral or spinal haemorrhage is a concern and this risk is

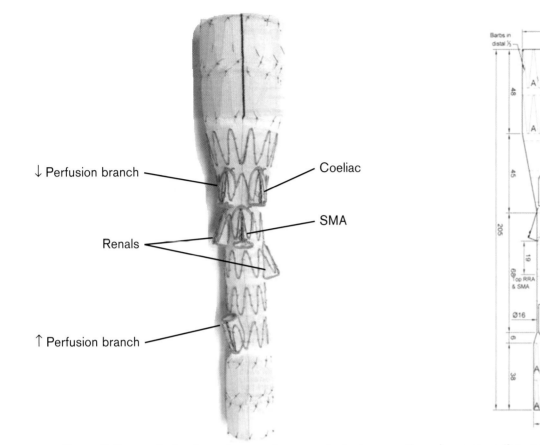

Figure 5. Sac perfusion branches are incorporated wherever there is room on the graft, with one upward and one downward-pointing branch. These perfusion branches are then closed percutaneously 3-5 days postoperatively using an Amplatzer® plug.

increased if fluid is withdrawn too rapidly; blood-stained fluid is an indication to withdraw the drain. Rapid withdrawal of a large volume of CSF can also result in coning and must be monitored carefully. Finally, there is a risk of infection which can have very serious consequences. For this reason the drain should be withdrawn within 3 days unless there is a strong indication to continue.

Temporary sac perfusion branches

For endovascular interventions, the greatest risk of paraplegia is following treatment of thoraco-abdominal aortic aneurysms with multibranched endografts, and runs at between 10% and 15%. Most often symptoms develop during the immediate postoperative period of cardiovascular instability. The trigger is hypotension, but the condition may not be reversed immediately by raising the blood pressure. In

one such case, Chuter reversed the paraplegia by inserting a stent alongside the aortic endograft to create a deliberate Type 1 endoleak [16]. Temporary postoperative sac perfusion through additional branches in the endograft has developed from this experience (personal communication). Two sac perfusion branches are incorporated into the endograft facing in opposite directions so that blood flows from one to the other through the sac rather than building up static pressure (Figure 5). This arrangement can also facilitate subsequent closure as one can easily be accessed from the other. The perfusion branches are closed with an Amplatzer® occlusion device usually 1 week following the aneurysm repair. Under local anaesthesia, temporary balloon occlusion enables the patient to report any adverse consequences, and if there are none, permanent closure is completed. If symptoms do develop, permanent closure can be delayed to allow more time for adjustment of the blood pressure or for a collateral circulation to develop. Further evidence of efficacy of this technique may obviate the need for spinal fluid drainage at the time of aneurysm repair.

Device-related complications

Two device-related complications are of concern following the endovascular repair of thoracic aneurysms. These are:

◆ conformability of endografts, or lack of it; and
◆ migration leading to endoleak.

Conformability

Stent grafts were designed originally as straight tubes and, while they functioned well in straight arteries, there were problems when they were required to conform to the curvature of the aortic knuckle. Two adverse consequences occurred, both extremely serious. First, there were reports of stents, particularly uncovered stents, eroding through the aorta at the proximal end of the device. Secondly, failure of apposition of the endograft to the wall on the inner curve of the arch occasionally resulted in collapse of the endograft and aortic obstruction. It is anticipated that these complications will not be associated with the latest generation of conformable endografts, but it is still too soon to know.

Migration and endoleak

Two circumstances increase the risk of stent graft migration: a large vacuous aneurysm sac with an endograft unsupported in a wide space and multiple endografts. A minimum three-stent overlap between contiguous endografts is needed to minimise the risk of late endoleak and need for secondary intervention.

Conclusions

Aneurysms of the arch of the aorta represent one of the greatest challenges to cardiac and vascular surgeons. While there is still some way to go, less invasive hybrid and wholly endovascular approaches have the potential to supercede conventional open surgery, involving extracorporeal bypass, with a lower risk of serious complications. For descending thoracic aneurysms, endovascular repair is established already as the method of choice for many patients. The most feared complication of both open and endovascular surgery for this condition is paraplegia. Manipulation of spinal cord perfusion pressure is effective in reducing the risk of paraplegia and sometimes in reversing it after it has occured. In the case of endovascular repair, temporary sac perfusion appears to be safe and may confer added benefit although its efficacy is, as yet, uproven.

Key points

◆ Treatment of aortic arch disease remains complex and challenging with a high risk of cerebrovascular complications.

◆ Evolution of arch branched device technologies is developing rapidly and holds a promise of safer treatment for future patients with arch aneurysms.

◆ Spinal cord injury is a serious complication of thoracic aneurysm repair. Established measures to minimise this risk are: maintenance of patency of the left subclavian and internal iliac arteries, avoidance of concomitant abdominal aortic aneurysm repair, avoidance of unnecessary exclusion of patent intercostal and lumbar arteries and control of spinal fluid and arterial blood pressures.

◆ Temporary postoperative perfusion of the aneurysm sac, and intercostal arteries arising from it, through sac perfusion branches is an interesting concept but as yet unproved as a device to prevent spinal cord ischaemia.

◆ Device-related complications associated with endovascular thoracic aneurysm repair may be reduced following the introduction of a new generation of conformable endografts.

◆ Generous overlap of contiguous endografts is essential to avoid migration and endoleak especially within a large aneurysm sac.

References

1. Ergin MA, Galla JD, Lansman SL, *et al*. Hypothermic circulatory arrest in operations on the thoracic aorta. *J Thorac Cardiovasc Surg* 1994; 107: 788-99.

2. Svensson LG, Blackstone EH, Rajeswaran J, *et al*. Does the arterial cannulation site for circulatory arrest influence stroke risk? *Ann Thorac Surg* 2004; 78: 1274-84; discussion 1274-84.

3. Strauch JT, Spielvogel D, Lauten A, *et al*. Technical advances in total aortic arch replacement. *Ann Thorac Surg* 2004; 77: 581-89; discussion 589-90.

4. Borst HG, Walterbusch G, Schaps D. Extensive aortic replacement using 'elephant trunk' prosthesis. *Thorac Cardiovasc Surg* 1983; 31: 37-40.

5. Svensson LG, Kim KH, Blackstone EH, *et al*. Elephant trunk procedure: newer indications and uses. *Ann Thorac Surg* 2004; 78: 109-16.

6. Baraki H, Hagl C, Khaladj N, *et al*. The frozen elephant trunk technique for treatment of thoracic aortic aneurysms. *Ann Thorac Surg* 2007; 83: S819-23.

7. Uchida N, Katayama A, Tamura K, *et al*. Long-term results of the frozen elephant trunk technique for extended aortic arch disease. *Eur J Cardiothorac Surg* 2010; 37: 1338-45.

8. Koullias GJ, Wheatley GH. State-of the-art hybrid procedures for the aortic arch: a meta-analysis. *Ann Thorac Surg* 2010; 90: 698-7.

9. Sugiura K, Sonesson B, Akesson M, *et al*. The applicability of chimney grafts in the aortic arch. *J Cardiovasc Surg* 2009; 50: 475-81.

10. McWilliams RG, Fearn SJ, Harris PL, *et al*. Retrograde fenestration of endoluminal grafts from target vessels: feasibility, technique, and potential usage. *J Endovasc Ther* 2003; 10: 946-52.

11. McWilliams RG, Murphy M, Hartley D, *et al*. *In situ* stent-graft fenestration to preserve the left subclavian artery. J *Endovasc Ther* 2004; 11: 170-4.

12. Sonesson B, Resch T, Allers M, *et al*. Endovascular total aortic arch replacement by *in situ* stent graft fenestration technique. *J Vasc Surg* 2009; 49: 1598-91.

13. Chuter TA, Schneider DB, Reilly LM, *et al*. Modular branched stent graft for endovascular repair of aortic arch aneurysm and dissection. *J Vasc Surg* 2003; 38: 859-63.

14. Buth J, Harris PL, Hobo R, *et al*. Neurologic complications associated with endovascular repair of thoracic aortic pathology: incidence and risk factors: a study from the European Collaborators on Stent/graft Techniques for Aortic Aneurysm Repair (EUROSTAR) Registry. *J Vasc Surg* 2007; 46: 1103-11.

15. Safi HJ, Hess KR, Randel M, *et al*. Cerebrospinal fluid drainage and distal aortic perfusion: reducing neurologic complications in repair of thoracoabdominal aortic aneurysm types I and II. *J Vasc Surg* 1996; 23: 223-8.

16. Reilly LM, Chuter TA. Reversal of fortune: induced endoleak to resolve neurological deficit after endovascular repair of thoracoabdominal aortic aneurysm. *J Endovasc Ther* 2010; 17: 21-9.

Case vignette Endograft repair of an aortic arch aneurysm

Peter L. Harris MD FRCS, Head of Multidisciplinary Endovascular Team
Jason Constantinou MD MRCS, Specialist Registrar in Vascular Surgery
Multidisciplinary Endovascular Team, University College London and University College London Hospital, London, UK

An 81-year-old, retired airline pilot, was found to have a complex thoracic aneurysm involving his aortic arch, whilst he was receiving treatment for superficial bladder cancer. His imaging (TeraRecon) showed a 65mm saccular aortic arch aneurysm, with two patent vertebral arteries (Figure 1).

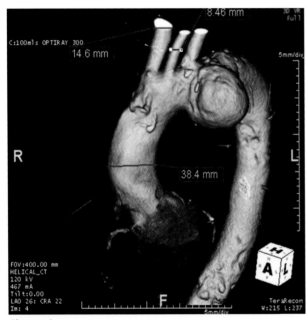

Figure 1.

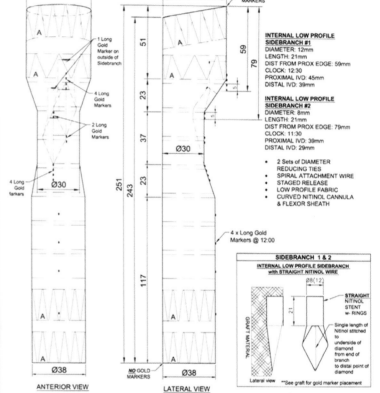

Figure 2.

He initially underwent a left common carotid to left subclavian artery bypass, and 5 weeks later his aortic arch aneurysm was repaired using a 24F custom branched arch endovascular device (Figure 2). This procedure involved a temporary 8mm Dacron® conduit sutured end to side to the right subclavian artery in the supraclavicular fossa. Completion angiography showed patency of all four supra-aortic vessels with total exclusion of the aneurysm sac (Figure 3).

The patient's postoperative intensive care stay was complicated by a minor stroke, which resolved completely. Despite an absence of major lung pathology, he remained ventilator-dependent and an EMG revealed bilateral phrenic nerve palsies with paradoxical movement of the diaphragm. Bilateral neck re-exploration showed the phrenic nerves to be intact, but without response on direct nerve stimulation. The phrenic nerve palsy was attributed to a pre-existing peripheral neuropathy that also affected his arms and legs. He was discharged back to his local hospital in preparation for discharge with home ventilation.

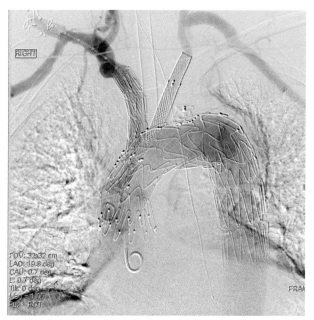

Figure 3.

Chapter 18 Acute and chronic aortic dissection

Robert Morgan MRCP FRCR, Consultant Vascular and Interventional Radiologist
Radiology Department, St George's NHS Trust, London, UK

Introduction

Acute aortic dissection is a major clinical emergency. Without treatment, the mortality rate after 48 hours is 36-72%, and up to 90% of patients die within 1 week [1]. The main causes of death are aortic rupture, aortic regurgitation, cardiac tamponade and malperfusion syndrome.

Aortic dissection has an incidence of 20 per million per year, occurs more frequently in men than women (3:1), and the peak incidence is between 40 and 70 years [2, 3] (Figure 1). Most patients are hypertensive and have aortic atherosclerosis, but other causes include Marfan syndrome, Ehlers Danlos syndrome, pregnancy and trauma. Aortic dissection is part of a spectrum of conditions referred to as Acute Aortic Syndrome (intramural haematoma, penetrating aortic ulcer, and traumatic aortic injury) [4].

While surgery remains the main therapy for aortic dissection involving the ascending aorta and proximal aortic arch, conservative therapy has been the preferred management for dissection involving the descending aorta, unless complications such as aneurysmal dilatation, aortic rupture or malperfusion occur. The development and insertion of endovascular stent grafts is becoming the standard of care for complicated aortic dissection involving the

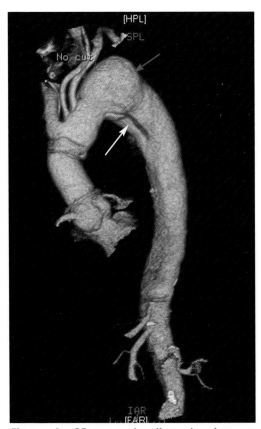

Figure 1. CT reconstruction showing an aortic dissection (white arrow) associated with some aneurysmal dilation of the proximal descending thoracic aorta (red arrow).

descending aorta and even some dissections that involve the aortic arch [5-8]. Despite considerable experience of this technique, endovascular treatment of aortic dissection is a treatment in evolution. Although there have been developments in device technology and modifications in procedural methods since the first reports of this technique 20 years ago, there is still room for further improvement to reduce the risk of complications.

Complications of endografting can be subdivided into procedural, early and late complications.

Procedural complications

Early procedural failure of open conversion is uncommon and has been reported in up to 4% of patients. The main procedural complications are listed in Table 1.

Table 1. Procedural complications and their management.	
Endograft movement	Insertion of additional endograft
Proximal Type 1 endoleak	Insertion of additional endograft
	Possible supra-aortic bypass may be required
Type 2 endoleak via the left subclavian artery	Embolise the left subclavian artery with an Amplatzer® plug or coils, electively or immediately
Rupture of the dissection flap	Prevent by not dilating endograft aggressively
	Treat by extending endograft coverage distally
Stroke 2%	Prevent by limiting manipulations in the aortic arch
	Prevent by performing elective subclavian bypass if this vessel will be covered by the endograft
Paraplegia 0.5-2%	Prevent by limiting endograft coverage of the aorta
	Prevent by not covering the left subclavian artery without prior bypass
	Treat by spinal drainage
Type A dissections 1-3%	Treat by urgent surgical repair
Iliac artery rupture 1-2%	Treat by immediate balloon tamponade and insertion of a covered stent
Insertion of endograft into the false lumen	Extend endograft coverage to upper abdomen
	May need to perform a percutaneous fenestration in the abdominal aorta

Movement of the endograft

Movement of the endograft during deployment may occur, particularly when deploying a device in the aortic arch. Movement is generally in the distal direction and is usually due to the windsock effect of the cardiac output on the partially opened endograft. The newest designs of endograft are increasingly resistant to this phenomenon, because they delay the complete release of the proximal end of the endograft until the remainder of the endograft has been deployed. The windsock effect can largely be prevented by reducing the systemic blood pressure below 100mmHg peak systolic pressure immediately before deployment of the proximal device.

If the endograft moves distally during deployment, insertion of an additional endograft proximally is usually required. For some reason, it is unusual for this second endograft to move during deployment, presumably because it is stabilized by the first.

Immediate endoleaks

Endoleak after thoracic endografting is classified in a similar manner to endoleaks after EVAR. Type 1 endoleak occurs at the proximal or distal attachment sites. In aortic dissection, a distal Type 1 leak at the distal graft attachment sites is almost unknown. Retrograde filling of the false lumen from natural fenestrations in the upper abdomen occurs frequently; however, these are not distal Type 1 endoleaks. Type 2 endoleaks are generally due to reversed flow into the aorta from intercostal arteries, or from the left subclavian artery if the origin of the vessel has been covered. A Type 3 leak occurs either at the connections between endografts, or as a result of a fabric tear in the graft material. Procedural Type 3 endoleaks are rare, mainly because endografts reline a relatively narrow true lumen rather than a capacious aneurysm sac. Similarly, procedural fabric tears are almost unknown, as are Type 4 leaks, due to graft porosity.

Proximal Type 1 endoleak

The common causes of a proximal Type 1 endoleak include an inadequate length of proximal landing zone, distal movement of an endograft during deployment (see previous section), and a very angulated aortic arch, where blood tracks along the underside of the endograft.

Inadequate landing zone

Type 1 endoleak due to an inadequate landing zone usually occurs after deployment of a device in the distal aortic arch, just beyond the left subclavian artery; this is the most common location for endograft deployment in aortic dissection. The ideal length of the proximal landing zone is 15mm, but there may not be 15mm from the main communication between the true lumen and the false lumen, and the left main subclavian artery. In order to avoid covering the left subclavian artery, it may be necessary to make do with a shorter landing zone, which increases the risk of a Type 1 endoleak. If this occurs, the only option is to extend the endograft proximally, and therefore possibly cover the origin of the left subclavian artery, and in some cases even the left common carotid and innominate arteries to achieve a seal. Although the left subclavian artery has been covered by endografts without prior subclavian bypass by many operators in the past, this practice is associated with an increased risk of stroke and paraplegia. Clearly in the setting of a procedural Type 1 endoleak, a decision must be made whether to proceed immediately with subclavian bypass and additional endograft insertion, or whether to reschedule the patient for an early elective procedure. Many operators might elect to wait and perform early elective subclavian bypass and additional endograft insertion. If additional left carotid or even innominate artery bypass is required to abolish a Type 1 endoleak, the pendulum swings even further towards rescheduling, and against proceeding immediately.

Distal movement during endograft deployment

As stated previously, when this occurs, treatment is by insertion of an additional proximal endograft.

Very angulated aortic arch

If a Type 1 endoleak occurs in this situation, it may resolve after gentle balloon moulding of the proximal end of the endograft. Balloon dilatation in the setting of aortic dissection is generally not performed because of concerns regarding rupture of the dissection flap. However, if the dilatation is limited to the normal non-dissected aorta at the proximal landing zone, the risk of rupture is theoretically reduced. If there is still a Type 1 leak after balloon moulding or if moulding is considered too hazardous, the only option is to extend endograft coverage proximally.

Type 2 endoleaks

Endoleaks due to filling of the false lumen by intercostal arteries are never seen during the procedure and there is no evidence that they ever require treatment. If the origin of the left subclavian artery has been covered, but not ligated surgically, late retrograde filling of the false lumen via the left subclavian artery may be seen at completion angiography. There is general consensus (though based on scientific fact) that these should be treated by embolisation, usually as a separate procedure, although some operators elect to proceed to

embolisation immediately. This involves catheterisation of the left brachial artery and embolisation of the proximal left subclavian artery using coils, or more commonly by deployment of a correctly sized Amplatzer® plug (Abbott).

Rupture of the flap

This is uncommon but may occur spontaneously during the procedure after release of the endograft. Flap rupture usually occurs as a result of strenuous balloon dilatation of the endograft in a relatively narrow false lumen in an attempt to produce a wider stented true lumen. This intervention is a mistake, is not necessary and, in the author's view, should never be performed. If rupture of the flap occurs, intended closure of the main communication by insertion of an endograft has inadvertently resulted in the iatrogenic creation of a much larger communication between the two lumens (Figure 2). The only option is to extend

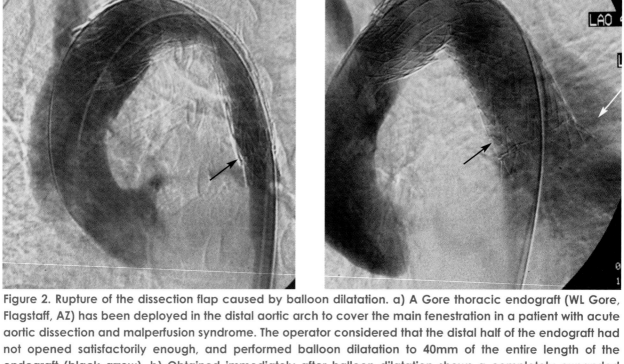

Figure 2. Rupture of the dissection flap caused by balloon dilatation. a) A Gore thoracic endograft (WL Gore, Flagstaff, AZ) has been deployed in the distal aortic arch to cover the main fenestration in a patient with acute aortic dissection and malperfusion syndrome. The operator considered that the distal half of the endograft had not opened satisfactorily enough, and performed balloon dilatation to 40mm of the entire length of the endograft (black arrow). b) Obtained immediately after balloon dilatation shows a completely expanded endograft (black arrow) and contrast passing freely into the false lumen at the lower end of the endograft (white arrow). Balloon dilatation had resulted in rupture of the dissection flap.

endograft coverage distally, usually to the upper abdominal aorta.

Stroke

The risk of stroke is around 2%, and seems less than after endovascular treatment of thoracic aneurysms. As the potential for treatment of stroke caused by thrombo-embolism is limited, operators should try to prevent stroke by limiting manipulations in the aortic arch, and by performing left carotid to left subclavian artery bypass if coverage of the left subclavian artery origin is expected.

Paraplegia

The risk of paraplegia after endovascular repair of thoracic dissection is around 0.5-2%. In general, the risk is reduced by limiting total endograft coverage of the aorta and avoiding covering the left subclavian artery without first performing carotid-subclavian bypass. If paraplagia occurs, immediate drainage of cerebrospinal fluid should be performed. The potential requirement for spinal drainage should be discussed with the anaesthetist before endografting, so that the procedure can be performed without delay, if needed, by someone experienced in the technique, thus limiting potential complications [9] (see Chapter 17).

Type A dissection

In patients with aortic dissection, the aortic wall even in the non-dissected part has an increased potential for further dissection. Catheter and guide wire manipulations in the aortic arch, the high radial force of a newly deployed endograft, or inflation of a balloon in the arch may all traumatize the intima and media sufficient to provoke further retrograde dissection. This occurs in around 1% of procedures (Figure 3). Retrograde dissection may only extend for a few centimetres, although most extend to the upper ascending aorta or as far as the aortic valve, with the potential to cause catastrophic aortic regurgitation, cardiac tamponade and death. The only treatment is urgent open surgical repair.

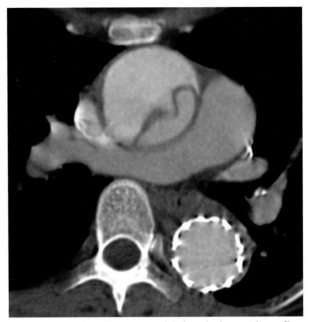

Figure 3. This CT scan obtained 4 weeks after endovascular repair of a Type B dissection shows a Type A dissection.

Iliac artery rupture

Iliac artery rupture is usually a complication following attempted endograft insertion through iliac arteries that are too small for passage of an endograft delivery catheter. The potential for rupture is also increased in calcified vessels. In general, the absolute minimum iliac artery diameter is 7.5mm, as most delivery systems are at least 22 French. Some device companies quote their delivery system calibre in inner rather than outer diameter, and operators must familiarize themselves with the individual characteristics of the devices that they wish to use. Rupture usually occurs in the external iliac artery, commonly at the origin. If rupture occurs, it is essential to retain guide wire access across the rupture. Even the most experienced of operators have difficulty attempting to bridge the two ends of the ruptured artery using catheter/guide wire techniques if guide wire access is lost. If rupture occurs, balloon tamponade of the proximal artery should be performed immediately to limit haemorrhage, followed by insertion of a suitable covered stent. Although peripheral stent grafts (e.g. Fluency® [Bard Angiomed, Karlsruhe, Germany]; Wallgraft™ [Boston Scientific Corp, Galway, Ireland]) are suitable, iliac limb components of many standard abdominal aortic endografts may also be used.

Inadvertent placement of an endograft in the false lumen

This unusual complication may occur if the operator has not made sure that guide wire access to the normal aorta above the dissection has passed through the true lumen of the dissected aorta, rather than the false lumen. It is standard practice to ensure that the catheter and guide wire pass through the true lumen of the thoracic aorta. This is generally achieved by performing a check angiogram in the upper abdomen and comparing the visceral arteries originating from the particular lumen that the catheter is located in, with the preprocedural CT scan. If the catheter is not in the true lumen, it must be redirected from below until true lumen position is achieved. If by mistake, an endograft is deployed passing from the true lumen proximally through the main fenestration into the false lumen, this inevitably increases the pressure in the thin-walled false lumen with an added risk of rupture. It also increases the risk of malperfusion if most of the visceral vessels are supplied by the true lumen. Should this avoidable complication occur, initial management is by extending endograft coverage distally to the upper abdomen (to reduce the potential for rupture of the thoracic aorta). After this, if angiography suggests evidence of poor perfusion of visceral or lower extremity arteries, a large fenestration must be created percutaneously between the two lumens in the abdominal aorta to improve perfusion of the true lumen.

Early complications

Early complications that occur within 30 days after endografting for aortic dissection are listed in Table 2. There is a substantial overlap with procedural complications.

In general, patients should undergo imaging by CT before they are discharged from hospital to detect any early complications, particularly Type 1 endoleak and retrograde Type A dissection. The management of these complications is as described in the previous section. Although paraplegia is usually manifest within a few hours of endografting, it may also occur a few days later, so vigilance for this complication and a readiness to intervene with spinal drainage should be maintained.

Late complications

Late complications that occur more than 30 days after the procedure are usually detected as a result of interval CT follow-up: performed usually at 6 months, 12 months, and annually thereafter. Most late complications relate to increasing aortic diameter, although some are intrinsic to the endografts themselves, and a small proportion of patients present with late aortic rupture. Causes of late complications and their management are presented in Table 3.

Table 2. Early complications and their management.	
Proximal Type 1 endoleak	Insertion of additional endograft
	Possible supra-aortic bypass may be required
Type 2 endoleak via the left subclavian artery	Embolise the left subclavian artery with an Amplatzer® plug or coils, electively or immediately
Paraplegia 0.5-2%	Treat by spinal drainage
Type A dissection	Treat by urgent surgical repair

Table 3. Late complications and their management.	
Increase in aortic calibre	
False lumen perfusion due to a proximal Type 1 endoleak	Extend proximal endograft coverage with/without supra-aortic bypass
False lumen perfusion due to Type 2 endoleak via intercostal arteries	Embolise by transarterial route or by direct puncture of the false lumen
Type 3 endoleak – fabric tear, endograft disconnection	Insert bridging endograft
False lumen perfusion from abdominal natural fenestrations	Close all fenestrations by hybrid procedure, branched endograft or open surgical repair
Abdominal aortic aneurysm	EVAR, hybrid procedure, branched endograft or open surgical repair
Iliac artery aneurysm	EVAR, peripheral and embolisation of the internal iliac artery. Iliac branched endograft
Aortic rupture – 3%	Consider if treatable by further endografting or open surgery
Endograft complications	
Endograft collapse	Supportive Palmaz® stent, additional endograft or open surgery
Stent strut fractures	Usually individual struts of little consequence Complete stent fractures require bridging endografts

Aortic rupture

This is uncommon, and usually occurs in patients who are not subject to follow-up or who miss CT appointments. If a patient survives long enough to reach hospital, immediate CT should be performed to assess whether management by additional endografting is feasible.

Increasing aortic diameter due to late proximal Type 1 leak

A late Type 1 endoleak may occur as a result of proximal extension of the dissection, proximal aneurysm formation, or more usually endograft movement, particularly in an angulated aortic arch. Endograft coverage should be extended proximally (see previous sections).

Increasing aortic diameter due to Type 2 endoleak

Late Type 2 endoleaks via the left subclavian artery should be embolised (see above) (Figure 4). Type 2 leak due to retrograde perfusion of the false lumen from intercostal arteries is very rarely associated with an increase in false lumen diameter, and the concept that this may occur at all is disputed. Nevertheless,

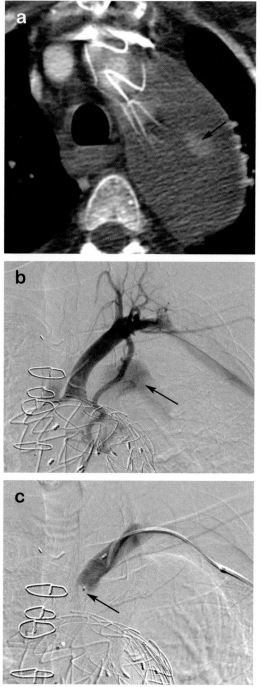

there are reports of the treatment of these Type 2 leaks either by a complex transarterial route, or by percutaneous direct puncture of the false lumen.

Increasing aortic diameter due to a late Type 3 endoleak

A leak may occur between two adjacent endografts as they separate, or a fabric tear may occur. In order for an increase in aortic calibre to occur, there also needs to be a local tear in the flap for the leak to perfuse the false lumen. Even though this undoubtedly occurs in some patients, late Type 3 leak is not a common cause of late aneurysm formation after aortic dissection. In the unlikely event of a Type 3 endoleak causing an increase in aortic diameter, insertion of an additional endograft is indicated.

Increasing aortic diameter due to perfusion of the false lumen via natural fenestrations in the upper abdomen

When all other causes of an increase in aortic diameter have been excluded or treated, perfusion and persistent pressurization of the thoracic false lumen through natural fenestrations in the upper abdominal aorta is the only remaining possible cause. There is evidence that false lumen perfusion in the thoracic aorta arising from fenestrations below the diaphragm is reduced at the level of the stented aorta compared with false lumen perfusion below the endografts, although this effect occurs less reliably in chronic, compared to acute dissections [10]. In view of this reduction in false lumen perfusion caused by the presence of an endograft in the adjacent true lumen, the first relatively straightforward option is to extend endograft coverage

Figure 4. Increasing false lumen diameter due to a Type 2 endoleak from the left subclavian artery. This patient underwent endovascular repair of a Type B dissection 6 weeks previously. The left subclavian artery had been covered by the endograft. Subclavian artery bypass had not been performed. a) This CT scan shows contrast in the false lumen (arrow) in the proximal descending aorta. b) The false lumen filling was considered to be secondary to retrograde flow from the left subclavian artery. Embolisation of the left subclavian artery was performed. After catheterisation of the left brachial artery, left subclavian arteriography confirmed passage of contrast into the false lumen via the left subclavian artery (arrow). c) The proximal left subclavian artery was embolised by deployment of a 14mm Amplatzer® plug (arrow).

of the true lumen to the upper abdomen. In a proportion of patients, this procedure prevents or slows any further increase in aortic diameter. At this time, there are few published data on the outcome of this practice, or which patients are likely to benefit.

If the aorta continues to expand, the only option is to close all communications between the true and false lumens in the abdomen or pelvis. This may be achieved by open surgical repair; however, hybrid procedures and branched endografts are now being used increasingly as less invasive alternatives. Hybrid procedures involve surgical bypass of the upper abdominal major visceral arteries followed by insertion of endografts to the distal aorta or into the iliac arteries depending on the anatomy and the presence of other additional distal fenestrations. In experienced hands, the outcomes of hybrid procedures compare favourably with open surgical repair. There is less experience of the use of branched aortic endografts in patients with aneurysmal dissections of the thoraco-abdominal aorta, compared with thoraco-abdominal aneurysms. However, early data are encouraging and the procedure offers a completely non-surgical solution to this problem. The technology is disadvantaged by high costs, and the length of time required to plan, manufacture and deliver devices.

Abdominal aortic aneurysm

Although the false lumen in the thoracic aorta may be stabilized, and even abolished, by endograft placement, the abdominal false lumen may continue to expand until there is either a thoraco-abdominal aneurysmal dissection, or an infrarenal aneurysm. Thoraco-abdominal aneurysmal dissections can be treated by hybrid procedures, branched aortic endografts or open surgery, similar to the previous section. Some purely infrarenal aneurysms can be treated by conventional EVAR, although this leaves the natural visceral fenestrations intact, with the potential to perfuse the infrarenal false lumen. In most cases, infrarenal EVAR is seldom adequate to stop aortic growth, but is used by some operators as a bridging procedure until a definitive solution, such as a hybrid procedure or a branched endograft solution can be instituted. For most patients, closure of all fenestrations similar to the previous section is required [11] (Figure 5).

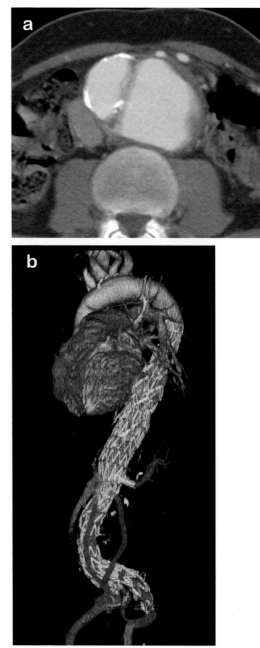

Figure 5. a) A patient with a chronic dissection, previously treated by placement of endografts in the thoracic aorta developed increasing size of the abdominal aorta. b) He was treated by a hybrid procedure in which all communications between the true and false lumen were closed by placement of endografts after visceral bypass of the superior mesenteric artery, coeliac artery and right renal artery. In this patient, a fenestration for the left renal artery is present in the aortic tube graft due to technical difficulties in performing bypass of the left renal artery.

Iliac artery aneurysm

If the dissection extends into the iliac arteries, the common and internal (though rarely the external) iliac arteries may dilate. Similar to aortic aneurysmal dissections, the management strategy involves closing all communications between the true and false lumen, possible embolisation of the internal iliac artery, and the placement of a supporting endograft in the true lumen. This may be limited to the iliac arteries, or may also require aortic endografting. Although there is a potential use for branched iliac endografts, there is little experience of their use in dissections.

Endograft collapse

Collapse of the proximal opening of a thoracic endograft is a very uncommon complication after endovascular repair for aortic dissection. Most reports of this phenomenon have involved relatively young patients, who have undergone endografting to treat traumatic aortic transection. Endograft collapse may be constant or it may be intermittent where the proximal end of the endograft opens and closes during the different stages of the cardiac cycle (fishmouthing) [12, 13].

Constant severe endograft collapse generally requires urgent intervention. There is some debate as to whether intermittent collapse requires treatment in all cases, or whether some completely asymptomatic patients can simply be observed. Treatment of endograft collapse is challenging; balloon dilatation is not effective. The main endovascular options involve placement of a supporting bare stent such as a Palmaz® stent (Johnson and Johnson, NJ) or extending endograft coverage more proximally in the aortic arch, although neither option is straightforward. Open surgery is a treatment option of last resort.

Conclusions

The majority of complications after endovascular repair of aortic dissection can be managed by additional endovascular manoeuvres, without the need for open surgery. Most procedural and early complications can be prevented (or predicted) by a critical assessment of the preprocedural images. Unfortunately, in general, late complications cannot be predicted and only a programme of indefinite follow-up can detect aortic expansion and its causes.

Key points

- Predict and prevent procedural and early complications by critical assessment of the preprocedural images and careful patient selection.
- Procedural Type 1 endoleaks should be treated on table if possible, although this may entail supra-aortic bypass if the proximal landing zone needs extending.
- Paraplegia may occur several days after endografting.
- Late expansion of the aorta usually requires closure of all of the communications between the true and the false lumen.
- Indefinite follow-up by CT is mandatory to detect late complications.

References

1.   Anangostopoulos CE, Prabhakar MJS, Kittle CF. Aortic dissections and dissecting aneurysms. *Am J Cardiol* 1972; 30: 263-73.

2.   Chavan A, Lotz J, Oelert F, *et al*. Endoluminal treatment of aortic dissection. *Eur Radiol* 2003; 13: 2521-34.

3.   Pate JW, Richardson RJ, Eastridge CE. Acute aortic dissection. *Ann Surg* 1976; 42: 395-404.

4.   Hagan PG, Nienaber CA, Isselbacher EM, *et al*. The International Registry of Acute Aortic Dissection (IRAD): new insights into an old disease. *JAMA* 2000; 283: 897-903.

5.   Eggebrecht H, Nienaber CA, Neuhauser M, *et al*. Endovascular stent-graft placement in aortic dissection: a meta-analysis. *Eur Heart J* 2006; 27: 489-98.

6. Williams DM, Lee DY, Hamilton BH, *et al.* The dissected aorta: percutaneous treatment of ischemic complications: principles and results. *J Vasc Intervent Radiol* 1997; 8: 605-25.

7. Nordon IM, Hinchliffe RJ, Loftus IM, *et al.* Management of acute aortic syndrome and chronic aortic dissection. *Cardiovasc Intervent Radiol* 2010; epub November 12.

8. Swee W, Dake MD. Endovascular management of thoracic dissections. *Circulation* 2008; 117: 1460-73.

9. Safi HJ, Estrera AL, Miller CC, *et al.* Evolution of risk for neurologic deficit after descending and thoracoabdominal aortic repair. *Ann Thorac Surg* 2005; 80: 2173-9.

10. Sayer D, Bratby M, Brooks M, *et al.* Aortic morphology following endovascular repair of acute and chronic type B aortic dissection: implications for management. *Eur J Vasc Endovasc Surg* 2008; 36: 522-9.

11. Song JM, Kim SD, Kim JH, *et al.* Long-term predictors of descending aorta aneurysmal change in patients with aortic dissection. *J Am Coll Cardiol* 2007; 50: 799-804.

12. Holt PJ, Johnson C, Hinchliffe RJ, *et al.* Outcomes of the endovascular management of aortic arch aneurysm: implications for management of the left subclavian artery. *J Vasc Surg* 2010; 51: 1329-38.

13. Hinchliffe RJ, Krasznai A, Schultzekool L, *et al.* Observations on the failure of stent-grafts in the aortic arch. *Eur J Vasc Endovasc Surg* 2007; 34: 451-6.

Chapter 19 Carotid intervention

David Williams MD FRCS, Endovascular Fellow, Sheffield Vascular Institute, Sheffield, UK
Duncan Drury MD FRCS, Specialist Registrar in Vascular Surgery, Sheffield Vascular Institute, Sheffield, UK
Jonathan D. Beard ChM MEd FRCS, Consultant Vascular Surgeon, Sheffield Vascular Institute and
Honorary Professor of Surgical Education, University of Sheffield, Sheffield, UK

Introduction

The best way to avoid the complications of a carotid intervention is to prevent the stroke occurring in the first place. Primary prevention will always be more cost-effective and best medical therapy (BMT), including good control of blood pressure, treatment of atrial fibrillation, antiplatelet agents, statins, good glycaemic control and smoking cessation support, must be offered to all at-risk patients. The evidence for any benefit from intervention for asymptomatic carotid disease remains unproven and will not be discussed further.

The justification for carotid endarterectomy (CEA) is based on the results of the North American Symptomatic Carotid Endarterectomy Trial (NASCET) [1] and the European Carotid Surgery Trial (ECST) [2].

Both trials demonstrated a benefit from surgery when compared to medical management alone for those with a significant carotid stenosis. Both trials were conducted over two decades ago, and the medical management of the patients would no longer be considered optimal. There is good evidence that modern BMT has improved outcomes, although the results of surgery have also improved, with registry data from the UK indicating a major adverse outcome rate of less than 2% [3].

More recent trials have compared CEA against carotid stenting (CAS). There have been six large randomised trials [4-9], including CAVATAS (which also included angioplasty and vertebral artery intervention), EVA - 3S, SPACE, ICSS as well as SAPPHIRE and CREST (which both included asymptomatic patients). The combined results (Table 1 and Figure 1) of these

Table 1. Combined results of the large randomised trials of stenting versus surgery.		
Complication	CEA	CAS
Death	27/3610 (0.75%)	36/3353 (1.1%)
Stroke	137/3822 (3.6%)	209/3708 (5.6%)
Myocardial infarction	47/3288 (1.4%)	27/2673 (1%)

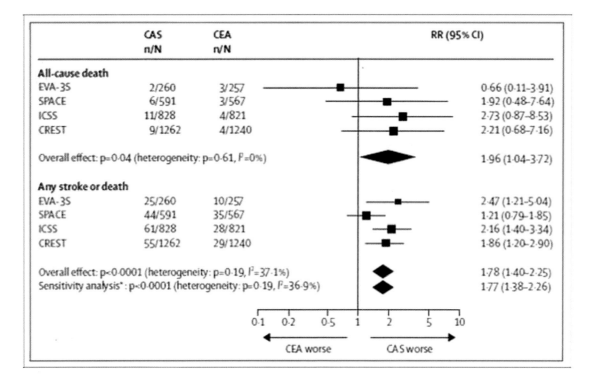

Figure 1. Forest plot comparing the stroke and death rates of the four largest trials of CAS vs. CEA for symptomatic carotid disease (50% of patients in CREST were asymptomatic). *Reprinted from the Lancet [10], with permission from Elsevier, © 2010.*

trials indicate that CAS has a better outcome for the complication of myocardial infarction, 27/2673 (1%) versus 47/3288 (1.4%), but CEA has a better outcome for stroke, 209/3708 (5.6%) versus 137/3822 (3.6%), and death, 36/3353 (1.1%) versus 27/3610 (0.75%) [10]. It also seems that CAS is less safe than surgery for the elderly, with an age cut-off between 70 and 80 years. Therefore, for the majority of symptomatic patients, CEA remains the safest option at the present time.

General prevention of complications

There are some general measures which are likely to reduce the complications of any carotid intervention.

Learning curves and workload

In most of the randomised trials, the surgeons had performed many CEAs whereas the interventionalists had performed few carotid stents. This is always a problem for new technology, but several of the trials used only experienced interventionalists and/or carefully selected centres on the basis of outcomes, and it is not surprising that no difference was found between the experienced and supervised centres. Registry data have shown worse outcomes when stenting is undertaken in less experienced centres, with major adverse events of 4-5.9% in centres performing <50 procedures, falling to 3% in centres with over 150 cases and continuing to fall to 1.56% for those having performed over 500 cases [11]. The same volume/outcome effect is seen for CEA and AAA repair. The implication is that complications can be reduced by restricting all interventional treatment to multidisciplinary teams working in centres with high volumes of work and independently audited results.

Best medical therapy

As well as being of vital importance for both primary and secondary prevention, BMT is also required to reduce the risk of peri-procedural complications. Trials of beta-blockers for coronary protection during major surgery have been inconclusive, but as good blood pressure control is important anyway, it seems sensible for all patients undergoing carotid intervention to be on a beta-blocker, unless contra-indicated.

Dual antiplatelet therapy with aspirin and clopidogrel has been shown by the Leicester group to reduce postoperative embolisation and thrombo-embolic events, to the extent that postoperative transcranial Doppler (TCD) monitoring is now unnecessary [12]. The pre-operative administration of statins significantly reduces the risk of peri-operative stroke, probably due to plaque stabilisation [13]. It seems sensible to commence all patients who have a TIA or stroke on a statin immediately, in case intervention is required.

Prevention and management of complications associated with CEA

Complications associated with CEA can be classified into remote, cervical and cerebral.

Remote complications

The GALA trial randomised 3526 patients to either local anaesthesia (LA), (n=1773), or general anaesthesia (GA), (n=1753). The primary outcome was stroke, death or MI between randomisation to 30 days postoperatively. The primary and secondary outcomes were similar: 4.8% for the GA group and 4.5% for the LA group [14]. Although there was no difference, the trial was not controlled for blood pressure and many high-risk patients were excluded.

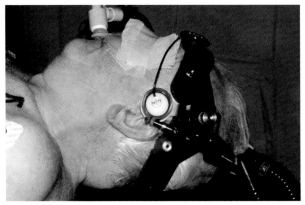

Figure 2. The general anaesthetic technique for CEA: patient paralysed and intubated with transcranial Doppler monitoring to help determine the need for a shunt (not always reliably). Many surgeons undertake CEA under local anaesthetic using a cervical block and intravenous sedation.

A cervical block is well tolerated by most patients and avoids the need for TCD monitoring (Figure 2). It also preserves cerebral autoregulation, which probably reduces shunt usage.

The CREST trial has demonstrated that the risk of periprocedural myocardial ischaemia (raised troponin) is higher for CEA than CAS. Raised troponin levels are associated with increased early and late mortality. As circulating catecholamine levels have been shown to be high during CEA under LA, it seems sensible to recommend CAS for patients with severe coronary artery/valve disease.

Cervical complications

The incidence of cranial nerve injury varies from 2.5-11.3%. The most common injury is a temporary neuropraxia of the facial, glossopharyngeal or vagus nerves due to traction, but rarely more significant and permanent nerve injuries are caused by diathermy or accidental nerve transection. Beasley and Gibbons [15] found no difference in cranial nerve injury between a retrojugular approach to the standard anterior approach. The advantage of the retrojugular approach is better access to the distal internal carotid artery, which can otherwise be obscured by the vagus and hypoglossal nerves. Although there was a slightly lower incidence of hypoglossal nerve injury, there was a higher incidence of accessory nerve injury. Careful dissection and identification, as well as avoidance of excessive diathermy and retraction, are important in reducing cranial nerve injury.

The haematoma rate in the surgery versus stenting trials varied considerably from 0.8-7%, possibly because of variable usage of combined antiplatelet agents. Although dual antiplatelet therapy increases the risk of wound haematoma, it also reduces the risk of cerebral embolism, and possibly also myocardial ischaemia. Meticulous haemostasis is the key to haematoma prevention. Bleeding from the suture line can be prevented with tissue glue. Fibrillar collagen rather than excessive diathermy can be used for haemostasis around the parotid and thyroid glands. There is no evidence that drains prevent haematomas. Reversal of heparin should be avoided as there have been reports that protamine may increase the risk of acute carotid occlusion.

A Cochrane review [16] has demonstrated that patch angioplasty significantly reduces ipsilateral stroke (RR 1.6% for patch plasty vs. 4.8% for primary closure). In addition, there is a reduction in the restenosis rate (4.8% for patch plasty vs. 18.6% for primary closure). There appears to be no significant difference between prosthetic or vein patch in terms of the risk of postoperative stroke and restenosis. Vein patches can blow out and prosthetic patches risk infection (Figure 3). A systematic review [17] of the literature on Dacron®

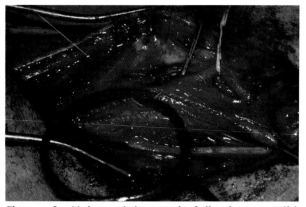

Figure 3. Vein patch repair following carotid endarterectomy. Here the carotid shunt is ready for removal, having been left in place until the patch is almost completed.

patch infection following carotid endartarectomy estimated the incidence of patch infection to be 0.25-0.5%. Soaking the Dacron® patch in rifampicin may reduce this risk.

The EVEREST trial [18] randomised 1353 patients to standard (n=675) or eversion endarterectomy (n=678). The early results showed no difference, but the later results showed that the risk of restenosis was significantly greater in the standard endartarectomy group at 4 years (9.2% vs. 3.6%, p=0.01).

Quality control on completion is recommended to avoid technical defects including intimal flaps, residual stenosis, kinking and thrombus. Intra-operative duplex ultrasound, arteriography or angioscopy can all be used. There have been no randomised controlled trials, but several series have reported reduced residual stenosis and stroke rates with the adoption of quality control measures [19].

Cerebral complications

The causes of peri-operative ischaemic stroke are clamping, cerebral embolisation and acute carotid occlusion. CEA has the advantage over CAS in that cerebral embolism can be reduced significantly or avoided (Figure 4). Measures include careful dissection (dissecting the patient off the carotid), early placement of a clamp on the distal ICA so that the brain is protected from emboli, complete removal of the carotid plaque with no residual fronds or flaps, adequate flushing to remove debris and thrombi, and declamping in the correct order (ICA back-bleed first and declamped last).

CAS has the advantage when it comes to the duration of carotid flow arrest. Even routine shunting results in a longer flow arrest time than CAS, unless cerebral protection with proximal balloon occlusion ± flow reversal is employed. However, a recent Cochrane review found no advantage for routine compared to selective shunting, or an advantage for any particular method of monitoring to select patients for selective shunting [20]. Cerebral ischaemia and the need for a shunt can often be avoided by ensuring a high per-operative blood pressure. This is also for cerebral embolism or bleeding. Catheter-directed thrombolysis or aspiration should be considered if the problem is cerebral embolism.

Hyperperfusion syndrome and intracranial haemorrhage have been reported after 0.4-14% and 0-1% of CEAs, respectively [21]. The diagnosis should be considered in any patient who develops postoperative symptoms of headache, photophobia, confusion or seizures, especially if they are hypertensive (Figure 5). Pre-operative blood pressure control and administration of IV beta-blockers such as labetalol or esmolol to maintain the postoperative BP below normal levels are good preventative measures. Vasodilators should be avoided as these can further increase cerebral blood flow. Specific treatment requires steroids, anti-epileptic drugs and ventilation.

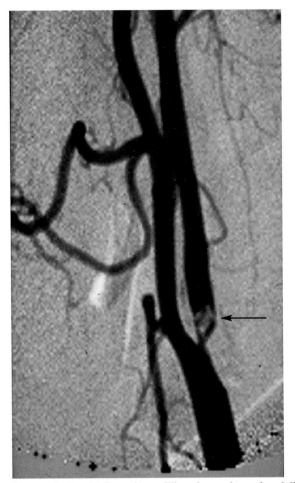

Figure 4. Fresh thrombus sitting in a stenosis at the origin of the ICA. This is best treated by careful dissection and early clamping of the distal ICA. This patient is not suitable for CAS.

important for good shunt flow. Failure of a shunt to restore a neurological deficit might indicate that the shunt is not working or that the problem is a cerebral embolus.

Despite the use of pre-operative antiplatelet agents and the intra-operative use of systemic heparin, acute occlusion of the carotid artery may occur in the peri-operative period. Any patient under GA who wakes with a new neurological deficit should be re-explored immediately and an intra-operative arteriogram obtained if no local abnormality is found. If a deficit occurs postoperatively, then an immediate duplex ultrasound scan is required. If the ICA is patent with no abnormality, then an urgent CTA is required to look

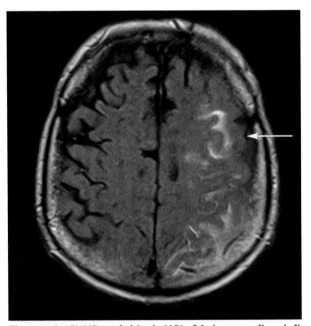

Figure 5. FLAIR-weighted MRI 24 hours after left carotid stenting showing changes consistent with cerebral hyperperfusion. Note the left hemispheric swelling with sulcal effacement, as well as the abnormal signal in the leptomeningeal space (arrow). The distribution of the signal changes is in the watershed territory between the left anterior and middle cerebral arteries.

Prevention and management of complications associated with CAS

Complications associated with CAS can also be classified into remote, cervical and cerebral.

Remote complications

Prophylactic anticholinergics are employed to block the effect of the baroreceptor stimulation that occurs during angioplasty/stenting but marked shifts in blood pressure and pulse can still occur. Some centres have used temporary pacing as a standard part of the procedure, whilst others use pacing if required. It seems sensible to ensure that an anaesthetist is present for high-risk patients.

CAS requires placement of a sheath in the common femoral artery (CFA), resulting in a significant puncture site in an artery which often has atherosclerotic changes. These patients are always treated with pre-operative dual antiplatelets and periprocedural heparin. Unsurprisingly, groin haematomas have been reported in 1.8-6% of cases and most centres therefore routinely use closure devices. Many radiologists use duplex ultrasound to select a non-calcified portion of CFA for catheterisation, as this reduces the risk of the closure device failing.

Cervical complications

Inability to gain access, place catheters and guide wires across the target lesion, or the demonstration of a non-treatable lesion occurred in 0.8-8% of patients in the large trials. Whilst patients can be selected for CEA on the basis of high-quality duplex ultrasound alone, this is unwise for CAS. Arteriography (conventional or MRA) is required to detect problems such as unfavourable aortic arch anatomy (Figure 6), and disease at the origin of the CCA or severe tortuosity (Figure 7). Acute stroke can occur during initial guide wire manipulation, especially if the anatomy is unfavourable. Analysis of the SPACE data showed that 10% of neurological events occurred during the navigation procedure.

Dissection can involve either the common (CCA) or internal carotid artery (ICA) and is usually caused by the guiding catheter or the introducer sheath during attempts to advance these devices whilst engaging the CCA. Early recognition is essential, as prompt anticoagulation can minimise the risk of stroke. A flow-limiting dissection requires gentle prolonged balloon dilatation or a stent. Spasm of the distal ICA is often caused by cerebral protection filters or the tip of the guide wire (Figure 8). Avoiding excessive movement of the wire or filter reduces the risk of spasm, which is treated with a vasodilator such as glyceryl trinitrate (GTN).

Plaque prolapse through the stent is a well-known complication of CAS, with an incidence ranging from

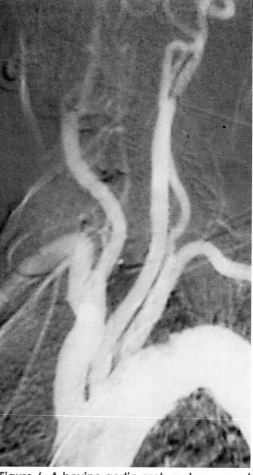

Figure 6. A bovine aortic arch makes cannulation of the carotid arteries more difficult and increases the risk of cerebral embolisation during guide wire manipulation. Patients for stenting should not be selected on the basis of a duplex scan alone.

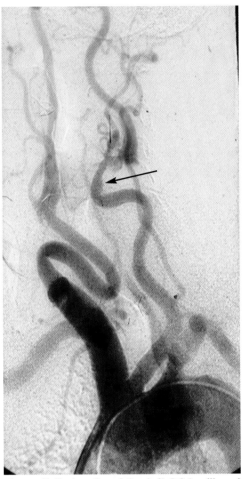

Figure 7. Tortuosity of the left CCA will make stenting of this left ICA stenosis difficult. Stenting will also increase the risk of kinking.

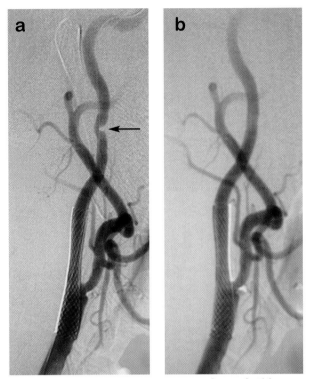

Figure 8. a) Spasm in the distal ICA (arrow). This can be caused by the guide wire or a filter device. b) The spasm resolved after the administration of nitrate.

0.2-4% [22]. The danger is that the prolapsed material can embolise or become a focus for thrombosis or restenosis (Figure 9). The risk of prolapse can be reduced by avoiding CAS in patients with high-risk echolucent plaques [23], and by using a closed-cell stent. Post hoc analysis of SPACE showed a higher adverse event rate for open-cell stents (5.6% closed versus 11% open). Significant prolapse can be treated by gentle balloon dilatation or placement of a second stent.

The reported incidence of restenosis varies depending upon the type of stent used and the length of follow-up (Figure 10). Open-cell stents seem to cause less restenosis, and are also more flexible, so less likely to cause kinking of the distal ICA [24].

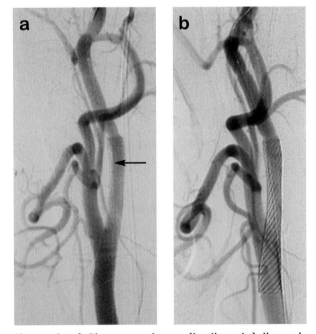

Figure 9. a) Plaque prolapse (toothpaste) through the open cells of a stent (arrow). This was treated with a second stent. b) The risk of plaque prolapse can be reduced by using closed-cell stents, and avoided by treating patients with echolucent plaques by endarterectomy instead.

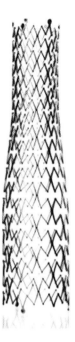

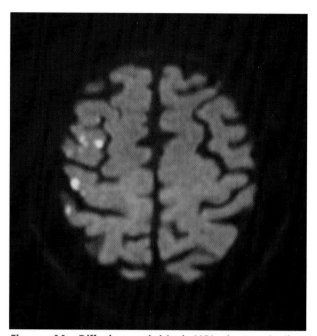

Figure 11. Diffusion-weighted MRI demonstrating multiple right cerebral micro-emboli 24 hours after right carotid stenting. There was no neurological deficit on clinical examination. Although these lesions may seem silent, there is concern that they can cause long-term cognitive impairment.

Figure 10. A stent designed specifically for the carotid artery. The Protege™ stent is made from self-expanding nitinol, with a tapered shape to fit the common carotid artery proximally and the internal carotid artery distally. It has an open-cell design which may reduce the rate of restenosis, but may be associated with a higher incidence of peri-procedural embolism.

CAVATAS is the only RCT with good long-term follow up thus far. Significant restenosis is twice as common after CAS compared to CEA, and is also associated with ipsilateral neurological events [25].

Cerebral complications

The biggest safety concern about CAS is the risk of cerebral embolisation. A number of anatomical, plaque morphology, procedural, device and patient-related factors have been identified which increase the likelihood of embolisation. Echolucent plaques have a higher risk of embolisation, as do patients who have existing ischaemic cerebral lesions. The large randomised trials have all reported twice as many strokes after CAS compared to CEA. The MRI substudy of the ICSS trial has shown that silent cerebral emboli occur five times more frequently after

CAS than after CEA [26], and there is increasing evidence that these micro-emboli can cause long-term cognitive impairment (Figure 11).

The initial response to the problem of cerebral embolism during CAS was to develop particulate filters that could be placed in the distal ICA. Although such filters do capture emboli, they can cause emboli as they are passed across the ICA stenosis. Despite many positive commercially sponsored trials, MacDonald *et al* have shown that filters do not reduce cerebral embolism [27]. Proximal balloon occlusion of the CCA combined with aspiration or reversed flow via an arteriovenous shunt seems a better method of cerebral protection. However, the best method of cerebral protection is probably a surgical clamp!

Cerebral hyperperfusion syndrome has an earlier onset following carotid artery stenting than after open surgery, usually occurring within 12 hours of the procedure. The incidence is lower than following CEA, but similar symptoms can also be caused by a shower of micro-emboli, contrast encephalopathy and cerebral haemorrhage [28]. A CT or MR head scan is required to determine the diagnosis, as treatment needs to be tailored to the cause.

Conclusions

At the present time, the safest carotid intervention for patients with symptomatic carotid disease remains CEA. However, modern BMT is much more effective in reducing the risk of a further stroke. This means that the advantage from any intervention may be reduced and the complication rate from any intervention probably needs to be less than 2% to remain cost-effective. The benefit of BMT and the low rate of complications associated with CEA make it difficult for CAS to compete, especially as it is an evolving technique. Any new trial of CEA versus CAS should also include a third arm, i.e. BMT alone. It seems likely that refinements in stent and cerebral protection technology will continue to erode the advantage of surgery, but applicability will be limited if the cost of consumables cannot be contained. Although CEA is safer than CAS in terms of stroke and death, it is associated with cranial nerve injury and a higher incidence of myocardial ischaemia and haematoma. The lowest rate of complications for any intervention will be obtained from multidisciplinary teams working in large-volume centres, who are able to offer all aspects of stroke treatment and who have independently audited outcomes. Patients must be fully informed of all the available treatment options and be involved in the decision-making process.

Key points

♦ Carotid artery intervention for stroke prevention in symptomatic patients is of proven benefit.

♦ Prevention is better than cure and all at-risk patients must be offered BMT intervention.

♦ On the basis of the current evidence, CEA is safer than CAS in terms of stroke and death, especially for elderly patients.

♦ CAS is associated with a lower risk of myocardial ischaemia, and also avoids the risk of cranial nerve injury.

♦ Cerebral emboli occur more frequently after CAS and may be associated with long-term cognitive impairment.

♦ Advances in stent and cerebral protection technology are likely to erode the advantage of surgery in the future.

♦ CAS seems a difficult technique to learn and simulation may play a role in training.

♦ The best results will come from multidisciplinary teams working in large-volume centres.

References

1. North American Symptomatic Carotid Endarterectomy Trial Collaborators (NASCET). Beneficial effect of carotid endarterectomy in symptomatic patients with high grade carotid stenosis. *N Engl J Med* 1991; 315: 445-53.

2. European Carotid Surgery Trialists' Collaborative Group (ECST). Randomised trial of endarterectomy for recently symptomatic carotid stenosis: final results of the MRC European Carotid Surgery Trial. *Lancet* 1998; 351: 1379-87.

3. UK audit of vascular surgical services and carotid endarterectomy. The Vascular Society of Great Britain and Ireland. July 2010 Public Report.

4. CAVATAS investigators. Endovascular versus surgical treatment in patients with carotid stenosis in the Carotid and Vertebral Transluminal Angioplasty Study (CAVATAS): a randomized trial. *Lancet* 2001; 357: 1729-37.

5. Mas JL, Trinquart L, Leys, D, *et al*, for the EVA - 3S Investigators. Endarterectomy versus angioplasty in patients with symptomatic severe carotid stenosis (EVA - 3S) trial: results for up to 4 years from a randomised, multicentre trial. *Lancet Neurol* 2008; 7: 885-92.

6. Eckstein H-H, Ringled P, AllenbergJ-R, *et al*. Results of the Stent Protected Angioplasty versus Carotid Endarterectomy (SPACE) study to treat symptomatic stenoses at 2 years: a multinational, prospective, randomised trial. *Lancet Neurol* 2008; 7: 893-902.

7. International Carotid Stenting Study Group. Carotid artery stenting compared with endarterectomy in patients with symptomatic carotid stenosis (International Carotid Stenting Study): an interim analysis of a randomised controlled trial. *Lancet* 2010; 375 (9719): 985-97.

8. Gurm HS, Yadav JS, Fayad P, *et al*, for the SAPPHIRE Investigators. Long-term results of carotid stenting versus endarterectomy in high-risk patients. *N Engl J Med* 2008; 358: 1572-9.

9. Brott TG, Hobson RW II, Howard G, *et al*, for the CREST Investigators. Stenting versus Endarterectomy for Treatment of Carotid-Artery Stenosis. *N Engl J Med* 2010; 363: 11-23.

10. Amarenco P, Labreuche J, Mazighi M. Lessons from carotid endarterectomy and stenting trials. *Lancet* 2010; 376: 1028-30.

11. Theiss W, Hermanek P, Mathias K, *et al*. Predictors of death and stroke after angioplasty and stenting: a subgroup analysis of the Pro CAS data. *Stroke* 2008; 39: 2325-30.

12. Sharpe RY, Dennis MJ, Nasim A, *et al*. Dual antiplatelet therapy prior to carotid endarterectomy reduces post-operative embolisation and thromboembolic events: postoperative transcranial Doppler monitoring is now unnecessary. *Eur J Vasc Endovasc Surg* 2010; 40: 162-7.

13. McGirt MJ, Perler BA, Brooke BS, *et al*. 3-hydroxy-3-methylglutaryl coenzyme A reductase inhibitors reduce the risk of perioperative stroke and mortality after carotid endarterectomy. *J Vasc Surg* 2005; 42: 829-36.

14. GALA Trial Collaborative Group. General anaesthesia versus local anaesthesia for carotid surgery (GALA): a multicentre, randomised controlled trial. *Lancet* 2008; 372: 2132-42.

15. Beasley WD, Gibbons CP. Cranial nerve injuries and the retrojugular approach in carotid endarterectomy. *Ann R Coll Surg Engl* 2008; 90: 685-8.

16. Bond R, Rerkasem K, AbuRahma AF, *et al*. Systematic review of randomised controlled trials of patch angioplasty versus primary closure and different types of patch materials during carotid endarterectomy. *J Vasc Surg* 2004; 40: 1126-35.

17. Knight BC, Tait WF. Dacron patch infection following carotid endarterectomy: a systematic review of the literature. *Eur J Vasc Surg* 2009; 37: 140-8.

18. Cao P, Giordano G, De Rango P, *et al* and collaborators of the EVEREST Study Group. Eversion versus conventional carotid endarterectomy: late results of a prospective multicentre randomised trial. *J Vasc Surg* 2000; 31: 19-30.

19. Dykes JR, Bergamini TM, Lipski DA, *et al*. Intraoperative duplex scanning reduces both residual stenosis and postoperative morbidity of carotid endarterectomy. *Am Surg* 1997; 63: 50-4.

20. Rerkasem K, Rothwell PM. Routine or selective carotid artery shunting for carotid endarterectomy and different methods of monitoring in selective shunting. *Cochrane Database Syst Rev* 2009: CD000190.

21. Naylor AR, Ruckley CV. The post carotid endarterectomy hyperperfusion syndrome. *Eur J Vasc Surg* 1995; 9: 365-7.

22. Roubin GS, New G, Iyer SS, *et al*. Immediate and late clinical outcomes of carotid artery stenting in patients with symptomatic and asymptomatic carotid artery stenosis; a 5-year prospective analysis. *Circulation* 2001; 103: 532-7.

23. Biasi GM, Froio A, Dietrich EB, *et al*. Carotid plaque echolucency increases the risk of stroke in carotid stenting. The imaging in carotid angioplasty and risk of stroke (ICAROS) study. *Circulation* 2004; 110: 756-62.

24. Bosiers M, de Donato G, Deloose K *et al*. Does free cell area influence the outcome in carotid artery stenting? *Eur J Vasc Endovasc Surg* 2007; 33: 135-41.

25. Bonati LH, Ederle J, McCabe DJH, *et al*, on behalf of the CAVATAS Investigators. Long-term risk of carotid restenosis in patients randomly assigned to endovascular treatment or endarterectomy in the Carotid and Vertebral Artery Transluminal Angioplasty Study (CAVATAS): long-term follow-up of a randomised trial. *Lancet Neurol* 2009; 8: 908-17.

26. ICSS-MRI Study Group. New ischaemic brain lesions on MRI after stenting or endarterectomy for symptomatic carotid stenosis: a substudy of the International Carotid Stenting Study (ICSS). *Lancet Neurol* 2010; 9: 353-62.

27. Macdonald S, Evans DH, Griffiths PD, *et al*. Filter-protected versus unprotected carotid artery stenting: a randomised trial. *Cerebrovasc Dis* 2010; 29: 282-9.

28. Buhk JH, Cepek L, Knauth M. Hyperacute intracerebral haemorrhage complicating carotid stenting should be distinguished from hyperperfusion syndrome. *Am J Neuroradiol* 2008; 27: 1508-13.

Dextran-induced haematoma after carotid endarterectomy

Frank C. T. Smith BSc MD FRCS FRCSEd, Reader & Honorary Consultant Vascular Surgeon
University of Bristol & Bristol Royal Infirmary, Bristol, UK

A 72-year-old lady underwent a left carotid endarterectomy for crescendo TIAs. Intra-operative transcranial Doppler (TCD) detected significant micro-embolisation and the patient was given intravenous dextran. Despite careful surgical haemostasis, the patient suffered a significant haematoma requiring postoperative decompression of the neck wound (Figure 1). The extensive haematoma extended into the retropharynx (Figure 2) and as far as the contralateral breast (Figure 3).

Dextran manufacture has now ceased. A randomised trial has suggested that a single 75mg dose of clopidogrel (administered the night before surgery in addition to daily 75mg aspirin) significantly reduces post-CEA embolisation [1]. Intra-operative TCD is no longer necessary.

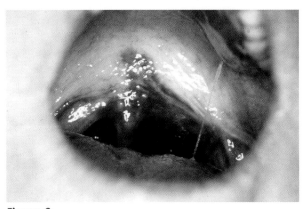

Figure 2.

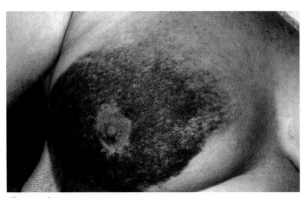

Figure 3.

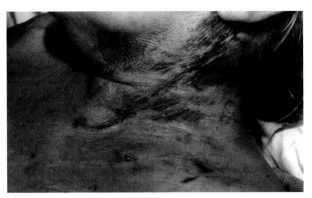

Figure 1.

Reference

1. Sharpe RY, Dennis MJ, Nasim A, *et al*. Dual antiplatelet therapy prior to carotid endarterectomy reduces post-operative embolisation and thromboembolic events: post-operative transcranial Doppler monitoring is now unnecessary. *Eur J Vasc Endovasc Surg* 2010; 40: 162-7.

Case vignette   Resection of a vagus nerve paraganglioma

Frank C. T. Smith BSc MD FRCS FRCSEd, Reader & Honorary Consultant Vascular Surgeon
University of Bristol & Bristol Royal Infirmary, Bristol, UK

A 68-year-old lady presented with a painless slowly enlarging mass at the level of the carotid bifurcation in the right side of the neck. A contrast CT scan confirmed a vascular blush in the mass which was contiguous with the carotid vessels (Figure 1). Surgery was undertaken for what was presumed to be a carotid body tumour.

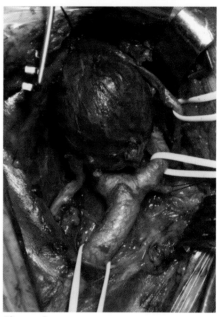

Figure 2.

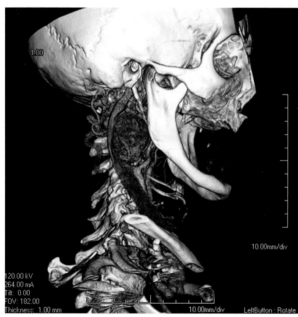

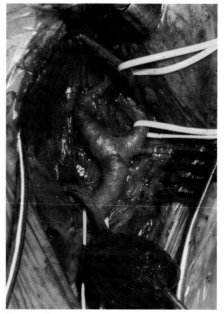

Figure 1.

At operation the mass was dissected free from the carotid vessels and a surgical tissue plane was developed relatively easily (Figure 2). However, during the dissection it became evident that the mass involved the vagus nerve, seen emerging from the distal aspect of the tumour (Figure 3).

The vagus nerve was sacrificed, but the hypoglossal nerve was preserved. On histological examination, the mass proved to be a paraganglioma of the vagus nerve. The patient sustained a unilateral vocal cord palsy which was subsequently treated by Teflon® injection.

Figure 3.

Chapter 20 Aorto-iliac and infra-inguinal surgery

Felicity Jane Meyer MA FRCS, Consultant Vascular Surgeon and Honorary Senior Lecturer
Norfolk and Norwich University Hospital, University of East Anglia, Norwich, UK

Introduction

The management of patients with aorto-iliac and infra-inguinal occlusive disease provides the mainstay of outpatient arterial vascular surgical practice. The majority of these patients are, however, treated conservatively with best medical therapy, and intervention is generally reserved for the treatment of patients with lifestyle-limiting symptoms of intermittent claudication or critical ischaemia (rest pain, gangrene or ulceration). This is because 80% of claudicants will either remain symptomatically stable or improve spontaneously without intervention [1]. In addition, even the very best reported patency rates for femoropopliteal bypass grafts are less than 90% [2, 3], and 1% of claudicants who undergo infra-inguinal surgery will require a major amputation [3]. Aorto-iliac interventions, whether surgical or radiological, carry a measurable mortality as well as a significant morbidity risk [4]. In essence, intervention for arterial occlusive disease is relatively difficult, occasionally dangerous and often does not provide the patient with the expected benefit. This chapter aims to help the reader deal with the complications associated with aortic, iliac or infra-inguinal intervention.

The aorto-iliac segment

Aorto-iliac surgery may be performed for patients with critical limb ischaemia or lifestyle-limiting claudication, where radiological intervention is either not feasible or has failed. Clamping of the aorta itself has significant physiological effects and aortic surgery is generally reserved for individuals with reasonable functional capacity. Extra-anatomical bypasses, such as femorofemoral crossover or axillofemoral bypasses are less physiologically demanding alternatives. With such high-risk surgery, it is important to understand the problems/operative complications which can occur and know how to overcome such difficulties with the minimum of detriment to the patient.

Clamp difficulties

Clamping difficulties usually arise because a vessel is too wide (Figure 1a), too calcified (Figure 1b) or disintegrates on clamping (Figure 1c). A useful trick to cope with either wide or heavily calcified arteries is to apply synthetic sleeves to ordinary clamps (e.g. Surg-I-Paw®, Scanlan). These covers are usually used for Crafoord or similar clamps, but applying them to ordinary DeBakey clamps, both increases the range

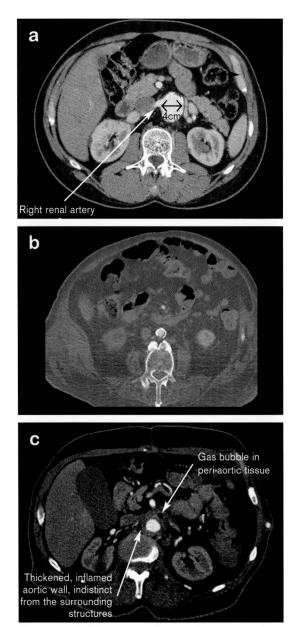

Figure 1. a) CT of the abdomen showing a wide aorta at the level of the right renal artery (clamp level). If the aorta has a diameter of ~3.5cm or more, as illustrated, a standard clamp cannot oppose its jaws adequately to occlude the vessel lumen. b) CT of the abdomen showing an infrarenal aorta with circumferential calcification. This tiny calcified aorta will not be compliant when a clamp is applied. The lumen, therefore, will not be occluded by clamping unless the arterial wall is disrupted. This may lead to uncontrollable haemorrhage. c) CT showing a thickened, inflamed aortic wall together with gas bubbles in the surrounding tissue. This infected aorta is liable to disintegrate on clamping. These findings are pathognomonic for arterial infection.

of the clamp and redistributes the force allowing ectatic or calcified arteries to be safely controlled (Figure 2). Another useful tip when suturing a heavily calcified artery is to apply fibrin sealant glue prophylactically before the clamp is released. This reinforces the artery around the stitch holes and may prevent tears.

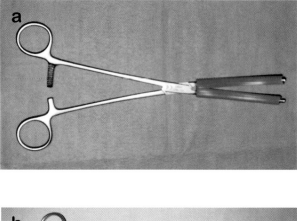

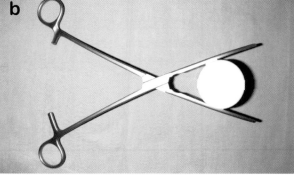

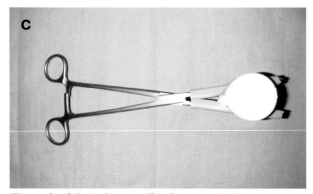

Figure 2. a) DeBakey aortic clamp and clamp covers applied. These are soft and non-traumatic to arterial tissues. b) An uncovered clamp is unable to clamp a 4cm object without inflicting significant damage. c) The covered clamp safely clamping the 4cm object with minimal risk of traumatic disruption.

Disintegration of the aorta or iliac arteries occurs either when a clamp is applied too vigorously or in the presence of infection (Figure 1c). An aortic compressor (Figure 3) or a thumb (the operating surgeon's or assistant's) can be applied while a suprarenal clamp is secured. In the presence of infection, however, particularly an infected juxtarenal aortic graft, it may be difficult to secure a suprarenal clamp. This may occur because of the presence of dense adhesions around a previous graft, an anastomotic pseudoaneurysm (Figure 4), or an active aortoduodenal fistula (Figure 5) that may bleed catastrophically if disturbed. For patients with such complications associated with previous grafting and for whom direct aortic clamping is deemed too much of a risk, a modification of a technique used in cardiothoracic surgery can be employed [5, 6]. The previous aortic graft is exposed and clamped proximally and distally, avoiding the fragile aortic tissues. A Prolene purse-string can then be sutured into the graft body and a hole cut in the middle of this purse-string. A large Foley urinary catheter can then be inserted into the hole and the purse-string tightened securely. The clamps can then be released and the catheter passed proximally until the balloon reaches the suprarenal aorta. The balloon can then be inflated and the suprarenal aorta is controlled from within. This technique can also be used for heavily calcified vessels.

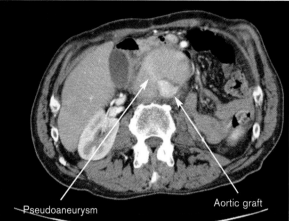

Figure 4. CT showing an anastomotic pseudoaneurysm complicating an infected aortic graft. There is contrast in the pseudoaneurysm where the aortic graft has become detached from the native vessel.

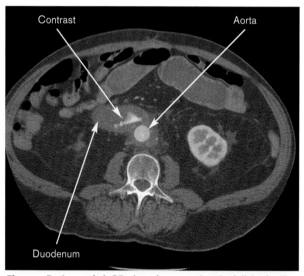

Figure 5. An axial CT showing contrast visible in the duodenum in an aortoduodenal fistula, indicating active bleeding from the aorta into the gut.

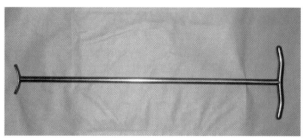

Figure 3. An aortic compressor.

Bleeding

Uncontrolled aorto-iliac bleeding is rapidly fatal. Aortic bleeding is best controlled with a clamp, but a balloon inserted from the femoral [7], brachial [8] or axillary [9] arteries can be used for temporary control during resuscitation. If there is persistent, generalised abdominal bleeding or ooze, intra-abdominal packing overnight is often helpful. Once all the anastomoses have been satisfactorily completed, intravenous protamine can be administered to reverse the heparin anticoagulation if required.

Iliac bleeding can occur as a result of percutaneous intervention or even spinal surgery and may not be recognised early, particularly as the haemorrhage may be retroperitoneal. In these cases, temporary percutaneous balloon tamponade followed by placement of a covered iliac stent is a quick and relatively easy solution [10].

Miscellaneous tips

When approaching the iliac vessels intra-abdominally, the small bowel may be stuck to or sitting in the pelvis, especially if there has been previous intestinal surgery. In this circumstance, putting the patient head down, as might be done for an anterior resection, instantly improves access. In addition, a pelvic retractor, such as a St Mark's deep pelvic retractor, may sometimes be useful.

The infra-inguinal segment

Infra-inguinal surgery is commonly performed for critical limb ischaemia: rest pain, gangrene or ulceration. These patients have often had several previous procedures, are frequently frail, elderly and malnourished, and may have infection either in their feet or in previous prosthetic grafts. All of these circumstances make reconstructive surgery technically difficult and liable to fail. Amputation, however, has a high morbidity and mortality and relatively few patients will walk again. Infra-inguinal reconstruction is, therefore, often the best available treatment option.

Clamping difficulties

Clamping difficulties in the infra-inguinal region can usually be managed in a similar way to those in the aorto-iliac segment. If it is not possible to clamp the common femoral artery, usually because of heavy calcification (Figure 6), there are at least two possible solutions. Firstly, if the groin is already open and there is a satisfactory portion of distal external iliac artery, the inguinal ligament can be divided to assist access. This is preferable to attempting to place a clamp on a proximal iliac vessel blindly, which often results in damage to the moderately sized veins which consistently cross anterior to the distal external iliac artery. The inguinal ligament can be divided for at least

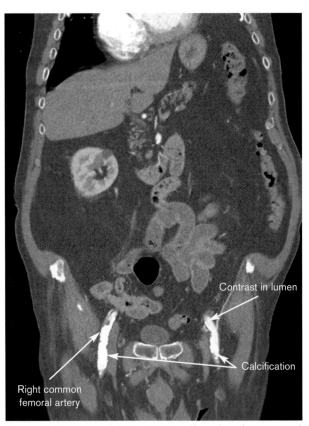

Figure 6. A coronal CT reconstruction showing normal contrast flowing through the common femoral arteries and extensive bilateral common femoral artery calcification.

a centimetre without any risk, to access the external iliac artery or any bleeding veins. If more extensive division is required, it should be repaired formally with non-absorbable sutures to prevent a pre-vascular hernia developing. If both the common femoral and the external iliac arteries are diseased, or an anatomical bypass is required from the common iliac to the common femoral arteries (Figure 7), the common or external iliac arteries can be accessed retroperitoneally via a modified Rutherford Morison skin incision and by dividing the muscles along the semilunar line.

Calcified occlusive plaque at any level, including occasionally the calf arteries, can be treated by performing a limited endarterectomy. If the standard available arterial clamps are too heavy, the distal calf arteries can usually be controlled with a double sling or a proprietary balloon occlusion catheter. A light titanium

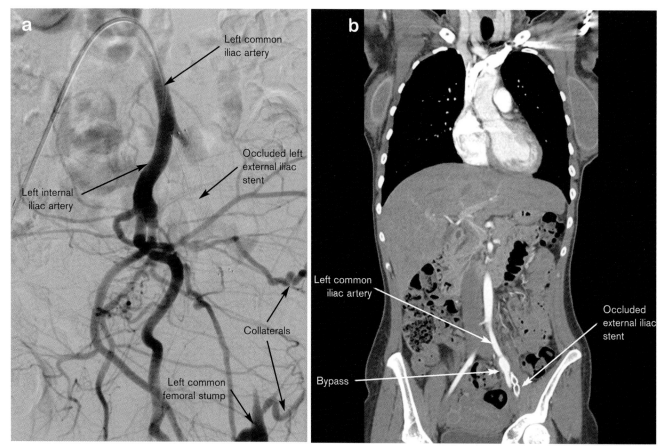

Figure 7. a) Oblique view of a digital subtraction angiogram with a catheter tip placed in the left common iliac artery showing an occluded left external iliac stent and common femoral artery. A short stump of the left common femoral artery is visible being supplied by large collateral arteries. **b)** Coronal CT reconstruction showing an anatomical iliofemoral bypass in the same patient. A reinforced Dacron® bypass was inserted between the left common iliac and common femoral arteries. The occluded stent can also be seen.

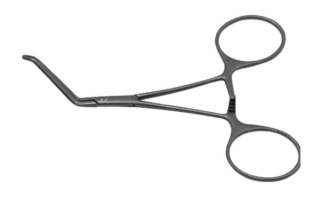

Figure 8. A titanium micro Kitzmiller clamp.

micro Kitzmiller clamp® (Figure 8) (Phoenix Surgical Instruments Limited), sometimes used in carotid surgery, is a useful alternative in these circumstances.

Bleeding

Bleeding in the infra-inguinal region is usually less immediately life-threatening than for aorto-iliac surgery. Uncontrolled intra-operative bleeding can arise, from an infected femoral pseudoaneurysm in an intravenous drug user. This is best prevented by controlling the iliac vessels via the modified Rutherford Morison approach before opening the groin. If the femoral bleeding occurs unexpectedly, firm pressure applied in the iliac fossa may be used to occlude the iliac system temporarily.

Suture-hole bleeding is a common problem with polytetrafluoroethylene (PTFE) grafts, which are commonly used in the infra-inguinal region. This can be minimised by using PTFE sutures, although many surgeons find them challenging to use. Topical haemostats such as Surgicel® (original or fibrillar, Ethicon) or Collatamp® (Eusa Pharma), which is also gentamicin-impregnated, are useful in this situation, as is fibrin sealant glue applied to the anastomosis prior to clamp release. Fibrin sealant glue can also be used to reinforce weak-walled arteries prior to suturing. Always remember the six Ps for haemostasis: patience, pressure, platelets, plasma, protamine and polymers (see Chapter 6).

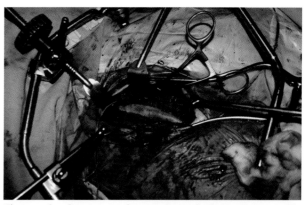

Figure 9. Common femoral endarterectomy with patch angioplasty made easier with a small Omnitract retractor.

Infra-inguinal bypass tips

Vascular patients are becoming increasingly obese [11] and the availability of assistants is often limited. A useful adjunct to operating in the groin in these circumstances is to use a FastSystem® Small Wishbone (paediatric or mini) Omni-Tract® retractor [12] (Figure 9). This allows extensive retraction of tissues,

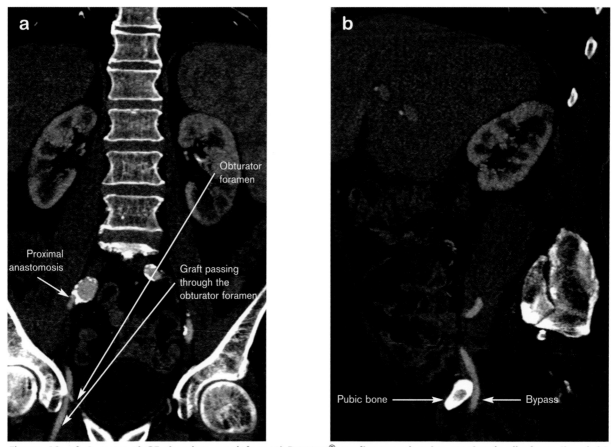

Figure 10. a) A coronal CT showing a reinforced Dacron® graft passed extra-anatomically from the right common iliac artery through the obturator foramen. This bypass was anastomosed distally onto the mid-thigh branches of the right profunda femoris artery. b) Sagittal view of the same bypass.

including the inguinal ligament, without assistance. It also allows a supervisor to train a more junior surgeon to perform the procedure.

If there is prolonged intra-operative common femoral artery occlusion, such as may arise in an aborted endovascular aneurysm repair in a heavily diseased iliofemoral segment, a large carotid shunt, such as a Javid™, can be used to restore flow to the lower limb while an endarterectomy or bypass is performed.

It may be necessary to bypass the groin, either because of infection or occlusion. In these circumstances, a graft can be passed through the obturator foramen, taking care to avoid the obturator vessels which lie anteriorly. Using this approach, it is possible to reach the distal superficial femoral artery or even the distal profunda branches and to avoid the inguinal region [13] (Figure 10). The distal profunda branches can also be accessed via the medial thigh [14]. Another lower limb extra-anatomical bypass is a lateral thigh femoro-anterior tibial prosthetic bypass (Figure

11). The reinforced graft is tunnelled laterally along the thigh thus avoiding the trauma of passing a large prosthetic bypass through the interosseous membrane.

If there is no obvious available long saphenous vein for a bypass in a patient where a prosthetic graft is undesirable, cephalic and basilic arm veins can be used. If the available arm vein is too short, smaller portions can be joined together to make a longer graft. Alternatively both small saphenous veins can be harvested and connected. If there is a disparity between an endarterectomised common femoral artery and these rather small reversed veins, the common femoral artery can be repaired with either a vein or prosthetic patch, and the vein graft sutured onto it through a small arteriotomy (Figure 12). If there is a

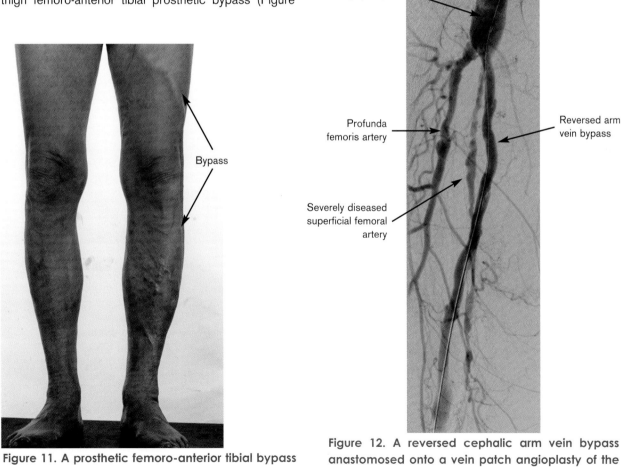

Vein patch angioplasty

Profunda femoris artery

Severely diseased superficial femoral artery

Reversed arm vein bypass

Bypass

Figure 11. A prosthetic femoro-anterior tibial bypass tunnelled along the lateral thigh.

Figure 12. A reversed cephalic arm vein bypass anastomosed onto a vein patch angioplasty of the common femoral artery. This graft is still functioning 3 years postoperatively.

long distal arteriotomy, a venous cuff can be used in a similar fashion. Both of these techniques reduce the calibre and compliance mismatch between the graft and the native arteries.

The distal vessels often have poor backflow, either because of spasm or disease. Spasm in any vessels can be treated with topical papaverine (up to 1ml of 40mg/ml papaverine solution). In patients with an acute thrombotic or embolic occlusion of distal vessels, this may be treated with Fogarty embolectomy using a small size 2F or 3F catheter. In the event of failure, or the clot is very distal, recombinant tissue plasminogen activator (rt-PA) can be infused directly into the affected vessel. If all else fails, an amputation may be necessary: it is better to lose a limb than a patient.

Conclusions

Arterial surgery is difficult and often hazardous and even the most competent vascular surgeons will occasionally face major challenges. For this reason, operations for occlusive vascular disease should only be performed for patients with critical ischaemia or where symptoms significantly impair quality of life. Meticulous pre-operative planning, particularly when performing an uncommon procedure, should reduce the risk of unexpected complications. When difficulties do arise, the principles of adequate control of the arteries both proximally and distally and of not opening a vessel without considering how it can be closed remain paramount to the maintenance of patient safety. Remember that approaches or instruments usually utilised in other vascular beds or in different areas of surgical expertise often provide an answer. A five-minute break away from the operating table may facilitate thought when problems occur. If all ideas run dry, it is always worth calling an experienced colleague sooner rather than later. They may well have faced the same situation before and have an elegant solution. If not, at least the problem has been shared and every possible avenue explored.

Key points

- Always consider conservative management.
- Plan difficult cases carefully.
- Control arteries and consider methods of closure before performing an arteriotomy.
- Remember the six bleeding Ps: patience, pressure, platelets, plasma, protamine, polymers.
- Use techniques and instruments from other specialities and different vascular procedures.
- Take a break and/or call for assistance.
- Never forget that complications happen to everyone.

References

1. Dormandy JA, Murray GD. The fate of the claudicant - a prospective study of 1969 claudicants. *Eur J Vasc Surg* 1991; 5: 131-3.
2. Watelet J, Cheysson E, Poels D. *In situ* versus reversed saphenous vein for femoropopliteal bypass: a prospective randomized study of 100 cases. *Ann Vasc Surg* 1986; 1: 441-52.
3. Goodney PP, Likosky DS, Cronenwert JL, Vascular Study Group of Northern New England. Predicting ambulation status one year after lower extremity bypass. *J Vasc Surg* 2009; 49: 1431-9.
4. Beard J. Which is the best revascularization option for critical limb ischemia: endovascular or open surgery? *J Vasc Surg* 2008; 48: 11S-6.
5. Erath HG, Stoney WS. Balloon catheter occlusion of the ascending aorta. *Ann Thorac Surg* 1983; 35: 560-1.
6. Cosgrove DM. Management of the calcified aorta: an alternative method of occlusion. *Ann Thorac Surg* 1983; 36: 718-9.
7. Greenberg RK, Srivastava SD, Ouriel K, *et al.* An endoluminal method of hemorrhage control and repair of ruptured abdominal aortic aneurysms. *J Endovasc Ther* 2000; 7: 1-7.
8. Okhi T, Veith FJ. Endovascular grafts and other image-guided catheter-based adjuncts to improve the treatment of ruptured aortoiliac aneurysms. *Ann Surg* 2000; 232: 466-79.

9.   Smith FG. Emergency control of ruptured abdominal aortic aneurysm by transaxillary balloon catheter. *Vasc Surg* 1972; 6: 79-84.

10.   Formichi M, Raybaud G, Benichou H, *et al*. Rupture of the external iliac artery during balloon angioplasty. *J Endovasc Surg* 1998; 5: 37-41.

11.   Khandanpour N, Armon MP, Foxall R, *et al*. The effects of increasing obesity on outcomes of vascular surgery. *Ann Vasc Surg* 2009; 23: 310-6.

12.   Chaudhuri A, Clarke JM. Extended femoral endarterectomy using the Omnitract retractor. *Ann R Coll Surg Engl* 2004; 86: 308.

13.   Shaw S, Baue AE. Management of sepsis complicating arterial reconstructive procedures. *Surgery* 1963; 53: 75-86.

14.   Nunez AA, Veith FJ, Collier P, *et al*. Direct approaches to the distal portions of the deep femoral artery for limb salvage bypasses. *J Vasc Surg* 1988; 8: 576-81.

Case vignette   Profunda bleeding

Felicity Jane Meyer MA FRCS, Consultant Vascular Surgeon and Honorary Senior Lecturer
Norfolk and Norwich University Hospital, University of East Anglia, Norwich, UK

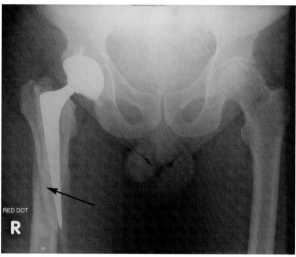

Figure 1.

A 62-year-old company chairman was admitted to the orthopaedic service with a femoral shaft fracture below a previous prosthesis (Figure 1). He was taken to theatre the following day and placed in a lateral decubitus position. The femoral component was replaced and encircling wires were fed around the femoral fracture; this resulted in profuse arterial bleeding. The vascular surgeon was called and the bleeding was controlled with pressure and blind suturing. The following day his haemoglobin had dropped and he had developed a swelling of his thigh. An arteriogram identified a bleeding profunda femoris branch (Figure 2), which was successfully embolised with coils (Figure 3). The patient went on to make a full recovery.

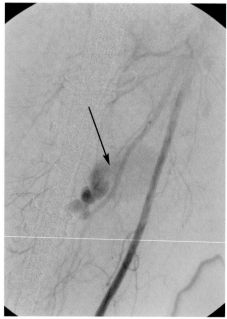

Figure 2.

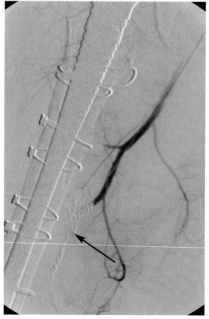

Figure 3.

Chapter 21 The diabetic foot

Frank C. T. Smith BSc MD FRCS FRCSEd, Reader & Honorary Consultant Vascular Surgeon
University of Bristol & Bristol Royal Infirmary, Bristol, UK

Introduction

With respect to avoiding complications in vascular surgery, the adage that if you had wanted to get to a particular place, you wouldn't have started from your current position is particularly apposite for the diabetic foot. Complications are best avoided by early recognition and prompt prevention of characteristic patterns of problems in this difficult clinical arena. Multidisciplinary treatment in fast-track or hot-foot clinics underpins successful management.

Diabetes affects approximately 3% of the UK population and treating diabetic complications accounts for approximately 9% of total NHS hospital costs [1, 2]. Foot problems account for more admissions than any other diabetic complication. Up to 5% of patients with diabetes will develop a foot ulcer in any year. Recurrence rates, even after ulcer healing, are high (up to 25%). The development of a diabetic foot ulcer is a poor prognostic indicator, preceding 75% of leg amputations. Diabetic foot problems are the most common cause of non-traumatic limb amputation, imposing a 13-fold risk increase [3]. It is believed that amputation could be avoided in up to 85% of diabetics, with better foot care.

Despite publication of strategies for prevention and management of diabetic foot problems in hospital, variation of inpatient care for diabetic foot problems persists. Approximately 100 people a week lose a leg through diabetes in the UK, and the amputation rate remains approximately 0.5% [4].

The 2011 NICE clinical guidelines draw attention to the fact that diabetic foot complications have a significant impact on patients' quality of life and require urgent attention [1]. Delay in diagnosis and management increases morbidity and mortality and contributes to higher amputation rates.

The diabetic foot is best managed in a multidisciplinary setting using a focused approach in a dedicated diabetic foot clinic, with integrated care. The multidisciplinary team will include diabetologists, podiatrists, diabetic nurse specialists, tissue viability nurses, orthopaedic and vascular surgeons, and orthotists. Access to diagnostic and interventional radiology services is essential. The clinic should have rapid access and one-stop diagnostic facilities so that patients with a newly developed ulcer or foot infection can be seen promptly.

Complications in the diabetic foot are characterised by the inter-dependent triad of ischaemia, neuropathy and infection. This chapter summarises problems arising as a consequence of these factors and suggests management approaches to avoid them.

Classification

For practical purposes the diabetic foot can be classified as neuropathic or neuro-ischaemic; ischaemia without some degree of neuropathy is rare. In the neuropathic foot, the blood supply is preserved and thus it is important to make the distinction between the two conditions since management differs.

It has been estimated that approximately 25-44% of diabetic foot complications are due to neuropathy, 10% are due to ischaemia, anf 45-60% are neuro-ischaemic. Neuropathy, neuro-ischaemia and ischaemia all predispose to infection which is often the presenting clinical feature.

Recognition of the foot at risk of ulceration is important. Diabetic patients should have annual screening to identify potential risk factors including callus formation and deformity. In the foot identified as at risk, regular specialist podiatry review is indicated. Advice about footwear and early off-loading of pressure points or an incipient ulcer with orthotics is essential, and may allow ulcer healing. In the early stages of development, pressure off-loading can be achieved by bed rest, reducing the oedema which inhibits healing. Care needs to be taken to avoid the development of new pressure-related ulcers and to use DVT prophylaxis. Early mobilization can be achieved using a total contact plaster cast.

Assessment

Assessment of the diabetic foot is based on history, clinical inspection, palpation and sensory testing. Footwear should also be examined. The eight principal clinical characteristics of the diabetic foot are listed in Table 1 [5].

Table 1. Clinical characteristics of the diabetic foot.

- Neuropathy
- Ischaemia
- Deformity
- Callus
- Swelling
- Skin ulceration
- Infection
- Necrosis

Edmonds and Foster have described six stages in the natural history of the diabetic foot (Table 2) [5]. Clinical assessment allows staging and subsequent management, as directed, to preventing progression from one stage to the next.

Table 2. Staging of the diabetic foot.

Stage	Clinical condition
1	Normal
2	High risk
3	Ulcerated
4	Infected
5	Necrotic
6	Unsalvageable

Neuropathy

Neuropathy affects up to 50% of patients with diabetes. This is a polyneuropathy, affecting the autonomic and somatic (sensory and motor) peripheral nervous systems.

Possible explanations include impaired vascular supply to the nerves or accumulation of sorbitol due to increased activity of the polyol pathway, potentially resulting in toxic effects including demyelination and impaired nerve conduction velocities.

Autonomic neuropathy may result in arteriovenous shunts in the microcirculation diverting nutrient blood away from the skin. Loss of normal skin moisture due to autonomic denervation of sweat glands leaves the skin dry and prone to developing cracks and fissures, which increases susceptibility to infection. Hair loss and nail deformities also form part of the spectrum of trophic changes in the diabetic foot.

Attenuation of the nociceptive reflex with diminished responses to noxious stimuli impairs the neuroinflammatory response and increases risk of injury due to sensory loss, particularly with respect to pain, pressure-related trauma and temperature.

Motor neuropathy leads to atrophy and wasting of the intrinsic muscles of the foot. This reduces digital stability at metatarsophalangeal joint level, resulting in exaggeration of the plantar arch (pes cavus) and toes being drawn up into the 'claw' position. In turn, the normal balance of the foot is altered, placing abnormal pressure loading on the metatarsal heads and tips of the toes (and the dorsal interphalangeal joints where these rub against footwear), which may cause ulceration. Other common joint deformities include hallux valgus, hallux rigidus and hammer toe. Formation of thick callus may precede ulceration at pressure points (Figure 1).

Deformity secondary to neuropathy also occurs in the Charcot foot. Here a painless and progressive degenerative arthropathy affects the joints of the foot and ankle. Loss of proprioception and sensation results in these joints being subjected to abnormal forces causing ligamentous and capsular damage which progresses to painless joint laxity and subluxation. Wear of articular surfaces, bony degeneration and collapse often result in severe foot deformity. Collapse of the medial longitudinal arch of the foot gives rise to the appearance of the rocker-bottom deformity (Figure 2).

Colour and temperature may range from hyperaemic and warm in the well-perfused neuropathic foot, to cool and pale when ischaemia coexists. The foot may appear pink even when there is significantly impaired arterial inflow, due to arteriovenous shunting in the microcirculation.

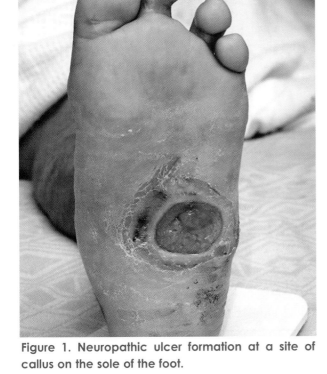

Figure 1. Neuropathic ulcer formation at a site of callus on the sole of the foot.

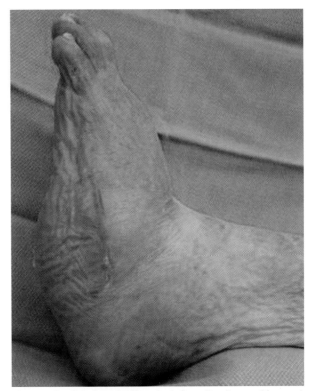

Figure 2. 'Rocker-bottom' deformity in a Charcot foot.

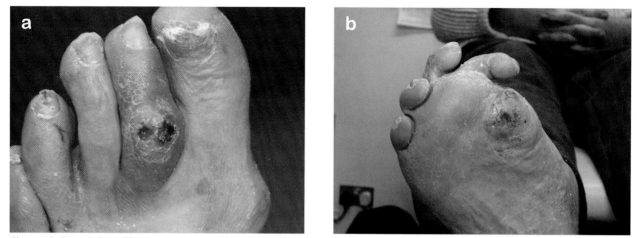

Figure 3. Toe deformities and neuropathic ulceration over a) dorsal interphalangeal joints and b) first metatarsal head.

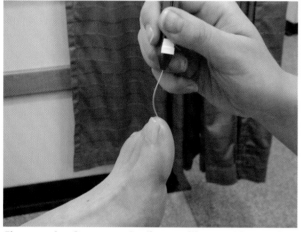

Figure 4. Sensory testing with a 10g nylon monofilament.

Examination for neuropathy should include assessment of colour and temperature of the foot. Trophic changes compatible with autonomic neuropathy should be sought. Deformities including claw toes and joint abnormalities (including crepitus) should be described (Figures 3a and b). Loss of pinprick sensation is a distinguishing feature of neuropathy. Use of a 10g nylon monofilament applied perpendicularly in a systematic pattern across the foot is a sensitive method of determining the extent of sensory impairment (Figure 4), but should not be relied on at sites affected by callus, which should be removed first (Figures 5a and b). Loss of vibration sense using a 128Hz tuning fork may be useful in distinguishing young patients at risk of developing

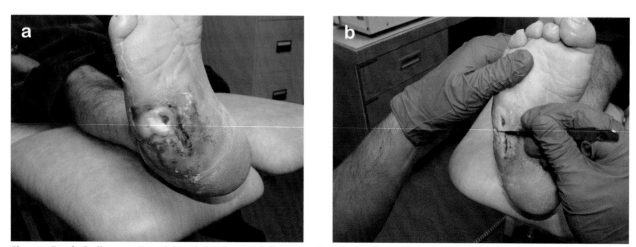

Figure 5. a) Callus on the side of the foot. b) This can be debrided without anaesthetic because the ulcer is neuropathic.

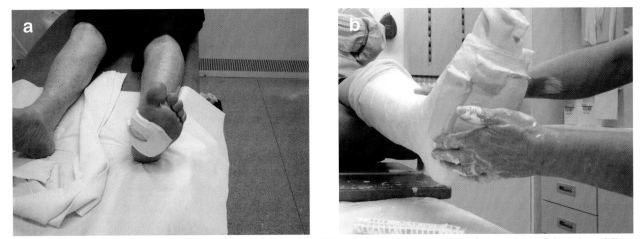

Figure 6. Off-loading of pressure from a stable neuropathic ulcer on the sole of the foot, using: a) local padding and b) a plaster cast.

further significant neuropathy. Absent ankle reflexes are a common finding. The degree of neuropathy may be quantified by neurothesiometry. Off-loading of pressure forms the mainstay of management in patients with neuropathic ulceration (Figure 6a and b).

Ischaemia

The most important principle in treating diabetic foot ischaemia is recognition that this occurs mainly as a result of macrovascular occlusion of the leg arteries due to atherosclerosis. Whilst microcirculatory dysfunction does occur in diabetes, the myth of small vessel disease as the main cause of diabetic foot ischaemia spawned a therapeutic nihilism culminating in excessive amputation rates. This approach is outdated and should be discouraged. Characteristic patterns of atherosclerosis in diabetic patients often principally affect the calf vessels, with relative sparing of the foot arteries (Figure 7). Microcirculatory changes, however, with localised capillary endothelial cell thickening, increased permeability, white cell margination and platelet aggregation may compound the effects of proximal arterial disease, leading to focal areas of skin ischaemia, predisposing to ulceration.

The prevalence of systemic atherosclerosis may be greater in patients with diabetes than those without. This increases the risk of concomitant coronary, cerebrovascular and renal artery disease and

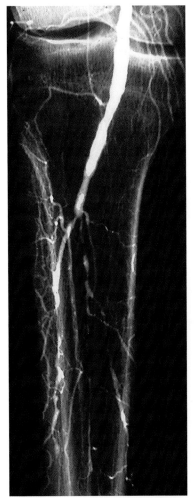

Figure 7. Angiogram demonstrating popliteal artery calcification and extensive diabetic calf vessel disease.

accompanying cardiovascular mortality. Diabetes has been identified as an independent risk factor for adverse cardiac events in patients undergoing major vascular surgery. Arterial reconstruction in diabetic patients is therefore accompanied by increased risk of cardiovascular morbidity and mortality.

Where arterial reconstruction is considered for critical ischaemia (threatened limb loss, rest pain or tissue loss), the ability to rehabilitate and walk postoperatively and the likelihood of return to home residence are primary considerations in terms of patient selection for surgery. In patients who are unlikely to do well after arterial reconstruction, early primary amputation may prove to be more appropriate (Figure 8). Less invasive endovascular procedures are employed with increasing frequency and may fend off or temporarily delay a need for arterial surgery.

Patients with salvageable foot ischaemia but with concomitant infection need to have the infection

controlled prior to definitive arterial reconstruction. Treatment with intravenous broad-spectrum antibiotics and debridement of overtly infected necrotic tissue (which may involve partial forefoot or digital amputation) should be undertaken as necessary, but a prolonged or protracted delay prior to definitive reconstruction should be avoided because this may result in extension of necrosis and further tissue loss. Digital amputation, drainage of abscesses and debridement of necrotic issue can often be done with minimal analgesia, or regional/anaesthesia in the profoundly neuropathic foot. Optimising medical treatment with respect to diabetic control (often difficult during septic episodes), use of appropriate antiplatelet agents, statins, ACE inhibitors and beta-blockers, in this interim, may reduce peri-operative cardiac mortality and morbidity.

Patients with proximal arterial disease may complain of claudication. Nocturnal cramps and lower limb dysaesthesia are not uncommon in diabetic patients, but should be carefully distinguished from classical claudication and ischaemic rest pain which, characteristically, occurs in the distal foot on elevation and may be relieved by dependency.

Skin colour may be dusky red due to arteriovenous shunting, or pale with evidence of blueness or mottling in acute ischaemia. The ischaemic foot will usually be cool (Figure 9). Palpation for posterior tibial, dorsalis pedis, popliteal and femoral pulses

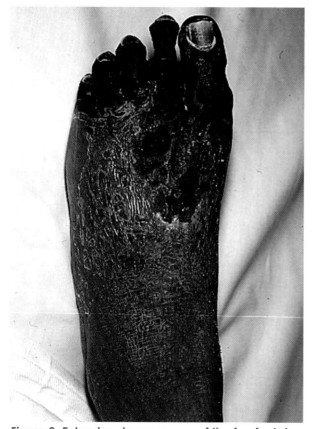

Figure 8. Extensive dry gangrene of the forefoot due to diabetic ischaemia.

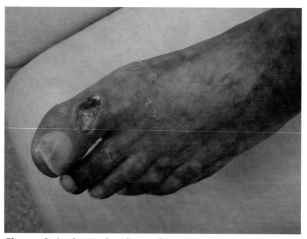

Figure 9. Ischaemic ulceration.

should be undertaken. It is not unusual for a popliteal pulse to be present in a diabetic patient with foot ischaemia largely due to calf vessel disease. Presence of palpable ankle or foot pulses makes significant foot ischaemia unlikely. A positive Buerger's test, with pallor and venous guttering on leg elevation, and rubor due to reactive hyperaemia, on dependency, suggests significant underlying peripheral vascular disease.

Initial investigations include measurement of ankle brachial pressure indices (ABPI) which may be reduced in ischaemia. However, the characteristic medial calcification that occurs in diabetic calf vessels

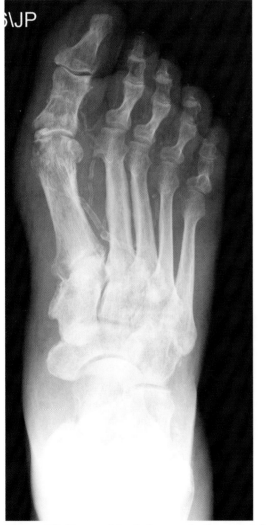

Figure 10. X-ray of foot demonstrating pedal artery calcification and osteomyelitis of the first metatarsophalangeal joint.

often renders them incompressible, resulting in a paradoxically elevated ABPI (Figure 10). In these patients other objective methods of assessing perfusion pressure, including digital artery pressure, pulse volume, $TcPO_2$ measurement, or empirical loss of ankle Doppler signal on leg elevation [6], may be useful. Arterial duplex imaging provides further useful information about the extent and sites of occlusive disease in the leg but is operator-dependent at the level of the tibial arteries and below.

When arterial reconstruction is considered, arteriography remains the investigation of choice for operative planning. Both inflow and run-off vessels, including the distal calf and pedal vessels, must be visualised. In recent years magnetic resonance angiography (MRA) has been employed increasingly to image the distal limb vasculature. However, resolution is not as good as that achieved with intra-arterial digital subtraction angiography (DSA) and images are prone to venous contamination. Gadolinium is used as a contrast agent and in patients with impaired renal function, it is associated with systemic interstitial fibrosis. DSA remains the standard in terms of quality of image resolution of the calf and pedal vessels but may be subject to under-filling artefacts and also carries a risk of contrast-induced acute kidney injury. Dependent Doppler is a useful adjunct to planning the site of an anastomosis in distal reconstruction, particularly when angiography is unhelpful due to underfilling of the calf vessels because of proximal disease.

Arterial reconstruction

The principles of arterial reconstruction for the ischaemic diabetic foot are similar to those employed for proximal disease. Good inflow and run-off are required. Vein is superior to prosthetic material as the latter is prone to infection when employed in situations involving ulceration, infection and tissue necrosis. There is no significant difference in patency between reversed and *in situ* vein grafts, in which the venous valves must be lysed with a valvulotome. However, when fashioning a graft anastomosis to a distal calf or pedal vessel, size disparity may render a non-reversed or *in situ* graft preferable to a reversed vein graft

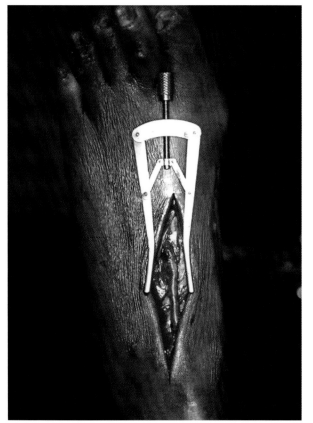

Figure 11. Femorodistal bypass to the dorsalis pedis artery using *in situ* long saphenous vein graft.

(Figure 11). Paradoxically the peroneal artery is relatively spared from occlusive calcification in diabetics, and should be considered as a potential site for run-off in distal bypass.

In diabetic patients the superficial femoral artery is often spared and the popliteal artery may provide a suitable site for the proximal graft anastomosis, shortening the procedure and reducing the risk of groin wound infection and the quantity of vein required. In cases of deficient or inadequate long saphenous vein, arm vein provides a satisfactory alternative. In the absence of suitable vein, when it becomes necessary to employ a small-calibre prosthetic graft as the bypass conduit to a distal vessel in the lower third of the calf, a Taylor vein patch, rather than a Miller cuff, is more likely to allow the graft anastomosis to lie flush with the native vessel. There is no convincing evidence of benefit in patency for one technique over the other in this situation.

Where the distal anastomosis might be threatened with exposure due to risk of infection or difficulty closing the skin, a lateral relieving incision can be performed with undermining of the intervening skin bridge to allow closure. This reduces the risk of anastomotic infection and secondary bleeding.

In the most experienced units, distal bypasses to pedal vessels have reported primary patencies, secondary patencies and limb salvage rates of approximately 57%, 63% and 78%, respectively, at 5 years, although patient survival at this interval was only 48.6% [7].

Endovascular intervention

Patients coming to arterial reconstruction will often already have had some sort of proximal endovascular intervention involving angioplasty and, or, stenting. Angioplasty is particularly suited to dilatation of short segment focal stenoses or occlusions less than 10cm in length and may be used as an adjunct to improve inflow prior to infra-inguinal distal bypass. There is little good evidence, however, in favour of one technique over the other in terms of outcome. Endovascular intervention is less invasive and less prone to the complications of surgery although surgery may confer longer benefit in terms of limb salvage and reduction of mortality [8].

Infection

Cracks and fissures in the skin may provide a portal for entry of bacteria giving rise to infection. Both impairment of the neurogenic inflammatory response and relative attenuation of the immune response due to hyperglycaemia predispose to infection, but these effects may also mask overt signs of infection and the extent of tissue involvement. The patient may be apyrexial and the white cell count is often not significantly elevated. Unexplained or persistent hyperglycaemia should raise clinical suspicion of occult infection.

Examination should include careful scrutiny of heels and between the toes for ulcers and fissures (Figure 12). Blisters and bullae may also provide breaks in the

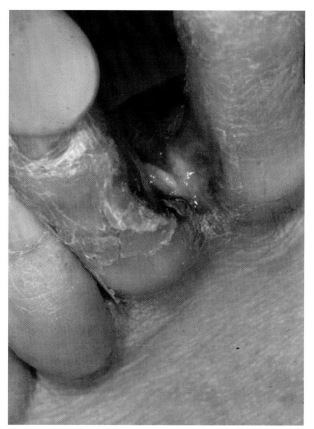

Figure 12. An inter-digital ulcer in a web space between the 2nd and 3rd toes.

Penetrating ulcers provide a track allowing the development of osteomyelitis. Ulcers should be probed to establish their depth and to determine whether bony involvement is likely (Figures 13a and b). This may necessitate preliminary debridement of superficial necrotic tissue. The area of infection observed on superficial foot inspection may belie the underlying extent of pathology, with extensive abscesses often tracking along deep tissue space planes (Figure 14). The patient may be unwell with systemic sepsis, and hyperglycaemia is often refractory. Gram-positive cocci are the most prevalent infecting bacteria, but gram-negative organisms and anaerobes may also be present.

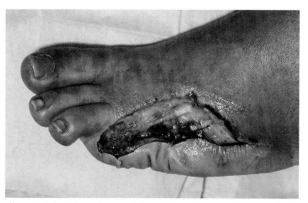

Figure 14. Extensive residual infection and necrosis in a patient who had already undergone toe amputations.

epidermal barrier. Overt signs of infection include swelling, warmth, induration and wet gangrene. Cellulitis and lymphangitis may be present.

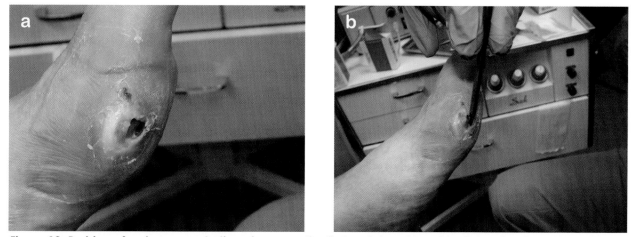

Figure 13. Probing of a deep penetrating ulcer over the first metatarsal head to determine the extent of bony involvement.

Plain radiographs of the foot are useful for demonstrating the extent of bony deformity in Charcot foot, joint effusions, osteomyelitis, gas and foreign bodies (incurred as a result of neuropathic insensitivity). MRI is also a sensitive and practical diagnostic modality and provides more anatomical information. When the presence of osteomyelitis is equivocal, a bone scan or white cell scan may occasionally be indicated.

Management of infection

Patients with limb-threatening infection require urgent hospital admission, immobilisation and intravenous broad-spectrum antibiotics, pending bacterial cultures from tissues and deep wound swabs. When sensitivities to antibiotics have been obtained, specific antimicrobial treatment should be targeted to avoid the development of antibiotic resistance. Hyperglycaemia should be controlled with intravenous fluids and an insulin sliding scale as necessary.

The presence of wet gangrene, necrotising fasciitis, deep abscesses and septic arthritis necessitates urgent surgery to debride necrotic and devitalised tissues and to incise and drain abscesses. Digital gangrene with spreading web-space infection may require open toe, ray or partial forefoot amputation. A principle of adequate surgical drainage is to undertake longitudinal incisions, opening up each tissue plane further than the corresponding deeper plane, in order to prevent persistence of residual pockets of pus. Tendon sheaths should be excised if infected.

Wounds are left open to achieve secondary closure, or loosely closed with interrupted sutures (allowing selective removal), with adequate drainage (Figure 15). In a patient who is severely unwell with extensive or life-threatening infection, a guillotine amputation will occasionally be the preferred and simplest form of definitive debridement, with resort to subsequent amputation revision when the patient is less sick.

The neuropathic diabetic foot with a good blood supply is generally forgiving of extensive debridement of necrotic tissue and amputation of ischaemic digits,

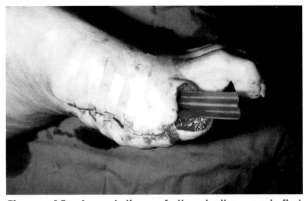

Figure 15. Amputation of the hallux and first metatarsal with loose wound closure and insertion of a corrugated drain.

and will often heal well, provided that bone, cartilage or tendon are not exposed. Even the most radical debridements may heal with good adjunctive wound care; vacuum dressings have proved particularly useful in this situation. Early re-exploration and further debridement of the wound may be needed if initial surgery is not extensive enough. It is also worth planning debridement to ensure conservation of any viable skin which may be useful in provision of a flap, improving the secondary healing rate.

When ischaemia is present, revascularisation will be necessary to promote healing. Occasionally in the presence of dry gangrene of a digit, particularly in an elderly or unfit patient, it may be feasible to allow a digit to mummify. Such digits will often separate spontaneously, but patients require careful surveillance to make sure that spreading infection does not occur in the interim.

Wounds should be irrigated thoroughly and packed with saline-soaked moist dressings which are changed frequently. Daily examination is necessary, with regular debridement of residual necrotic tissue.

There is little strong evidence to support one type of dressing over another, but negative pressure wound therapy (vacuum-assisted closure), has made a major contribution to managing foot wounds [9]. There is evidence that negative pressure dressings increase the proportion of wounds healed, the rate of wound healing and, potentially, result in fewer re-amputations. Portable devices permit an early return home.

There is little evidence for the use of larvae, growth factors, electrical stimulation, dermal substitutes or hyperbaric oxygen in the treatment of patients with non-healing wounds. These therapies should only be used in the context of clinical trials [1]. For extensive tissue loss in patients with good blood supply, more complex reconstructions should be considered, including free tissue transfer (Figure 16).

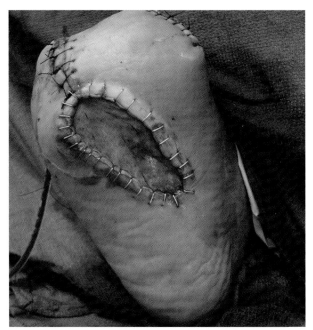

Figure 16. Transmetatarsal amputation of the forefoot and split-skin grafting over a healing sole defect in a diabetic patient with clean wounds, who had undergone prior revascularisation.

Conclusions

The diabetic foot is one of the most common and debilitating complications of diabetes. Improvement of clinical outcomes requires increased awareness of potential problems and early recognition of the foot at risk. Reduction in amputation rates is most likely to be achieved by focused management in multidisciplinary diabetic foot clinics with prompt and appropriate responses to the threatening triad of neuropathy, infection and ischaemia.

Acknowledgements

I thank Professor Clifford P. Shearman and Mr John F. Thompson for kindly providing some of the illustrations used in this chapter.

Key points

- Diabetic foot complications are the most common cause for lower limb amputation in the UK.
- Early identification of diabetic patients at risk of developing foot complications is essential if amputation rates are to be decreased.
- Diabetic patients at increased risk of developing lower limb complications can reduce this risk by participating in a foot care programme that provides foot care education, podiatry (including minor surgical procedures) and, where required, protective footwear.
- Patients with diabetic feet are best managed in a focused multidisciplinary diabetic foot clinic with integrated care.
- In people with diabetes who develop foot ulceration, prompt intervention can minimise their risk of subsequent disability and amputation.
- The infected foot in a diabetic patient is a surgical emergency and requires assessment, treatment with antibiotics, drainage and debridement within 24 hours.
- Foot revascularisation should subsequently be considered in those patients with significant arterial disease.
- In some patients with extensive disease, or those who are unlikely to rehabilitate, primary amputation may provide a more practical and safer alternative to extensive vascular reconstruction.

References

1. Diabetic foot problems: inpatient management (NICE Clinical Guideline 119). www.nice.org.uk/guidance/CG119. NICE clinical guideline. Draft, November 2011. http://www.nice.org.uk/nicemedia/live/11989/52429/52429.pdf.

2. National Service Framework for Diabetes: Standards. Department of Health, 2001. http://www.dh.gov.uk/prod_consum_dh/groups/dh_digitalassets/@dh/@en/documents/digitalasset/dh_4058938.pdf.

3. Boulton AJM, Vileikyte L, Ragnarson-Tennvall G, Apleqvist J. The global burden of diabetic foot disease. *Lancet* 2005; 366 (9498): 1719-24.

4. Putting feet first. Commissioning specialist services for the management and prevention of diabetic foot disease in hospitals. Diabetes UK, 2009. http://www.diabetes.org.uk/Documents/Reports/Putting_Feet_First_010709.pdf.

5. Edmonds ME, Foster AVM. *Managing the diabetic foot,* 2nd ed. Blackwell Publishing, 2005.

6. Smith FCT, Shearman CP, Simms MH, Gwynn BR. Falsely elevated ankle pressures in severe leg ischaemia: The Pole Test - an alternative approach. *Eur J Vasc Surg* 1994; 8: 408-12.

7. Pomposelli FB, Kansal N, Hamdan AD, *et al.* A decade of experience with dorsalis pedis artery bypass: analysis of outcome in more than 1000 cases. *J Vasc Surg* 2003; 37: 307-15.

8. Adam DJ, Beard JD, Cleveland T, *et al.* BASIL Trial Participants. Bypass versus Angioplasty in Severe Ischaemia of the Leg (BASIL): multicentre randomised controlled trial. *Lancet* 2005; 366 (9501): 1925-34.

9. Armstrong DG, Laver LA, Diabetic Foot Study Consortium. Negative pressure wound therapy after partial diabetic foot amputation: a multicentre randomised controlled trial. *Lancet* 2005; 366 (9498): 1704-10.

Chapter 22 **Thoracic outlet surgery**

John F. Thompson MS FRCSEd FRCS, Consultant Surgeon
Exeter Vascular Service, Peninsula College of Medicine and Dentistry, Exeter, UK

Introduction

Surgery for thoracic outlet syndrome (TOS) is a satisfying area of modern vascular practice. The patients are usually younger than those with occlusive or aneurysmal disease and the condition can have a major impact on their quality of life. Serious sequelae of TOS include neurological disability, pulmonary embolus, ischaemia and even limb loss. On the other hand, the complications of surgery, although uncommon, are potentially serious [1].

Selection of patients

TOS is relatively rare so it is vital to make the right management decision at the outset. Redo surgery is difficult and potentially dangerous, so the first intervention should be the definitive one. The retrospective criticism "did the patient actually need the intervention in the first place?" is to be avoided at all costs. The history, clinical examination and relevant investigations should be compiled meticulously so as to build a case either supporting or refuting the diagnosis. In cases of neurological TOS (N-TOS) especially, there may be no clear black and white diagnosis.

Key points when taking the history include:

◆ take time in clinic and listen carefully;

◆ go back to basics: TOS symptoms are worse with the arm elevated and are usually relieved by dependency or rest;

◆ some patients demonstrate illness behaviour out of frustration in not being given a diagnosis, even after consulting several specialists;

◆ apart from the well-known symptoms of classic venous, arterial or neurological TOS there are other characteristic features;

◆ these include a typical and pathognomonic ipsilateral occipitofrontal headache, sensory blunting (asbestos hands), facial or neck pain and subjective difficulty in swallowing;

◆ patients with TOS point to their supraclavicular fossa if asked where the problem arises;

◆ N-TOS patients point to the palmar aspect of their hands in the ulnar nerve distribution, whereas those with radiculopathy point to the dorsum;

◆ nerve compression syndromes are worse premenstrually.

Secondary diagnoses, such as subluxation of the shoulder, may co-exist with TOS as a result of under-use of the limb, so if in doubt obtain a second opinion. Double crush phenomena, such as coexistent carpal tunnel syndrome, may confuse the diagnosis, and some conditions such as diabetes or uraemia may sensitise nerves. Other common co-existing conditions include cervical radiculopathy, degenerative disc disease and especially the occupationally related upper limb disorders (cumulative motion disorders).

Key points in the examination include:

- look at the patient's posture, especially for kyphosis and protracted shoulders;
- the supraclavicular fossa may be convex rather than concave if a cervical rib or band is present and the subclavian pulse may be well above the clavicle;
- examine the cervical spine fully and look for abnormal motion segments;
- Tinel's test over the plexus and percussion tenderness over the clavicle are helpful. Passive elevation of the clavicle provides relief;
- percussion over the mid-trapezius is characteristically very painful; leave until last;
- exclude ulnar and median nerve entrapment;
- examine the hand carefully for intrinsic muscle wasting.

Pulse changes

Pulse changes in TOS are important, but must be taken in context. In our experience, the Roos test (slow, gentle finger clenching with both arms in the surrender position) is usually positive in a matter of seconds in true cases, in that it reproduces the patient's symptoms. The pulse usually disappears consistently in cases of arterial TOS (A-TOS) and re-appears on dependency with a whoosh of reperfusion. In venous TOS (V-TOS), the artery is often affected asymptomatically, but few patients complain of brachial ischaemia on elevation. Venous collaterals increase in size around the shoulder and the arm becomes suffused.

In cases of a cervical rib leading to N-TOS or A-TOS, the pulse may not be affected by assuming the Roos position because the artery can lift out of the wedge formed by the cervical rib and scalenus anterior tendon (Figure 1). Nonetheless, painful C8/T1 paraesthesia is provoked by this manoeuvre.

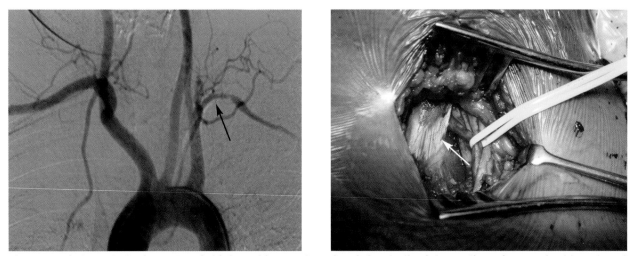

Figure 1. a) The subclavian artery is high arching and wedged due to the intersection of a cervical band and the scalenus anterior tendon (arrow). Plain X-ray appearances were normal. b) Showing the operative findings – the arrow shows the band at the edge of the left scalenus anterior muscle.

Duplex scanning

Our initial enthusiasm for duplex scanning has been replaced by selective use with the following lessons:

♦ in difficult cases, patients can be scanned in positions known to provoke their symptoms, such as playing their musical instrument;
♦ in cases of subclavian aneurysm, CT angiography now provides better anatomical data to plan reconstruction. The subclavian artery is shadowed by the clavicle making duplex scanning difficult;
♦ in N-TOS, compression of the subclavian artery is a useful indication that the lowest trunk of the plexus is also compressed;
♦ in cases of effort thrombosis, it is easy to insonate a prominent collateral rather than the main subclavian vein.

Electromyography (EMG)

There is now no doubt that EMG can confirm the diagnosis of N-TOS. Key features include a decrease in the sensory action potential of the median antebrachial cutaneous nerve (C8, T1) and abnormal F-wave conduction. It is, however, most important to identify other diagnoses such as carpal tunnel syndrome and to obtain a baseline before surgery (to protect the surgeon).

Magnetic resonance imaging

MR imaging is most useful to exclude cervical root compression, but it may miss small cervical ribs or bands. For this reason, we favour plain X-rays of the cervical spine (PA and lateral) to distinguish between cervical ribs and rudimentary first ribs.

Documentation and consent issues

It is well known that consent for surgery is a continuous process and that the consent form is only a small part of this process. Key areas arising from cases of litigation in TOS include:

♦ making the wrong diagnosis (assuming the cervical rib was the problem);
♦ not providing alternative advice (such as advising a body builder to cut down on exercise);
♦ not providing the option of positive conservative management such as physiotherapy, postural advice, a change of occupation or weight loss;
♦ not allowing enough time for such advice to take effect before operating;
♦ neurovascular damage;
♦ uncontrolled haemorrhage.

It no longer matters that the consent form mentions, for example, nerve or vessel injury. The assumption is that in any properly performed operation such damage cannot occur, so that if it does the operation must have fallen below an acceptable standard. This argument has already been tested in cases of bowel injury during laparoscopy.

We would strongly recommend copying patients into all correspondence and that such letters should be full, detailed and contain all the options available, as well as the implications of not having surgery.

Choice of approach

In general it is advisable for the surgeon to be familiar with a both a supraclavicular approach as well as the transaxillary route. Planning is vital and an escape route should be available. Some features of each approach are shown in Table 1.

One important pitfall is a failure to recognise developmental variants at the root of the neck. Any rib arising from the downward sloping transverse process of C7 is a cervical rib and a cervical spine X-ray is, therefore, essential in order to count the vertebrae. A rudimentary first rib may look exactly like a cervical rib, except that it arises from the transverse process of T1. It may articulate or even fuse with the second rib, which can obscure the operative view from below. Difficulty in resecting this 'pseudo' cervical rib may result in a brachial plexus injury (Figure 2).

Complications related to the different approaches to the thoracic outlet are classified as generic or

Table 1. Advantages and disadvantages of the operative approach for the management of patients with TOS.

	Transaxillary	Supraclavicular
Access to artery	Good for decompression	Essential for reconstruction
Access to vein	Good for decompression	Limited without infraclavicular incision
Access to C8/T1 root	Very good	Very good
Access to upper plexus	Poor	Excellent
Cervical/rudimentary 1st rib	Must take first rib first	Better visibility
Redo surgery	Previous supraclavicular approach	Previous transaxillary surgery
Wound implications	Intercostobrachial nerve paraesthesia	Supraclavicular nerve paraesthesia

specific. The surgeon must be fully trained or proctored before embarking on this area. A good assistant, an experienced nurse and a vascular/thoracic trained anaesthetist are vital for these procedures, and facilities to open the chest in an emergency must be available if required. Poor positioning of the patient can make the transaxillary operation virtually impossible and the appropriate instruments are essential. Lighting must be of good quality; we recommend the Vital Vue™ light source

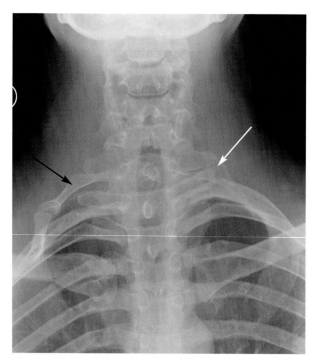
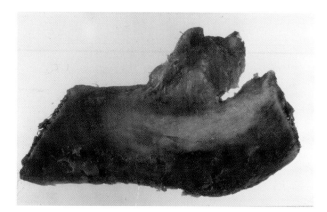

Figure 2. a) Fully articulated right cervical rib (black arrow) with shorter rib on the left (white arrow). If a transaxillary resection is planned, the first rib must be resected initially, to gain safe access. b) Initial resection specimen, seen from below.

(Covidien, UK) and often use an HD laparoscopic stack with a 30° scope to guide surgery and for teaching. A blood group and antibody screen should be obtained for transaxillary and re-do cases.

Supraclavicular approach

Problems encountered during this operation (and ways to avoid them) include:

◆ poor access: place an inflatable bag vertically between the scapulae with the head on a ring and the shoulders drawn caudally;

◆ suprascapular allodynia: divide the supraclavicular nerves cleanly and do not use diathermy;

◆ scar formation and recurrent TOS: divide the deep cervical fascia and scalene fat pad close to the clavicle and reflect superomedially. Wrap the plexus in the fat pad on closing. Wash out with warm saline on closure and avoid haematoma by meticulous haemostasis;

◆ phrenic nerve palsy: avoid excessive neuromuscular blockade and use a nerve stimulator until experienced. The phrenic nerve is tiny and is at risk during scalenectomy;

◆ chylothorax: if chyle appears in the thoracic duct area, ligate the leak with a fine monofilament suture. Remember the possibility of a right-sided thoracic duct;

◆ subclavian artery bleeding: the artery is thin-walled and must be treated with care. Ligate and divide the thyrocervical trunk in continuity before mobilizing;

◆ brachial plexus injury: do not separate the trunks of the plexus, avoid excessive traction and do not trust an inexperienced assistant. Use bipolar diathermy. A chronically compressed lower trunk looks yellowish, like a tendon and does not always respond to a nerve stimulator! The suprascapular nerve is very variable and can arise high. The thin long thoracic nerve can be lower than expected;

◆ inadequate resection of a cervical or first rib (Figure 3): fully expose the neck of the rib and protect the plexus with a Langenbeck retractor. Use Kerrison's neurosurgical rongeurs from a laminectomy set and a plastic spinal Yankhauer

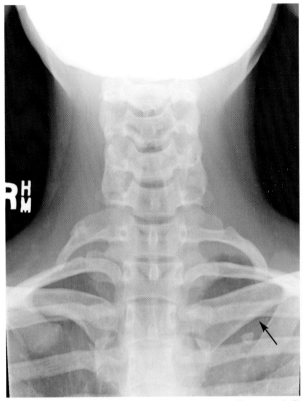

Figure 3. Inadequate cervical rib resection on left side – supraclavicular route (arrow).

sucker to clear bleeding and always maintain vision;

◆ subclavian vein bleeding: the vein is at risk during supraclavicular first rib resection and whilst trimming a prominent scalene tubercle. We recommend a separate infraclavicular approach to the first costochondral junction in difficult cases. A retractor can be placed over the vein whilst it is divided under vision.

Transaxillary first/cervical rib resection

A detailed description of the operation can be found elsewhere [2]. Problems encountered include:

◆ difficult access: place the patient on a vacuum mattress in the half lateral position with their carefully padded arm fully supported in a large L-shaped bar that can be elevated. An illuminated Deaver retractor, Vital Vue™ and laparoscopic assistance are useful. Do not proceed up into the axilla until the dissection has reached the fascia of the chest wall, where a clear, avascular plane is encountered. Divide the intercostobrachial nerve neatly if it lies across the operative field. Divide the superior intercostal vessels before elevating the arm, which opens up the costoclavicular angle;

♦ winged scapula: the long thoracic nerve can lie anteriorly and should be avoided;

♦ poor vision: pack the wound at intervals to keep the field dry and divide the intercostal muscles last to avoid oozing and bleeding from the first intercostal artery, which does not lie in a subcostal groove. The neurovascular structures should remain in clear vision throughout;

♦ pneumothorax: it does not matter if the pleura is breached when reflecting the suprapleural membrane and packing it with a swab. The wound is closed with a vacuum drain to re-inflate the lung;

♦ C8/T1 root damage: avoid diathermy in the depths of the wound and do not use a lipped retractor. The posterior rib resection should be performed under direct vision and the nerve protected using a paddle. Do not try to divide too far back as the rib stump can be nibbled back afterwards. Bone nibblers should be used with great care – never blind;

♦ inadequate resection: the posterior first rib stump should be 2cm behind the C8/T1 root. The anterior resection should be to the costal cartilage, which requires complete disconnection of the subclavius tendon (Figure 4);

♦ bleeding: bleeding from intercostal arteries can be controlled by careful diathermy or use of a 5mm endoscopic clip applicator. The Vital Vue™ irrigation facility is very useful in this respect. Bleeding from the internal mammary artery can be challenging. If it does occur, the artery can be found arising from the proximal subclavian artery and clipped. If packing does not stop the bleeding, there may be a need for thoracoscopic clipping which is straightforward if undertaken immediately;

♦ postoperative bleeding or tension pneumothorax: these patients must be

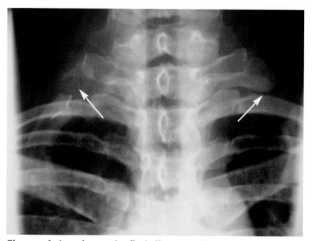

Figure 4. Inadequate first rib resection on both sides (arrows).

assumed to have had a thoracotomy and should be nursed on a specialist vascular or thoracic ward.

Complications and the Paget-Schroetter syndrome

Paget-Schroetter syndrome (PSS) or effort thrombosis of the axillosubclavian venous system, often affects young athletes or manual workers. It is usually due to hypertrophy of the pectoral girdle muscles combined with repetitive upper limb movement. The complications of the primary thrombosis include pulmonary embolus in about 10% and approximately 30-40% develop a post-thrombotic limb with disabling venous hypertension. A review of the condition can be found elsewhere [3]. The issues regarding consent and documentation described above are especially important because this condition is often treated urgently. Several complications may occur during the management of PSS:

♦ missed diagnosis: many patients with PSS are never referred to vascular specialists. The thrombus should be less than 2-3 weeks old for treatment to be successful;

♦ inappropriate treatment: older patients, the non-dominant arm affected, exceptional circumstances leading to the thrombosis and an otherwise sedentary lifestyle should lead to a recommendation of conservative management with anticoagulation for 3 months;

♦ failure to explain the whole package: it is pointless to undergo thrombolysis with its attendant risks of stroke, bleeding and catheter-related complications (quoted at 1% in this fit, young group) unless the vein is to be decompressed and treated by venoplasty;

♦ failure of lysis: successful lysis involves embedding the catheter in the clot proximal to collateral veins, via a sheath placed in the basilic vein. Heparin should be infused through the sheath side arm to prevent pericatheter thrombosis and continued after the lysis catheter has been removed;

♦ immediate rethrombosis following rib resection can be caused by:
  - inadequate venolysis at surgery (the whole axillosubclavian vein must be freed of constriction);
  - attempts at pre-operative venoplasty (it is best to wait until the rib has been removed); and
  - finally, a well-established collateral venous circulation that steals blood (due to longstanding symptoms) (Figure 5);

♦ postoperative bleeding: patients who have had lysis and heparin are at increased risk of

bleeding which may require chest drainage. We have had a case of serious intrathoracic bleeding following the use of rt-PA to try and re-open an early postoperative thrombosis;

♦ treatment failure: persistent venous hypertension should be treated conservatively in the first instance in an attempt to build up collaterals. If this fails after a year or so, a brachial arteriovenous fistula can be fashioned to increase the size of the collaterals. The fistula is reversed after several months.

Complications and re-do surgery

In good hands, the results of re-do surgery can be excellent. Patient selection is once again vital. In our experience it is important to distinguish between persistent and truly recurrent TOS. The history is important and, in our series, recurrent TOS generally occurs within 6 months of the operation. Important questions that should be asked include the following:

♦ was the diagnosis correct in the first place?
♦ bearing in mind the powerful placebo effect of surgery (30-35%), did the first operation actually work?
♦ is the current problem something new (such as a frozen shoulder or tension headache)?
♦ are the recurrent symptoms typical for TOS?
♦ is this a complex regional pain syndrome?

On examination the principles described above still apply. Upper limb neural tension tests can be used to diagnose scar tissue binding the plexus. The outreach test (imagine reaching deep into a cupboard) is also helpful. Investigations should include electromyography, plain X-ray for bony re-growth and contrast studies if arterial reconstruction is contemplated.

Before considering re-do surgery, conservative treatment should be pursued aggressively and second opinions sought. The increased risk of complications should be discussed. In general, the approach should be through virgin tissue if possible; a skilled assistant is essential. Nerve stimulation is useful when dissecting through scar tissue and the operating microscope can be helpful. The most dangerous part

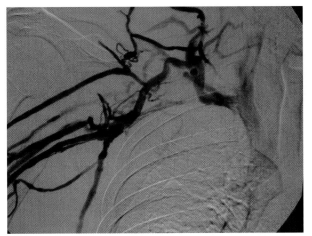

Figure 5. Well-established collateral circulation in a patient with Munchausen's syndrome pretending to have painful upper limb swelling. Rib resection would result in immediate re-thrombosis of the subclavian vein. Treatment was psychiatric advice.

of a redo operation occurs during the dissection of the subclavian artery from a first rib stump or scarred scalene muscles. The peri-arterial plane can be obliterated (very different from the femoral artery) and spectacular bleeding can occur.

Classically, the approach to a bleed from the left subclavian artery is via a fourth space thoracotomy

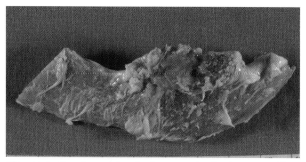

Figure 6. Previous aborted supraclavicular resection of cervical rib leading to ectopic new bone formation surrounding the brachial plexus. Resection specimen after lengthy re-do surgery.

and for a right-sided bleed a median sternotomy is recommended. We have had recourse to the latter on one occasion; the patient lost two blood volumes, required internal cardiac massage and was left with a phrenic nerve palsy. Bleeding during a recurrent left subclavian aneurysm repair was controlled in one case by passage of a Fogarty catheter via the aneurysm, followed by oversewing of the artery distal to the vertebral origin and carotid-brachial bypass. The patient developed a chylothorax which responded to an ultralow fat diet.

Re-do surgery is demanding, time consuming and potentially dangerous. It is, therefore, vitally important to get the first operation right (Figure 6).

Conclusions

Thoracic outlet surgery is an extremely satisfying area of vascular practice. However, there are many potential pitfalls and useful tricks of the trade. The best advice is to avoid failing in the first place.

Key points

- Select patients for operation very carefully.
- Look for secondary or alternative diagnoses and ask for a second opinion, where necessary.
- Consider a period of conservative management.
- Document the case very carefully and copy the patient in all correspondence.
- Surgery is not for the occasional operator.
- Correct positioning, instrumentation and assistance are essential.
- Avoid the need for re-do surgery by performing an anatomically adequate first procedure.

References

1. Leffert RD. Complications of surgery for thoracic outlet syndrome. *Hand Clin* 2004; 20: 91-8.
2. Thompson JF. Transaxillary first rib resection. In: *Vascular and Endovascular Surgical Techniques*. Greenhalgh RM, Ed. London: WB Saunders, 2001: 279-82.
3. Thompson JF, Winterborn RJ, Bays S, *et al*. Venous thoracic outlet compression and the Paget-Schroetter syndrome. A review and recommendations for management. *CVIR* 2011; 34: 903-10.

Case vignette Paradoxical venous thoracic outlet syndrome

John F. Thompson MS FRCSEd FRCS, Consultant Surgeon, Exeter Vascular Service, Peninsula College of Medicine and Dentistry, Exeter, UK
Mark Whyman MB BS FRCS MS, Consultant Surgeon, Cheltenham General Hospital, Cheltenham, UK
Garrett McGann FRCR, Consultant Radiologist, Cheltenham General Hospital, Cheltenham, UK

A 24-year-old female teacher presented with worsening symptoms of left upper limb venous hypertension interfering with her work. She had a history of childhood injuries to her arm including a forearm fracture sustained during a fall on her outstretched hand.

Her symptoms were unusual in that they were worse during dependency and she could relieve the swelling by supporting the arm in an abducted position. This led to an initial presumed diagnosis of lymphoedema and she was informed that nothing definitive could be done. She was seen by a vascular surgeon, who suspected venous thoracic outlet syndrome (V-TOS). There were no neurological or arterial symptoms.

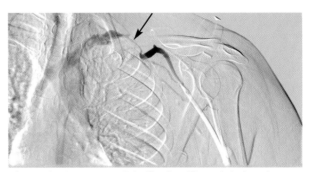

Figure 2. Venogram (via the basilic vein) showing an unusual appearance of the proximal subclavian vein (arrow).

On examination there were prominent venous collaterals about the shoulder at rest, but on stress testing (repeated finger clenching in the surrender position) there was none of the expected increase in the size of the collaterals.

Plain X-rays of the thoracic outlet were normal (Figure 1). She was investigated further with venography (Figure 2), which revealed an unusual obstruction of the proximal subclavian vein at the level of the first rib. The obstruction was relieved by elevation of the upper limb.

CT (Figure 3) revealed a prominent exostosis at the costochondral junction that was further delineated by surface rendered views (Figure 4).

The vein was decompressed via a left transaxillary approach. The first rib was divided anterior to the costochondral junction and immediately behind the lesion. This enabled a clear view of the subclavian vein, artery and the lowest trunk of the brachial plexus, so that the remaining part of the first rib could be

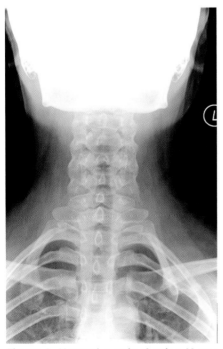

Figure 1. Normal cervical spine X-ray.

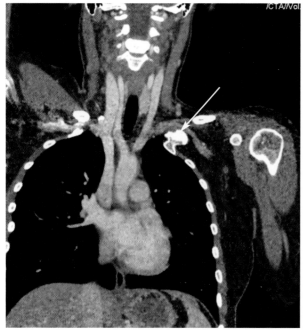

Figure 3. CT venography demonstrating exostosis at the left first costochondral junction (arrow).

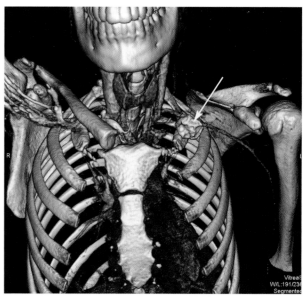

Figure 4. Surface rendered CT further illustrating the exostosis (arrow). The subclavian artery lay behind the lesion and was not compressed.

resected safely. Histology of the lesion confirmed a benign ecchondroma.

Following surgery, she was discharged on the third postoperative day with complete resolution of her symptoms. She returned to work successfully.

Positionally related upper limb symptoms in an otherwise fit young patient strongly suggest an entrapment syndrome. Venous entrapment may lead to upper limb DVT with a risk of post-phlebitic limb. There is still an important role for contrast venography in the diagnosis and treatment of V-TOS.

Chapter 23   Endoscopic thoracic sympathectomy

Rakesh Kapur MBBS MS FRCS (Glasg) FRCS (Gen Surg) PCME (Postgrad Cert in Med Edu)
Specialist Registrar in Vascular Surgery
Shane MacSweeney MA MB BChir MChir FRCSEng, Consultant Vascular Surgeon
Department of Vascular and Endovascular Surgery, Nottingham University Hospital, Nottingham, UK

Introduction

A review of the published literature confirms that endoscopic thoracoscopic sympathectomy (ETS) is a safe and effective operation for hyperhidrosis, with an enviably high success rate of over 95% and substantial improvement in quality of life [1, 2]. Yet the internet has many websites vilifying ETS (e.g. www.truth aboutets.com, www.etsandreversals.yuku.com) run by patients who view themselves as victims of avoidable surgery. They highlight lack of adequate informed consent, and list numerous known (and several unconfirmed) complications of the procedure. This emphasises the vital importance of careful patient selection; ETS should only be offered to patients with debilitating symptoms in whom conservative treatments have failed, and after thorough, carefully documented pre-operative patient counselling about the possible complications. These patients are often young, with many years to cope with any resulting complications that result. Hyperhidrosis (excessive sweating) is the commonest indication for ETS, and although not dangerous, it can be extremely debilitating with a major impact on quality of life. As the years go by patients continue to be aware of any complications, while the memory of their original complaint may recede (Table 1).

Table 1. Clinical illustration 1.
A computer engineer suffered from such severe palmar hyperhidrosis that her rubber gloves would fill up with sweat, spilling over and damaging the circuitry. She was delighted after her successful sympathectomy and had some mild compensatory hyperhidrosis around the trunk which she agreed was much less troublesome than her palmar hyperhidrosis. A few years later she came back complaining about the compensatory sweating. After a reminder about how bad the original problem had been, she agreed that the current symptoms were far preferable. This illustrates the problem that patients have to live with side effects in the long term whereas as time goes by, the memory of the original symptoms may fade.

Indications

Historically, thoracic sympathectomy has been performed for many dubious indications such as idiocy, epilepsy, goitre and glaucoma. In 1920, Kotzareff was the first to use it to treat hyperhidrosis. The endoscopic version of thoracic sympathectomy was popularised by Goren Claes and Christer Drott in Sweden in the late 1980s.

In Nottingham, as in most UK centres, ETS is done for palmar, and palmar combined with axillary hyperhidrosis, and occasionally for facial blushing in carefully selected patients. The palmar hyperhidrosis should be debilitating (Table 2 and Figure 1), and other conservative measures such as antiperspirants, iontophoresis and botulinum toxin need to have been considered. Generalised hyperhidrosis, for example, due to thyrotoxicosis should have been excluded. Botulinum toxin injections are effective, but painful in the hands, and many patients do not find them a viable long-term option for palmar hyperhidrosis, unlike for axillary hyperhidrosis where they are the treatment of choice.

Table 2. Clinical illustration 2.
A 42-year-old woman had a back office job, and had always wanted to set up her own business but was afraid to do so because of palmar sweating. She could not face the embarrassment of having to shake hands with clients, give presentations and deal with the public directly. Following her sympathectomy, she set up a successful business.

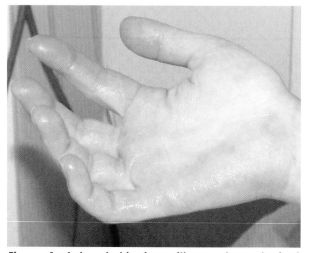

Figure 1. A hand dripping with sweat – a typical patient with hyperhidrosis.

Facial flushing, in which sudden facial flushing occurs in stressful situations, needs to be distinguished from causes of a red face/skin conditions such as rosacea; menopausal flushing is self-limiting. A dermatological opinion can be helpful. Cognitive behaviour therapy may be helpful for some patients. It is easy to trivialise the significance of facial flushing, but if severe, it can have a major impact on quality of life, employment and social function (Table 3).

Table 3. Clinical illustration 3.
A middle-aged man with severe facial flushing requested sympathectomy. He worked on an oil rig and had been teased at work to the extent that he had lost his job. He wanted to give his daughter away at her wedding but was terrified that he would embarrass himself and her by flushing. With some misgivings his sympathectomy was carried out, the wedding went well and he eventually got a new (and better) job.

Other indications for ETS

Other indications for which ETS is sometimes used are:

- secondary Raynaud's disease;
- other vasospastic disorders such as acrocyanosis, causalgia: T2-5 ablated;
- thoracic splanchnicectomy for splanchnic pain (pancreatic carcinoma/chronic pancreatitis): T4-10 ablated;
- reflex sympathetic dystrophy;
- upper extremity ischaemia (digital arteriosclerosis, Buerger's disease, intravenous drug users with severe ischaemia due to accidental intra-arterial injection of drugs;
- angina pectoris: intractable angina.

Quality of life (QoL) following sympathectomy

Most authors merely refer to a subjective improvement in patients' symptoms, or better patient satisfaction levels postoperatively. However, more objective and validated QoL tools to assess postoperative improvement in symptoms are available. The Short-Form 36 is a generic QoL measure which has been used to evaluate patients with hyperhidrosis before and after ETS. The Hyperhidrosis Disease Severity Scale (HDSS) is a qualitative measure of the effect of patients' symptoms on their daily activities. The Dermatology Life Quality Index (DLQI) is another practical, validated questionnaire for assessing QoL in patients with hyperhidrosis and a variety of other dermatological conditions. Transepidermal water loss (TEWL) measurements provide an indirect, but quantitative measure of sweating, and have been used to provide objective evidence of improvement in QoL after ETS [3]. De Campos *et al* have developed a detailed, objective questionnaire of their own to assess symptom severity in patients with hyperhidrosis, and improvement after ETS [4].

The published literature on QoL confirms that good outcomes after ETS for hyperhidrosis are obtained only in patients with severe symptoms. The worse the pre-operative QoL among patients undergoing ETS to treat hyperhidrosis, the better the postoperative QoL will be [5].

Technique

There are a variety of options for general anaesthesia. A double-lumen endobronchial tube has the advantage of facilitating single-lung ventilation and providing excellent visualisation. The disadvantage is that it is more unpleasant for the patient and more complex for the anaesthetist, with the possibility that an inexperienced anaesthetist may inadvertently place both sides of the double-lumen tube in one main bronchus. Cameron has described three deaths in patients who had double-lumen tube anaesthesia; they had an uneventful operation on the first side, but had problems with falling oxygen saturations on the other side, culminating in prolonged hypoxia and brain death [6]. The alternative to a double-lumen tube is standard endotracheal or laryngeal mask ventilation. These are simpler anaesthetic techniques but may produce less good visualisation for the surgeon.

As a result of the complications mentioned above, it has been argued that only one side should be done at a time. However, most patients will require ETS on both sides to obtain satisfactory relief of their symptoms, and there is ample evidence from the literature of very large numbers of bilateral sympathectomies being performed with extremely low complication rates [7]. A sensible option is to perform a bilateral sympathectomy when indicated, unless there is any concern from the anaesthetist or surgeon during the operation on the first side.

Standard practice is to insert carbon dioxide into the thoracic cavity to aid visualisation of the thoracic chain; it is important to inflate slowly to keep the pressure and volume to the minimum necessary for adequate visualisation. Rapid insertion of carbon dioxide creates an iatrogenic tension pneumothorax.

With respect to operative technique, the main choice of port position lies between two axillary ports (or one axillary operating port which allows visualisation and instrumentation through the same port) and one axillary and one infraclavicular port, inserted through the second intercostal space in the midclavicular line. Although the infraclavicular approach allows ready instrumentation of the thoracic chain, it produces an unsightly scar, particularly in women, and also risks injury to intrathoracic structures. The authors prefer to use two 5mm axillary ports; it is important that they are positioned far enough apart to avoid clashing between the scope and diathermy hook. The first port insertion is always a time of potential risk, particularly if there are unrecognised pleural adhesions. We have found the Visiport™ (Covidien) very helpful as it allows full visualisation during port insertion. The second port can then be inserted under direct vision with the scope through the first port site. Careful gentle movements and always keeping the diathermy hook under vision reduce the risk of inadvertent injury to intrathoracic structures.

Sympathectomy in the prone position has been described and allows very good visualisation as the lungs fall forward away from the sympathetic chain, but adds unnecessary complexity to the anaesthetic.

The authors' practice is to divide the sympathetic chain with a diathermy hook on the neck of the rib at a level determined by the indication (see below). It is not necessary to resect the sympathetic chain.

Complications

Compensatory hyperhidrosis

This is not a complication *per se*, but a normal consequence of sympathectomy, and occurs to some degree in almost all patients [8, 9]. They should be warned to expect it. Since ETS abolishes sweating in the denervated area, the body compensates by increased sweating from other regions, such as the back, lower chest and abdomen, the perineum, and legs. Although most people consider this less debilitating than palmar hyperhidrosis, and many will not mention it unless asked specifically, in approximately 1-2% of the patients it can be severe and disabling, and cause them to regret having the procedure. It is essential that patients are aware of this complication before agreeing to surgery, and that they know sympathectomy is designed to be irreversible (Table 4). It is not possible in advance to predict who will develop compensatory hyperhidrosis.

Table 4. Clinical illustration 4.

A nurse underwent a sympathectomy for severe hyperhidrosis unresponsive to other treatment modalities. She was delighted with her dry hands but suffered from severe compensatory sweating around the groin which was inconvenient and embarrassing. She agreed that she had been warned about hyperhidrosis and that she had been unlucky, rather than misinformed. A very detailed and frank discussion of the potential drawbacks is essential. This should be documented clearly in the case notes and in the letter to the general practitioner, which could be copied to the patient, if appropriate.

There is contradictory evidence in the literature on which level of sympathectomy achieves the best results, while minimising the incidence of compensatory hyperhidrosis [8, 10, 11]. Many authors recommend a T2 sympathectomy for palmar hyperhidrosis, although others suggest a T4 sympathectomy as being superior to other levels. It is difficult to compare the available studies, as there is marked heterogeneity with respect to study population and entry criteria, and lack of uniform definitions with regards to outcome. A T2 sympathectomy is necessary for facial flushing; however, T3 and T2 sympathectomies are equally effective for palmar sweating but T3 division is associated with less severe compensatory sweating [11]. A meta-analysis of publications between 2000 and 2010 showed that single-level ablation was as effective as multiple-level ablations, and had the minimum incidence of compensatory hyperhidrosis. The authors identified T3 ablation as best in terms of efficacy and minimum side effects [12]. The authors prefer to avoid T2 when performing sympathectomy for palmar hyperhidrosis.

There is also controversy regarding the type and method of resection of the sympathetic chain. While there is consensus that division of the sympathetic chain yields equally good results compared to resection, some authors claim that clipping the chain is better than dividing it because it significantly reduces the incidence and severity of compensatory and gustatory hyperhidrosis, and is potentially reversible, although the evidence is not convincing.

Gustatory sweating

Facial sweating when eating, particularly in response to spicy or acidic food is common, and occurs in up to 32% after ETS. The mechanism is not understood.

Recurrence of sweating

Recurrence of the original symptoms due to nerve regeneration or nerve sprouting can occur within the first year after surgery, but regeneration may start years after sympathectomy. Zacherl reported a recurrence rate of 7% at a median 16 years of follow-up [13].

Uncommon complications

Failure

This occurs in approximately 1-5% of patients. The common reason is failure to divide the sympathetic trunk because it could not be visualised, usually due to pleural adhesions, or an opaque or thickened pleura (Table 5). Rarely, there are anatomical abnormalities such as an azygos lobe. On occasions the sympathetic trunk is identified incorrectly.

Table 5. Clinical illustration 5.
On insertion of a scope into the chest cavity of a man with no previous history of lung disease, dense vascular pleural adhesions were encountered and the procedure was abandoned. A further attempt as a joint procedure with the thoracic surgeons was also unsuccessful. Surgeons who undertake ETS should be prepared to abandon the procedure if there are significant hazards.

Bleeding

This can occur in up to 5% of procedures but is usually minor. Life-threatening bleeding from subclavian vessels or injury to the heart is extremely rare, but a few cases have been described in the literature. Major bleeding may need a thoracotomy, and the operating surgeon should be capable of proceeding.

Blind port placement can potentially be complicated by lung, heart, and major vascular injuries. Routine insertion of the first port under direct vision (see technique) reduces the risk of major organ/vascular injury.

Pain

Chest pain, chest hypersensitivity, arm pain, paraesthesias of the upper limb and the thoracic wall, and recurrent pain in the axillary region have all been described. Intra-operative intrapleural analgesia using bupivacaine can help reduce postoperative pain. Using a 5mm rather than 1cm port causes less postoperative discomfort, particularly in women with narrow intercostal spaces.

There is no significant association between the type of scalpel (electric vs. harmonic scalpel) used for sympathectomy and the severity of postoperative pain [14].

Pneumothorax (Figure 2)

Pleural gas on a postoperative chest X-ray usually represents residual carbon dioxide used for insufflation which is rapidly absorbed and is of no clinical significance. Pneumothorax is usually managed expectantly, but in about 2% of cases requires insertion of a chest drain. Pneumothorax can also result from underlying lung injury, particularly following a more extensive resection, e.g. T5-11. Full re-inflation of the lung under direct vision and avoiding excessive

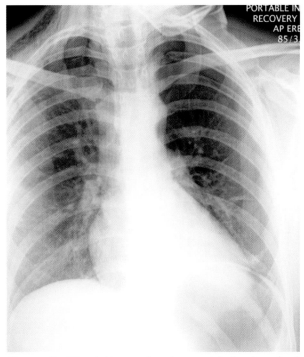

Figure 2. Chest X-ray showing a bilateral apical pneumothorax more marked on the left. There is also some surgical emphysema on the right. No treatment was needed.

insufflation can both reduce the amount of residual carbon dioxide.

Harlequin syndrome

Harlequin syndrome, named after the traditional harlequin mask (Figures 3 and 4), is a consequence of incomplete ETS, so that the sympathetic fibres are successfully transected on one side but remain intact on the other. This results in unilateral sweating and flushing on the untreated side of the upper thoracic region of the chest, neck and face. In some patients, the symptoms may be minimal, but in others, they may be exaggerated by a compensatory increase in sweating and flushing as a result of the contralateral sympathectomy.

Rare complications

Infection
Infection is rare after ETS.

Horner's syndrome (Figure 5)
This occurs after about 1% of procedures and is characterised by a triad of symptoms: anhidrosis, ptosis and meiosis. About two thirds will recover spontaneously over time, and some of the remainder will not require treatment if the eyelid droops only slightly. If treatment is required for severe ptosis, surgical correction is feasible.

Formal resection of the sympathetic chain is associated with a significantly higher risk of Horner's syndrome than simple division [15]. The further away the dissection is from T1, the less is the chance of Horner's syndrome. Hence, preserving T1-2 and confining sympathectomy to T3-4 significantly reduces the risk.

It has been claimed that using scissors rather than diathermy to divide the sympathetic chain reduces the likelihood of Horner's syndrome but this is not supported by evidence.

Chylothorax
This has been reported (<1%) due to inadvertent injury to the lymphatics.

Brachial plexus injury
This is also extremely rare.

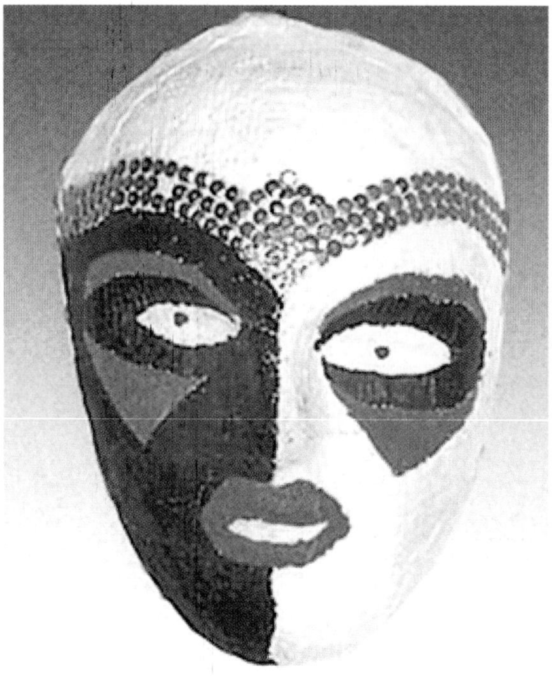

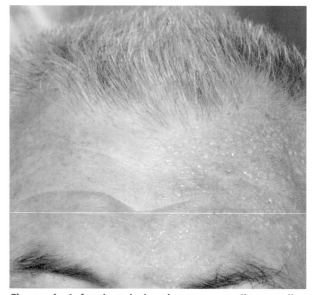

Figure 4. A forehead showing no sweating on the side with successful sympathectomy and intense sweating on the untreated side (Harlequin syndrome).

Figure 3. A Harlequin mask.

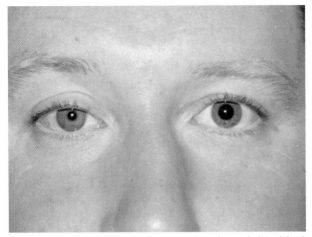

Figure 5. Horner's syndrome showing right-sided ptosis and meiosis. *Courtesy of Mr. M. G. Wyatt, Freeman Hospital, Newcastle upon Tyne, UK.*

Mortality

No death following ETS has ever been reported in the literature, but nine anecdotal fatalities are known, five resulting from major intrathoracic bleeding and three from anaesthetic mishap [6].

Anaesthetic complications

Hypoxemia, hypotension, transient bradycardia, and re-expansion pulmonary oedema have all been rarely described. One patient had a cardiac arrest during use of the diathermy.

Conclusions

ETS is an elegant, simple and effective operation. In order to minimise the risk of dissatisfaction, very careful selection and full and frank discussion of the potential complications are needed with every patient. The risk of complications can be minimised by careful anaesthetic and surgical technique, yet complications can occur even in the best of hands. It is important to maintain perspective and remember that ETS has been shown to be effective and to produce major improvements in quality of life. While it is very important to advise patients carefully there is also a risk of becoming so risk averse that patients are denied an effective treatment. Flushing and sweating can have a huge long-term negative impact on people's lives. ETS is extremely effective and can transform lives for the better.

Patient information on ETS is available at http://www.circulationfoundation.org.uk/vascular_disease/endoscopic_sympathectomy.

Key points

- Careful pre-operative counselling of the risks and benefits, particularly the risk of compensatory hyperhidrosis, is essential.
- Symptoms should be debilitating and alternative treatment methods such as iontophoresis/botox should have been considered.
- Patients should be aware that the operation is designed to be irreversible.
- The worse the pre-operative symptoms the greater the benefit of surgery.

References

1. Cerfolio RJ, De Campos JR, Bryant AS, *et al*. The Society of Thoracic Surgeons expert consensus for the surgical treatment of hyperhidrosis. *Ann Thorac Surg* 2011; 91: 1642-8.

2. Henteleff HJ, Kalavrouziotis D. Evidence-based review of the surgical management of hyperhidrosis. *Thorac Surg Clin* 2008; 18: 209-16.

3. Tetteh HA, Groth SS, Kast T, *et al*. Primary palmoplantar hyperhidrosis and thoracoscopic sympathectomy: a new objective assessment method. *Ann Thorac Surg* 2009; 87: 267-74; discussion 274-5.

4. de Campos JR, Kauffman P, Werebe Ede C, *et al*. Quality of life, before and after thoracic sympathectomy: report on 378 operated patients. *Ann Thorac Surg* 2003; 76: 886-91.

5. Wolosker N, Yazbek G, de Campos JR, *et al*. Quality of life before surgery is a predictive factor for satisfaction among patients undergoing sympathectomy to treat hyperhidrosis. *J Vasc Surg* 2010; 51: 1190-4.

6. Ojimba TA, Cameron AE. Drawbacks of endoscopic thoracic sympathectomy. *Br J Surg* 2004; 91: 264-9.

7. Bachmann K, Standl N, Kaifi J, *et al*. Thoracoscopic sympathectomy for palmar and axillary hyperhidrosis: four-year outcome and quality of life after bilateral 5mm dual port approach. *Surg Endosc* 2009; 23: 1587-93.

8. Liu Y, Yang J, Liu J, *et al*. Surgical treatment of primary palmar hyperhidrosis: a prospective randomized study comparing T3 and T4 sympathicotomy. *Eur J Cardiothorac Surg* 2009; 35: 398-402.

9. Lyra RM, De Campos JRM, Kang DWW, *et al*; Sociedade Brasileira de Cirurgia Torácica. Guidelines for the prevention, diagnosis and treatment of compensatory hyperhidrosis. *J Bras Pneumol* 2008; 34: 967-77.

10. Li X, Tu Y, Lin M, *et al*. Endoscopic thoracic sympathectomy for palmar hyperhidrosis: a randomized control trial comparing T3 and T2-4 ablation. *Ann Thorac Surg* 2008; 85: 1747-51.

11. Yazbek G, Wolosker N, Kauffman P, *et al*. Twenty months of evolution following sympathectomy on patients with palmar hyperhidrosis: sympathectomy at the T3 level is better than at the T2 level. *Clinics* 2009; 64: 743-9.

12. Deng B, Tan QY, Jiang YG, *et al*. Optimization of sympathectomy to treat palmar hyperhidrosis: the systematic review and meta-analysis of studies published during the past decade. *Surg Endosc* 2011; 25: 1893-901.

13. Zacherl J, Huber ER, Imhof M, *et al*. Long-term results of 630 thoracoscopic sympathicotomies for primary hyperhidrosis: the Vienna experience. *Eur J Surg* 1998; 580: 43-6.

14. de Campos JR, Wolosker N, Yazbek G, *et al*. Comparison of pain severity following video-assisted thoracoscopic sympathectomy: electric versus harmonic scalpels. *Interact Cardiovasc Thorac Surg* 2010; 10: 919-22.

15. Wait SD, Killory BD, Lekovic GP, *et al*. Thoracoscopic sympathectomy for hyperhidrosis: analysis of 642 procedures with special attention to Horner's syndrome and compensatory hyperhidrosis. *Neurosurgery* 2010; 67: 652-6.

Chapter 24 Varicose veins

Jonothan J. Earnshaw DM FRCS, Consultant Vascular Surgeon
Gloucestershire Royal Hospital, Gloucester, UK

Introduction

Treatment of varicose veins is the commonest intervention in vascular surgery; upwards of 50,000 procedures occur in the UK every year [1]. Although major complications are rare, when they do occur they cause a disproportionate amount of anxiety and concern, since most interventions are for symptomatic, but uncomplicated varicose veins. The risk of complaints and litigation is higher after varicose vein treatments than other general surgery procedures [2]. Sometimes it is a relatively minor complication, or a less than desirable outcome that can produce litigation, as a result of unrealistic patient expectations. Until a decade ago, the only treatments for varicose veins were surgery and liquid sclerotherapy. A number of new treatments, including endovenous thermal ablation and foam sclerotherapy, have now entered the market place [3, 4]. This has expanded the number of potential complications and the difficulty in obtaining informed consent from patients, many of who arrive with overoptimistic and unrealistic expectations fuelled by glossy advertisements from the internet.

Consent

There should be no apology for highlighting the issue of consent at the very beginning of a chapter in avoiding complications. The main cause for dissatisfaction after varicose vein procedures is a failure of communication. The patient and the surgeon should have the same aspirations and expectations from any intervention. As numerous therapeutic modalities are now available and treatment plans may be complex, patients should be counselled by someone who understands the condition and who is aware of all the various options for treatment and their risks. It is no longer acceptable for a patient with varicose veins to be counselled by an inexperienced junior surgeon. The pre-operative management should involve a well-documented history and examination, including risk factors such as previous deep vein thrombosis (DVT) and/or potential risk factors for postoperative DVT. The clinical examination should include the use of a hand-held Doppler and may also include duplex imaging, as an increasing number of vascular specialists are familiar with their use. The clinical stage of venous disease should be documented using the CEAP score, and it may even be helpful to include quality of life assessment. In the UK, patients undergoing treatment for varicose veins will all complete a Patient Reported Outcome Measure (PROM) assessment before the intervention, and then again after 3 months, as part of treatment evaluation.

Whereas treatment for varicose veins in the presence of active or healed varicose ulceration (CEAP 5/6) is evidence-based [5], the majority of patients request treatment for symptomatic, uncomplicated varicose veins (CEAP 2/3). Although there is good evidence that treatment in these circumstances improves quality of life, and at a cost below the threshold accepted by the National Institute for Health and Clinical Excellence [6], there is an increasing reluctance to offer these procedures widely in the NHS, leading to implicit rationing [1]. In this circumstance, clear documentation of the options for treatment, including no intervention or compression therapy should be recorded in the medical records, together with a summary of the debate about the risks and benefits of treatment with respect to the indications. An information sheet should be supplied and recorded in the notes as having been given. Procedures should also be in place to ensure that written consent is obtained before any intervention, and is taken by someone with specialist knowledge. As is so often the case, accurate documentation is of great importance. Although most hospitals now have their own information sheets, copies of approved information sheets can be obtained from the Vascular Society/Circulation Foundation website (www.vascularsociety.org.uk).

Diagnosis

One of the major components of good care is accurate diagnosis of the cause of venous insufficiency [7]. In many cases, for primary uncomplicated varicose veins, the use of a hand-held Doppler can give adequate information to plan intervention. Several randomised trials have suggested that improved results are obtained by formal pre-operative duplex imaging. The largest of these studies involved non-vascular specialists, some of who made a clinical diagnosis without even using the Doppler [8]. This may have contributed to the poor results in the control (no duplex) group, and it may well be the case that an experienced vascular specialist can make the diagnosis of the source of

truncal reflux in most patients with the hand-held Doppler alone. For clinicians who use selective duplex imaging before surgical intervention, the following categories are agreed as specific indications:

◆ previous DVT;
◆ recurrent varicose veins;
◆ small saphenous varicose veins;
◆ any unusual appearance or confusing symptoms;
◆ non-truncal reflux on hand-held Doppler.

Nevertheless, best practice includes formal duplex imaging, since this occasionally demonstrates unexpected findings, such as old deep vein damage that might shape decisions about thromboprophylaxis. Most modern endovenous treatments require pre-operative duplex imaging for treatment planning, which in many cases is done by the individual vascular specialist at the initial consultation. Diagnostic ultrasonography does, however, require expertise and should therefore only be done by an individual who has been through a formal training programme, with accreditation [9].

Reducing recurrence

Whilst recurrence is not strictly a complication after varicose vein treatment, from the perspective of the patient it is one of the most important outcomes and can therefore be a cause of disappointment (and litigation). A number of alternatives to standard surgery now exist: various novel stripping techniques such as cryo-stripping; targeted surgery with saphenous preservation (CHIVA or ASVAL methods); thermal ablation techniques (laser or radiofrequency) or ultrasound-guided foam sclerotherapy [3, 4]. The impetus for the development of novel techniques came from the perceived high recurrence rates after standard surgery. Specialisation has largely removed the risk of inadequate surgery that was blamed for high recurrence rates in the 1990s. Duplex-guided surgery and CHIVA have reduced recurrence rates in longitudinal studies [8, 10], but they do not overcome the trauma of surgery in the groin for saphenofemoral disconnection which most vascular surgeons agree causes the neovascularisation that is the prime reason for recurrence [11]. Endovenous thermal ablation techniques avoid surgical trauma, which minimises neovascularisation, and also have the advantage of reduced postoperative pain and thus improved recovery times. Perhaps their major advantage is that they can be done under tumescent local anaesthesia, thus avoiding the need for general anaesthesia, and taking the treatment of varicose veins out of the operating theatre and into an outpatient setting. This goes some way to offsetting the costs of the equipment needed for ablation techniques. Foam sclerotherapy is the least effective technique at obliterating major truncal incompetence. On the other hand it is the cheapest method and is easily repeatable; where cost is an issue it can be an appropriate first-line intervention [12].

All the above methods of treatment for varicose veins have been shown to improve quality of life, and therefore there is justification for their routine use [13]. Most vascular specialists now offer at least one alternative to standard surgical treatment, and they must be aware of the others and be prepared to counsel patients appropriately. Treatment can be individualised to the patient's requirements and personal circumstances. Exaggerated claims of efficacy should, however, be avoided; for example, claims of improved recurrence rates from modern techniques should not be made until there is better evidence from formal randomised trials currently under way. It should, however, be noted that many existing trials were not powered to examine late outcomes, and meta-analysis of the available material may be needed. There should be no reluctance to refer a patient onwards if the most appropriate treatment is only available in another clinic.

Major complications of interventions for varicose veins

The three major complications of varicose vein treatments are deep vein thrombosis, nerve damage and infection. These can occur after any of the different treatments and are not specific to any one.

Deep vein thrombosis (DVT)

DVT is actually very rare after routine intervention for varicose veins. It is related to underlying risk factors such as obesity and, most importantly, previous DVT. Patients are often confused that the presence of varicose veins themselves is a risk for DVT and seek treatment particularly if they are about to go on a long haul flight. In this situation reassurance alone is often satisfactory.

Before treatment, particularly surgery, patients should undergo a risk assessment using NICE guidelines, which should be recorded in the case notes [14]. There are no controlled trials to inform the approach to thromboprophylaxis in patients undergoing intervention for varicose vein surgery. Whilst some surgeons have a blanket policy of thromboprophylaxis for all patients, there is support for a selective policy where low-risk individuals having unilateral treatment with procedures lasting less than 30 minutes avoid thromboprophylaxis, which of course has its own risks of bruising. The role of thromboprophylaxis for new endovenous treatments is not yet established, but some specialists would offer people in higher-risk categories, particularly if they have had previous DVT, a single peri-operative injection of low-molecular-weight heparin. In contrast to varicose vein surgery, patients who have a modern endovenous treatment including both endothermal ablation and foam sclerotherapy have routine ultrasound follow-up. Occasional femoropopliteal DVT is diagnosed, but another concerning finding is a tongue of thrombus at the level of, or protruding into the femoral or popliteal vein at the top of an occluded truncal vein. This is termed endovenous heat-induced thrombosis (EHIT) and four classes are recognised:

- Class 1: thrombus to the level of the deep vein, without protrusion;
- Class 2: protrusion into the deep system, with <50% luminal occlusion;
- Class 3: protrusion into the deep system, with >50% luminal occlusion;
- Class 4: protrusion into the deep system, with total deep venous occlusion.

Most clinicians prescribe a short course of anticoagulation for patients with EHIT Classes 2 and 3 to prevent extension of the thrombus into the deep veins. Total deep venous occlusion should be treated as a DVT with formal anticoagulation.

For those at moderate risk of DVT, a single injection of low-molecular-weight heparin at the time of the procedure is mandatory. Patients at higher risk, in particular those with previous DVT, should be warned explicitly of the risk of recurrent DVT at the time of the intervention, and they may be suitable for additional mechanical compression devices. Whilst there is no scientific evidence of further benefit, prophylaxis may be continued until the patient is fully mobile by teaching patients to self-inject low-molecular-weight heparin at home. It remains controversial how to manage women who are taking hormone replacement or oestrogen-based contraception. Whilst some clinicians recommend stopping these medications for

1 month before intervention to reduce the risk of DVT, this has no evidence base, and in fact the potential complications of unexpected pregnancy probably outweigh the risks of DVT. An acceptable alternative is simply to ensure they get adequate thromboprophylaxis at the time of treatment. All patients should be encouraged to be as mobile and active as possible early after intervention for varicose veins, of whatever type.

Patients sometimes present with tender varicose veins due to thrombophlebitis. Whilst this is usually treated conservatively with anti-inflammatory painkillers and gentle compression, it has become apparent that extensive thrombophlebitis can progress to DVT. There should be a low index of suspicion for arranging a duplex scan to rule out DVT in this situation. Thrombophlebitis is also a complication of all techniques for treating varicose veins, and both the management, and the index of suspicion for DVT are the same (Figure 1).

Nerve damage

After standard varicose vein surgery, and any secondary procedures after endovenous ablation, cutaneous nerve damage related to the phlebectomy incisions is very common. Warning about local sensory loss should be an explicit part on the consent form. In most people it is transient and improves with patience. More serious is traumatic damage to named nerves, which is much rarer, and occurs almost exclusively after surgery. It is said to be more common in small saphenous varicose vein surgery where the sural nerve and common peroneal nerves are particularly at risk [15]. However, in a recent prospective trial involving over 200 procedures, there was only one report of damage to the sural nerve and this was transient [16]. Major nerve injury is very debilitating and is one of the frequent causes of litigation after varicose vein surgery. After endovenous thermal ablation, there is anecdotal evidence of increased risk to the saphenous and sural nerves with distal punctures, and care should be taken, particularly in patients with less extensive veins. Neuropraxia is also reported after treatment of localised perforating veins with thermal ablation.

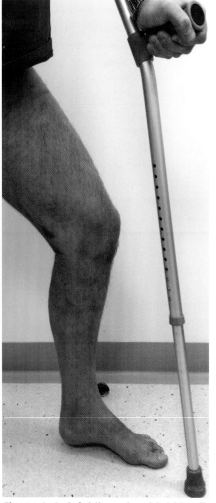

Figure 1. **Painful thrombophlebitis after varicose vein surgery. This required hospital admission, and the patient walked with a crutch for 2 weeks. No DVT was evident on duplex imaging.**

Infection

Severe infection is a rare complication after varicose vein surgery. It is even more uncommon after endovenous procedures that do not involve an incision in the groin. A single randomised trial has suggested that antibiotic prophylaxis can reduce the rate of infection after varicose vein surgery although the cost benefit of this blanket treatment in low-risk patients may not be worthwhile [17]. Clearly where there are risk factors for infection such as obesity, or open wounds including varicose ulceration, good antiseptic techniques to clean the skin and a dose of antibiotic prophylaxis would seem sensible.

Specific procedures

Endovenous thermal ablation

This can be done using laser or radiofrequency energy, and the aim is to produce controlled heating inside the vein to denature the proteins in the venous wall and thus cause thrombosis and obliteration. Many of the early complications of this technique were related to the temperature required to denature the vein, causing burns to any overlying skin or nerve that runs adjacent to the vein. The advance in treatment is to use tumescent local anaesthesia. The vein is surrounded with an injection of a dilute solution of local anaesthetic and saline which has analgesic effects but also acts as a thermal buffer to reduce the risk of burn injury. Although burns should be excessively rare in endovenous ablation techniques, the treatment of a very superficial truncal vein (or segment) can present a difficult challenge. Even a very superficial vein can often be pushed over 10mm from the skin surface with judicious use of tumescent anaesthesia. However, where a segment of truncal vein remains very superficial, the use of alternative techniques, such as avulsion, or injection sclerotherapy may be necessary, in addition to thermal ablation. It is also important to remember to keep the laser fiber within the sheath on withdrawal to prevent a skin burn at the entry site.

The randomised trials that compare laser and radiofrequency suggest that early postoperative pain is more common after laser ablation, which is thought to be due to the fact that laser, particularly using forward firing fibres, may perforate the vein wall causing a localised haematoma [18]. Anecdotally, pain after laser ablation occurs 3-5 days after the procedure, although newer radial laser fibres and higher wavelengths (1470nm) are purported to cause less post-procedure pain. Other complications include the development of small telangiectatic veins at the site of catheter entry or along the course of the ablated truncal vein, though these can also occur after phlebectomy with any venous intervention, including sclerotherapy (Figure 2).

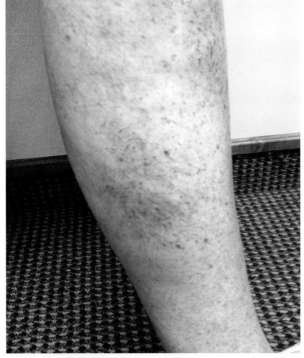

Figure 2. Telangiectatic matting at the site of a previous phlebectomy incision. This can occur after any varicose vein procedure, and is more common in people with existing spider veins, who should be warned pre-operatively.

Foam sclerotherapy

Ultrasound-guided foam sclerotherapy techniques can now be used to treat the majority of varicose veins with occlusion rates of 75-90% after 6 months [19-21]. The aim is to use sclerosant to damage the endothelium to cause permanent vascular occlusion.

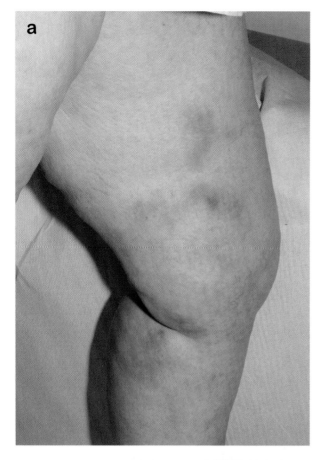

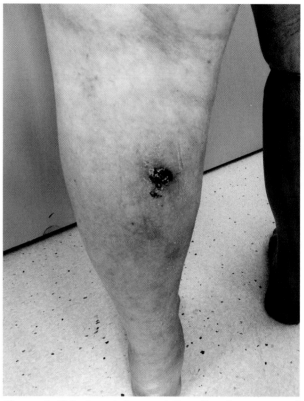

Figure 4. Skin breakdown at the site of an area of thrombophlebitis that became infected.

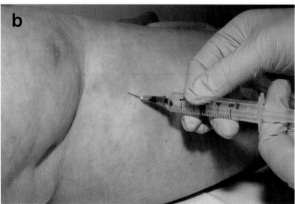

Figure 3. a) Painful phlebitis in the thigh and calf 3 weeks after foam sclerotherapy. b) Aspiration of liquefied thrombus from the calf provides immediate relief.

The process involves a degree of thrombophlebitis and therefore this can hardly be regarded as a complication, although in people with large varicose veins the inflammation can be quite extreme. If the patient is reviewed 2-4 weeks after the foam

sclerotherapy, it is often possible to aspirate a little dark liquefied thrombus from a tender area of phlebitis with immediate symptom improvement (Figure 3). Very rarely, the area of phlebitis can break down to produce skin ulceration (Figure 4). Most patients also develop a degree of skin discolouration with a brown stain over the occluded vein. This is usually mild and settles with time and is probably related to the depth of the vein beneath the surface of the skin. It may also be caused by extravascular leakage of foam, and highlights the importance of ensuring the needle remains within the target vein during injection. It can, however, occur after any treatment for varicose veins (Figure 5). Understanding the cause of these suboptimal results may lead to refinements of foam technique, and help minimise the risks.

Most series report a small proportion of patients who develop eye symptoms within half an hour of sclerosant foam injection. Patients describe blurred vision, usually not complete loss of vision, similar to the aura of migraine, and often followed by headache,

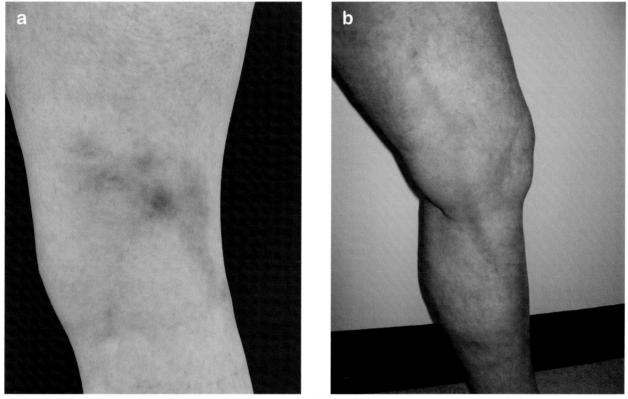

Figure 5. Skin staining after: a) foam sclerotherapy; and b) radiofrequency ablation.

raising the possibility of common aetiology. Symptoms are usually transient, and seldom last more than 30 minutes. No treatment is necessary as long as the symptoms resolve; it is probably worth recommending patients wait at least half an hour before going home after foam treatment, particularly if they might be driving. A very few cases of focal neurological ischaemia lasting longer than 30 minutes have been described. The well-known report in the literature occurred where 30ml of foam was injected into the varicose veins; foam was then seen in the carotid arteries on duplex imaging, presumably as a result of its passage across a patent foramen ovale (PFO) [22]. Since 10% of people have a PFO, passage of small amounts of sclerosant and air must be common. This is easily demonstrated on dynamic echocardiography. Yet even when bubbles were detected in the middle cerebral artery using transcranial Doppler monitoring after foam sclerotherapy, magnetic resonance imaging showed that vascular occlusion did not occur, suggesting visual symptoms are an electrical rather than an occlusive phenomenon [23]. Restricting the

overall volume of foam injected to 12ml reduces the incidence of blurred vision. An alternative is to use carbon dioxide instead of air to mix with the sclerosant. Other authors recommend occluding the saphenofemoral junction or more particularly the saphenopopliteal junction (or perforator sites) whilst injecting foam to prevent its immediate transfer into the deep veins. Dynamic echocardiogram studies have suggested that whilst this does reduce micro-embolisation for the duration of the compression, once compression is relaxed a bolus of sclerosant and gas is released [24]. It has also been suggested that people should be screened for a PFO, and foam sclerotherapy treatment withheld in those with a positive scan. Yet PFO is common and the problem of blurred vision is rare, meaning that many people would be denied foam sclerotherapy if this was an exclusion criterion. In addition, PFO can be quite difficult to diagnose accurately without sophisticated testing. Foam sclerotherapy has been adopted in many centres, and in many countries. Large numbers of patients have been treated, with an excellent safety profile, leading to NICE approving its general use, subject to close follow-up [25].

Varicose ulceration

Treatment of any superficial venous disease is indicated in patients with open or recently healed varicose ulcers [26]. Multilayer graduated compression is the principal first treatment; a large randomised trial of superficial venous surgery showed that surgical correction of superficial incompetence did not affect initial healing, but it had a significant effect on reducing subsequent recurrence [5]. Patients with a varicose ulcer are often elderly and frail, and surgical treatment under general anaesthesia can pose challenges and extra risks. Ambulant treatment under local anaesthesia using endothermal ablation or foam sclerotherapy are good choices; foam is emerging as a standard of care in these patients with low complications and low ulcer recurrence rates [27, 28].

Conclusions

Although the majority of patients who have treatment of their varicose veins are delighted with the results and the improvements in their symptoms and quality of life, a few are disgruntled by complications or a less than optimal outcome. Most litigation is the result of a failure of communication: pre-operatively a misunderstanding about what can be achieved and likely outcomes, and postoperatively a failure to explain complications sympathetically and realistically. A pre-operative discussion with an expert, good information sheets and careful pre-operative consent build on thorough pre-operative investigation and diagnosis and high-quality therapy. It is incumbent upon the modern vascular specialist to keep up to date with novel technology. It is no longer acceptable to offer only varicose vein surgery, and most clinicians should offer at least one alternative. This means learning about the novel therapies, securing training and accreditation, where required, and clinicians never using methods with which they are not completely familiar. Attention to detail is the best method to avoid complications and to improve outcomes.

Acknowledgements

I am grateful to Ian Franklin and Manj Gohel for their advice in preparing this manuscript, and to Ian for his permission to use Figure 5b.

Key points

- Although complications are rare after treatment for varicose veins, they are fertile ground for complaints and litigation.
- Good pre-operative communication and the use of information sheets are fundamental preparations for treatment.
- Counselling and consent should be undertaken by a specialist familiar with modern varicose vein treatments.
- New treatments for varicose veins have individual complication profiles, that require individual methods of prevention.
- The increase in technology has improved options for the patient but has placed increasing demands on knowledge and training for each vascular specialist.

References

1. Lim CS, Gohel MS, Shepherd AC, *et al*. Secondary care treatment of patients with varicose veins in National Health Service England: at least how it appeared on the National Health Service website. *Phlebology* 2010; 25: 184-9.

2. Campbell WB, France F, Goodwin HF. Medicolegal claims in vascular surgery. *Ann R Coll Surg Engl* 2002; 84: 181-3.

3. Campbell WB. Varicose veins and their management. *BMJ* 2006; 333: 287-92.

4. De Maeseneer M. The endovenous revolution. *Br J Surg* 2011; 98; 1037-8.

5. Gohel MS, Barwell JR, Taylor M, *et al*. Long-term results of compression therapy alone versus compression plus surgery in chronic venous ulceration (ESCHAR): randomised controlled trial. *BMJ* 2007; 335: 83-7.

6. Michaels JA, Brazier JE, Campbell WB, *et al*. Randomized clinical trial comparing surgery with conservative treatment for uncomplicated varicose veins. *Br J Surg* 2006; 93: 175-81.

7. Coleridge-Smith P, Labropoulos N, Partsch H, *et al*. Duplex investigation of the veins in chronic venous disease of the lower limbs: UIP consensus document. Part 1. Basic principles. *Eur J Vasc Endovasc Surg* 2006; 31: 83-92.

8. Blomgren L, Johansson G, Emanuelsson L, *et al*. Late follow-up of a randomized trial of routine duplex imaging before varicose vein surgery. *Br J Surg* 2011; 98: 1112-6.

9. Berridge DC, Lees T, Earnshaw JJ. The VEnous INtervention (VEIN) Project. *Phlebology* 2009; 24 suppl 1: 1-2.

10. Pares JO, Juan J, Tellez R, *et al*. Varicose vein surgery: stripping versus the CHIVA method: a randomized controlled trial. *Ann Surg* 2010; 25: 624-31.

11. Winterborn RJ, Foy C, Earnshaw JJ. Causes of varicose vein recurrence: late results of a randomized controlled trial of stripping the long saphenous vein. *J Vasc Surg* 2004; 40: 634-9.

12. Gohel MS, Epstein DM, Davies AH. Cost effectiveness of traditional and endovenous treatments for varicose veins. *Br J Surg* 2010; 97: 1815-23.

13. Rasmussen LH, Lawaetz M, Bjoern L, *et al*. Randomized clinical trial comparing endovenous laser ablation, radiofrequency ablation, foam sclerotherapy and surgical stripping for great saphenous varicose veins. *Br J Surg* 2011; 98: 1079-87.

14. National Institute for Health and Clinical Excellence. Venous thromboembolism: reducing the risk. NICE Clinical Guideline 92. www.nice.org.uk/guidance/CG92.

15. Sam RC, Silverman SH, Bradbury AW. Nerve injuries and varicose vein surgery. *Eur J Vasc Endovasc Surg* 2004; 27: 113-20.

16. O'Hare JL, Vandenbroeck CP, Whitman B, *et al*. A prospective evaluation of the outcome of small saphenous varicose vein surgery with one-year follow-up. *J Vasc Surg* 2008; 48: 669-74.

17. Mekako AI, Chetter IC, Coughlin PA, *et al*. Randomized clinical trial of co-amoxiclav versus no antibiotic prophylaxis in varicose vein surgery. *Br J Surg* 2010; 97: 29-36.

18. Shepherd AC, Gohel MS, Brown LC, *et al*. Randomized clinical trial of VNUS Closure Fast radiofrequency ablation versus laser for varicose veins. *Br J Surg* 2010; 97: 810-8.

19. Jia X, Mowatt G, Burr JM, *et al*. Systematic review of foam sclerotherapy for varicose veins. *Br J Surg* 2007; 94: 925-36.

20. O'Hare JL, Parkin D, Vandenbroeck CP, *et al*. Mid-term results of ultrasound-guided foam sclerotherapy for complicated and uncomplicated varicose veins. *Eur J Vasc Endovasc Surg* 2008; 36: 109-13.

21. Darvall KA, Bate GR, Adams DJ, *et al*. Duplex ultrasound outcomes following ultrasound-guided foam sclerotherapy of symptomatic primary great saphenous varicose veins. *Eur J Vasc Endovasc Surg* 2010; 40: 534-9.

22. Forlee MV, Grouden M, Moore DJ, *et al*. Stroke after varicose vein foam injection sclerotherapy. *J Vasc Surg* 2006; 43: 162-4.

23. Regan JD, Gibson KD, Rush JE, *et al*. Clinical significance of cerebrovascular gas emboli during polidocanol endovenous ultra-low nitrogen microfoam ablation and correlation with magnetic resonance imaging in patients with right to left shunt. *J Vasc Surg* 2011; 53: 131-7.

24. Hill D, Hamilton R, Fung T. Assessment of techniques to reduce sclerosant foam migration during ultrasound-guided sclerotherapy of the great saphenous vein. *J Vasc Surg* 2008; 48: 934-9.

25. National Institute for Health and Clinical Excellence. Ultrasound-guided foam sclerotherapy for varicose veins (interventional procedures overview), April 2009. http://www.nice.org.uk/guidance/index.jsp?action=download&o=43966 (accessed 22/7/11).

26. van Gent WB, Wilschut ED, Wittens C. Management of venous ulcer disease. *BMJ* 2010; 341: 1092-6.

27. O'Hare JL, Earnshaw JJ. Randomised clinical trial of foam sclerotherapy for patients with a venous leg ulcer. *Eur J Vasc Endovasc Surg* 2010; 39: 495-9.

28. Pang KH, Bate GR, Darvall KA *et al*. Healing and recurrence rates following ultrasound-guided foam sclerotherapy of superficial venous reflux in patients with chronic venous ulceration. *Eur J Vasc Endovasc Surg* 2010; 40: 790-5.

Chapter 25 Vascular malformations

Manj Gohel MD FRCS, Specialist Registrar in Vascular Surgery & Honorary Lecturer
Michael Jenkins BSc MS FRCS FEBVS, Consultant Vascular Surgeon & Honorary Senior Lecturer
St Mary's Hospital, Imperial College London, London, UK

Introduction

Although a number of definitions and classifications have been proposed, the term vascular malformation refers to a wide range of conditions characterised by abnormal development of one or more components of arterial, venous, capillary or lymphatic systems. As a result of the huge diversity of presentations, these conditions are managed by multiple medical teams with numerous treatment approaches. The management of patients with vascular malformations presents specific challenges and treatments are associated with unique risks and complications. The aim of this chapter is to summarise the types of vascular malformation, available treatment options and to highlight specific difficulties and complications that may be encountered, with suggestions for getting out of trouble.

Vascular malformations

Classification of vascular malformations

The classification of vascular malformations is the source of considerable confusion and controversy. A number of esoteric pathophysiological and haemodynamic classification schemes have been published. However, perhaps the most pragmatic involves defining the lesion as low flow or high flow,

with further sub-classification according to the tissue components involved. Although any combination of vascular and lymphatic components may be affected, over half of all lesions are venous (Figure 1) and these along with arteriovenous, and lymphovenous malformations represent the majority of lesions encountered. As described in the classification by Mulliken and Glowacki [1], vascular malformations are considered a separate entity from haemangiomas, which are characterised by hyperplasia of vascular endothelial components. Numerous types of haemangioma are recognised, including capillary (port-wine stain) and cavernous (strawberry naevus). Infantile haemangiomas often present in early childhood and are typically associated with proliferative, resting and regressive phases.

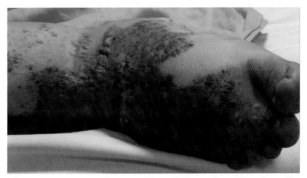

Figure 1. Vascular malformation (predominantly venous) affecting right lower limb and foot.

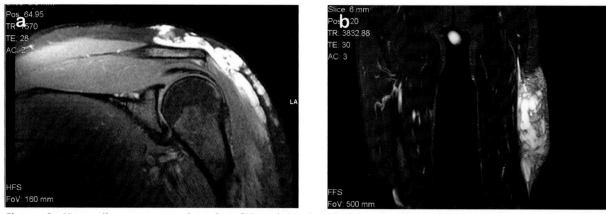

Figure 2. Magnetic resonance imaging (T2-weighted with fat saturation) demonstrating low-flow vascular malformations affecting the: a) shoulder; b) lateral thigh.

Clinical assessment and investigation

Clinicians should maintain a high index of suspicion and consider the diagnosis of vascular malformation when assessing any coloured skin or soft tissue lesion. A palpable thrill would indicate an arterial component. In addition, the precise location, extent of the lesion and level of symptomatology and disability should be assessed and documented. Formal photography of lesions is recommended as a baseline evaluation against which post-intervention appearances may be compared. A detailed examination should be performed to identify other lesions or associated abnormalities, as vascular malformations are commonly seen as part of a wider clinical syndrome (such as Parkes-Weber, Klippel Trenauney or Mafucci syndromes).

Colour duplex ultrasound is an excellent non-invasive investigation to confirm the presence of a vascular malformation and determine whether the lesion is low flow or high flow. The location and number of feeding arteries may also be clearly visualised. However, cross-sectional imaging is mandatory in all but the smallest of vascular malformations as the deep extent of lesions may be impossible to determine from examination or duplex alone. In the limbs, lesions may breach the fascial layers and involve muscles or bones. Magnetic resonance imaging is widely used as vascular lesions appear hyperintense, and are clearly visible on T2-weighted images with fat saturation [2] (Figure 2). Additional investigations such as digital subtraction angiography may have a role in selected cases, particularly where embolisation of a feeding artery may be an option. For high-flow lesions, angiography is probably the optimal investigation in order to identify the nidus of the lesion as well as the presence and anatomy of micro or macro fistulae.

Natural history and management strategies

The majority of low-flow lesions have a relatively benign natural history. Symptoms and complications are most commonly seen in very extensive lesions, or malformations with a significant arteriovenous shunt. In extreme cases, high-output cardiac failure may ensue. The importance of multidisciplinary evaluation and management cannot be overemphasised for this patient group. Vascular surgeons, specialist nurses, plastic surgeons, interventional radiologists, psychologists, camouflage specialists and other health professionals all have a potential role [3]. Treatments should begin with conservative measures and compression therapy, with escalation as required. Vascular malformations with ulceration or bleeding generally require surgical excision, whereas injection sclerotherapy may be particularly suitable for venous and other low-flow malformations [4]. Commonly used treatment options include:

- conservative management (including analgesia, camouflage treatments and psychological therapy);
- compression therapy;
- injection sclerotherapy;
- embolisation procedures (either as stand-alone treatment, or before surgical excision);
- surgical excision (partial or complete);

◆ other surgical procedures (such as vasoconstrictive suturing techniques).

Specific pitfalls and complications

Clinicians managing patients with vascular malformations may encounter a number of challenges before, during and after treatment. These include: pitfalls in diagnosis, expectations from treatment, skin necrosis and other ischaemic complications, complications of embolisation, complications of laser treatment, bleeding complications and damage to adjacent structures.

Pitfalls in diagnosis

Problems may be encountered through either misdiagnosis of other conditions or inadequate characterisation of vascular malformations. The possibility of soft tissue malignancy should always be considered and actively excluded, particularly with firm or rapidly enlarging lesions [5]. For lesions confirmed as vascular malformations, multimodal investigation is usually necessary to define the precise components of the lesion in order to guide management. Inadequate investigation, or simply labelling all lesions as arteriovenous malformations may lead to inappropriate treatment plans and a higher risk of complications and recurrence. For example, in patients with a venous malformation of the leg, deep veins should be assessed in detail as deep venous aplasia or hypoplasia may be seen and would influence the choice of treatment offered. It should be noted that invasive investigations such as angiography are usually only performed for symptomatic lesions where treatment is being considered. In patients with thrombocytopaenia and a vascular malformation, clinicians should be aware of the Kasabach-Merritt syndrome, characterised by platelet trapping within a proliferative haemangioma. The condition is an indication for urgent treatment of the lesion, as it can result in disseminated intravascular coagulation and multi-organ failure.

Expectations from treatment

The patient's expectations from treatment should match those of the treating clinician. Patients seek treatment for a variety of reasons, ranging from minor cosmetic concerns, to life-threatening complications such as bleeding or cardiac failure. The clinician should make a specific effort to identify the precise symptoms and patient concerns, as well as the specific medical risks associated with the vascular malformation, before developing a treatment plan in conjunction with the patient. The specific aims of treatment should be clear (e.g. removal of lump, reduction of pain, improved cosmetic appearance) and agreed with the patient prior to intervention. The impact of symptoms should not be underestimated, as chronic pain and depression are common in this patient group. Patients should understand that for extensive lesions, the best that can be achieved is often palliation, rather than cure.

Addressing cosmetic concerns is an extremely difficult challenge. As lesions are usually congenital, patients with vascular malformations are often young and concerned about their appearance. The patient should be warned that the cosmetic appearance after surgical excision of vascular malformations may be worse than the initial lesion. In addition to a scar (which may be very large), severe contour asymmetry or cavitation may result, particularly for deep lesions involving muscle. As with other conditions associated with significant physical disfigurement, psychologists may have a role in helping patients to live with large or prominent lesions.

Skin necrosis and other ischaemic complications

Skin necrosis after injection sclerotherapy
Cutaneous necrosis is a specific concern after injection sclerotherapy and in published reports, may occur in up to 5% of treated patients. The degree of necrosis may range from a small area of skin to extensive necrosis of musculocutaneous compartments. Injection sclerotherapy is used for low-flow (usually venous) malformations (Figure 3), and the greatest risk factor for skin necrosis is the proximity of the lesion to the surface of the skin. Lesions located on the dorsum of the hand or foot may be at particular risk. The use of large volumes of sclerosant may also increase the risk; the sclerosant type (ethanol, sodium tetradecyl sulphate, foam) is probably of less importance. The authors favour the use of smaller volumes of sclerosant, accepting that a larger number of treatments may be required. In recent years, the use

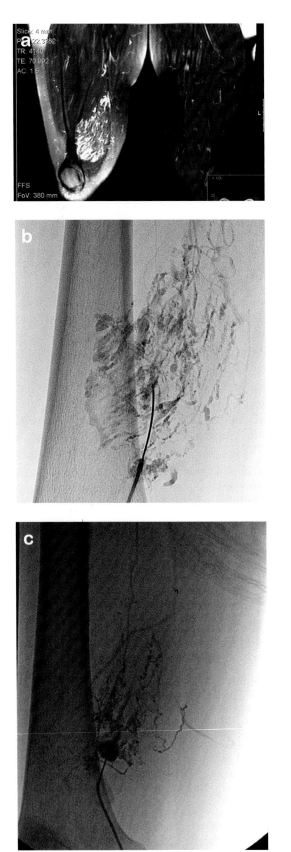

of foam sclerosant has increased and studies have suggested that efficacy may be higher, and volumes injected may be lower, using foam in comparison to liquid sclerosant. However, the choice of sclerosant should be made individually, guided by the personal experience and preference of the clinician. The number of sclerosant injections required for venous malformations in published studies varies dramatically (from 1 or 2 to over 20), reflecting the heterogeneity of lesions treated and variations in clinician preference. The authors prefer an interval of at least 6 weeks between treatment sessions.

In order to reduce the risk of cutaneous necrosis, detailed imaging and discussion in a multidisciplinary forum are essential components of management. Patients should undergo multimodal imaging prior to MDT discussion. If the lesion is slow flow and the option of sclerotherapy is considered, then the risk of skin necrosis is assessed on the basis of the clinical examination and imaging. These multidisciplinary assessments form the basis of subsequent discussions with the patient and their family. In many hospitals an experienced interventional radiologist carries out injection sclerotherapy procedures under ultrasound and fluoroscopic guidance. Adequate image guidance is essential, as a number of authors have reported inadvertent arterial or subcutaneous injection of sclerosant.

Skin necrosis after other treatments

During surgical excision of vascular malformations, care should be taken to avoid devascularisation of skin flaps. For extra-fascial venous malformations, *en bloc* excision of skin is often necessary. For the excision of extensive lesions, the early involvement of plastic surgeons can optimise measures for skin closure. Skin necrosis may also occur after vasoconstrictive suturing techniques for large vascular malformations (such as purse string or 'Popescu' plicating sutures), although these procedures are not in common use. It should be noted that painful thrombophlebitis is very common after minimally invasive and surgical treatments, and may be the mechanism of action (as with injection sclerotherapy). Emptying of venous lakes before injection may reduce the extent of thrombophlebitis and improve treatment efficacy. Patients should be warned that thrombophlebitis might last for several weeks.

Figure 3. Low-flow vascular malformation affecting the vastus medialis muscle treated with injection sclerotherapy. a) MRI image before intervention. b) First injection treatment. c) Significant improvement on imaging at second treatment after 8 weeks.

Complications of embolisation

Embolisation of feeding arteries in arteriovenous malformations may result in cutaneous or digital necrosis. Careful treatment planning on the basis of good quality digital subtraction angiography, and avoidance of embolisation in very distal lesions affecting the limbs, may reduce the risk of such complications. Radiologists with extensive experience of selective and super selective catheterisation should perform embolisation procedures. As arteriovenous malformations may have multiple shunts, specific target vessels for embolisation should be carefully planned. Occlusion of the main feeding artery may be undesirable, as the lesion may be rendered inaccessible for further embolisation while distal collaterals may continue to form. Although uncommon, the risk of paradoxical embolisation should always be considered in lesions where large arteriovenous connections are present.

Complications of laser treatment

Laser therapy (particularly pulsed light laser) has become popular for the treatment of capillary or intradermal malformations. This technique is usually reserved for flat port-wine stain lesions rather than deeper malformations with venous lakes. Although generally safe, laser treatment should be avoided in patients with darker skin pigments (Fitzpatrick skin types IV, V and VI) as burns and pigment loss are much more common. Moreover, patients should be warned that numerous treatments (often more than six) might be required to see significant results [6]. Camouflage or cosmetic therapy should be considered for all patients with a port-wine stain as significant advances have been made in this field in recent years.

Bleeding complications

Bleeding represents the most feared of complications from vascular malformations. Lesions that ulcerate or bleed usually require intervention, often with surgical excision. A number of pre, peri and postoperative strategies may be employed to reduce the risk of bleeding. The principles of bloodless surgery, a concept developed for transfusion avoidance, should be applied to this patient group.

Pre-operative

Pre-operative assessment should include detailed evaluation of clotting and platelet function, and all drugs that may predispose to bleeding (antiplatelet or anticoagulants) should be stopped where possible. Adequate planning is essential to ensure the optimal skill mix and availability of equipment and blood products during the procedure. Pre-operative imaging-guided marking of the extent of the lesion to be excised, and key vessels or other anatomical landmarks, may be of assistance. Particularly with very extensive lesions, the operative plan should be defined clearly before surgery. Embolisation of feeding arteries should always be considered prior to embarking on surgical excision as the extent of the resection and blood loss may be reduced significantly.

Intra-operative

Tourniquets and cell-salvage devices should be employed wherever possible. Surgical technique should be optimised to minimise blood loss and the use of haemostatic dissecting aids (such as the harmonic scalpel or Ligasure™ tissue fusion device) should be considered. Large lesions may be best managed with staged procedures to reduce the risk of massive blood loss during a single procedure.

Postoperative

The surgical team should remain vigilant to the possibility of postoperative bleeding and monitor the output from surgical drains and inspect the surgical site regularly. Following significant intra-operative blood loss, aggressive correction of thrombocytopaenia or coagulopathy is imperative.

Damage to adjacent structures

As vascular malformations may be associated with considerable distortions of normal anatomy, the risk of damage to nerves and other local structures is greater than surgical procedures for other pathologies. The inherent difficulties in maintaining a bloodless surgical field further add to the risk. The risk of nerve injury is greatest during the surgical treatment of head and neck, and upper limb vascular malformations. Nerves and other important anatomical structures should be identified on pre-operative imaging where possible and surgical teams should refresh their familiarity with local anatomy, particularly when treating vascular malformations in unusual locations. During surgery, identification and control of important vessels and nerves should be part of the operative plan (Figure 4).

Conclusions

The effective management of patients with a vascular malformation is dependent on detailed imaging and treatment planning within a multidisciplinary team. Careful assessment of the patient's symptoms and level of disability is essential, as treatment strategies may be complex and complications are common. Conservative management is often the most appropriate approach. Injection sclerotherapy is an effective and minimally invasive treatment for patients with low-flow vascular malformations, although very superficial lesions may be best treated with surgical excision due to the risk of skin necrosis [7]. Haemorrhage and nerve damage are significant risks associated with surgical excision. Percutaneous management is likely to remain the mainstay of treatment for vascular malformations, although further efforts are needed to develop new treatment modalities for this complex spectrum of conditions.

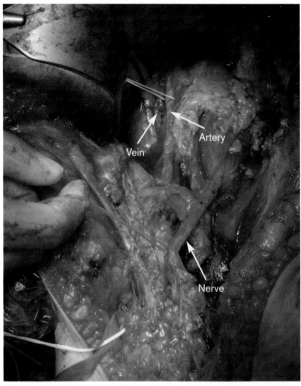

Figure 4. Intra-operative photograph after resection of a large vascular malformation demonstrating control of femoral vessels and nerve in the left iliofemoral region.

Key points

- Detailed multimodal imaging and a multidisciplinary approach are essential components in the modern management of patients with vascular malformations.
- The symptoms should be assessed carefully and the patient's expectations from treatment should match those of the treating clinician.
- Most low-flow vascular malformations can be managed with conservative measures or injection sclerotherapy.
- The risk of complications may be reduced with careful planning.

References

1. Mulliken JB, Glowacki J. Hemangiomas and vascular malformations in infants and children: a classification based on endothelial characteristics. *Plast Reconstr Surg* 1982; 69: 412-22.
2. Alomari A, Dubois J. Interventional management of vascular malformations. *Tech Vasc Interv Radiol* 2011; 14: 22-31.
3. Lee BB, Do YS, Yakes W, *et al*. Management of arteriovenous malformations: a multidisciplinary approach. *J Vasc Surg* 2004; 39: 590-600.
4. Dompmartin A, Vikkula M, Boon LM. Venous malformation: update on aetiopathogenesis, diagnosis and management. *Phlebology* 2010; 25: 224-35.
5. Wambeek N, Munk PL, O'Connell JX, *et al*. Popliteal vascular malformation simulating a soft tissue sarcoma. *Skeletal Radiol* 1999; 28: 532-5.
6. Carvalho NT, Ribas-Filho JM, Macedo JF, *et al*. Laser treatment of venous malformations. *Rev Col Bras Cir* 2010; 37: 345-50.
7. Gloviczki P, Duncan A, Kalra M, *et al*. Vascular malformations: an update. *Perspect Vasc Surg Endovasc Ther* 2009; 21: 133-48.

Chapter 26 Renal transplant, vascular access and dialysis

David C. Mitchell MA MS FRCS, Consultant Vascular and Transplant Surgeon
Southmead Hospital, Bristol, UK

Introduction

The biggest problem encountered in vascular access surgery is establishing secure access for the patient requiring dialysis. Managing this in both a timely and effective way is a significant challenge for clinical teams and patients [1].

Patients who require urgent dialysis and who do not have established permanent access usually require the insertion of a central venous catheter. These are a major cause of blood-borne sepsis in the dialysis population. Patients commencing haemodialysis with a central vein catheter are more likely to die than those starting with a fistula or access graft. In addition, patients may suffer complications from the insertion of such catheters. Long-term use is associated with fibrin cuff formation and major vein stenosis (Figure 1), which may prevent formation of permanent access in the limbs drained by these veins. Avoiding the use of central venous dialysis catheters forms the mainstay of planning around provision of vascular access in western health care systems. This principally relates to the reduction of sepsis.

The alternatives to central venous catheters are an autologous arteriovenous (AV) fistula, or a prosthetic arteriovenous access graft where no suitable vein is

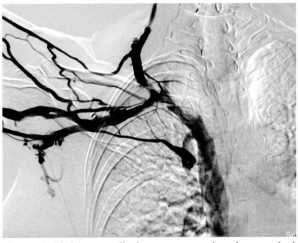

Figure 1. Right upper limb venogram showing central vein stenosis following prolonged central venous catheter use.

available. It is widely accepted that a fistula is the ideal form of access, as this is the most sepsis-resistant and least likely to thrombose of all the access options. Fistulas are more difficult to establish than grafts and take longer to mature before they can be used; advance planning is therefore an important element of a vascular access service. Grafts are regarded as a second line of access as they have a higher thrombotic rate (80% at 1 year versus 15% for fistulas) and are more prone to becoming infected [2, 3].

The complications associated with vascular access surgery can be broadly divided into those related to flow (either too much or not enough), thrombosis, or problems related to infection. Other complications will be discussed separately.

Problems related to blood flow

Thrombosis

Dialysis patients depend on their vascular access for dialysis and to stay alive. Any problem with this access represents a major life event and often causes significant distress. Thrombosis of the access site requires prompt intervention if this access is to be maintained. This is particularly true of arteriovenous fistulas where a fibrotic reaction in the vein wall occurs quite quickly after thrombosis and can lead to loss of the fistula despite attempts at recanalisation. Attempts to salvage a thrombosed AV fistula should ideally be undertaken within 24-48 hours. For vascular access grafts this is not a problem and grafts are amenable to salvage up to several weeks after thrombosis.

Early identification of thrombosis allows early intervention and services should be designed to ensure that interventions can proceed with minimal delay. If the patient is on a surveillance programme and there is a known stenosis within the graft or fistula, catheter-directed thrombolysis with simultaneous angioplasty may be sufficient to re-establish flow and salvage the fistula.

If this is not the case, then the options for treatment are direct surgical intervention or a trial of thrombolysis followed by either angioplasty or surgery as appropriate, subsequent to recanalisation. An endovascular approach is preferable as it allows the patient to recommence dialysis immediately. Open surgery often necessitates exposure of the graft or fistula and this imposes a delay of some days before the access can be used, necessitating insertion of a central line for dialysis.

The technique for thrombolysis is to insert a butterfly needle into the middle of the thrombosed fistula, or two if the fistula is more than four or five inches long. A

bolus of 2.5mg of recombinant tissue plasminogen activator (rt-PA) is injected followed by an infusion running at a rate of 0.5-1mg of rt-PA per hour. If successful, this will produce lysis and some flow within 4-6 hours. It is probably not sensible to persist beyond 6 hours as this may lead to haemorrhagic complications.

If flow is re-established, the next step is usually an ultrasound scan. This can detect any stenoses of the fistula and allows for planning of angioplasty to re-establish a good flow rate and to allow for continued dialysis. If thrombolysis is not successful, a surgical approach is usually indicated. For fistulas the problem is usually a stenosis between the needling sites or around the arterial anastomosis; initial surgical attempts are therefore directed towards the arterial anastomosis. Anastomotic stenoses are best treated by reconstructing the anastomosis. Stenotic segments in mid-fistula can be dilated on table, or resected if short. Longer mid-fistula stenosis may require formal bypassing.

The most common cause of graft thrombosis is a stenosis at the venous anastomosis and therefore initial surgical efforts should be directed towards the venous end of the graft. Graft thrombectomy can often be achieved with a Fogarty catheter from the venous end achieving a good inflow. The procedure of choice for managing a venous stenosis at the top end of an access graft has not been formally tested, but it is the author's opinion that patching is less successful than extending the graft to a segment of normal vein an inch or two beyond the original anastomosis.

Problems related to low flow

It is known that grafts and fistulas are more likely to thrombose with low flow and that dialysis efficacy is impeded by low flow within grafts or fistulas due to re-circulation. Re-circulation occurs when the flow is low in the fistula/graft and the dialysis machine re-circulates some of the same blood continuously. This can be measured; increasing proportions of re-circulation can indicate a problem with the access. Ideally access grafts and AV fistulas should have a flow of at least 600ml per minute to allow for blood to be circulated through the dialyser at about 300ml per minute without excessive re-circulation [4].

Most units now undertake some form of surveillance of their vascular access procedures, although there is little evidence that this extends the life of an AV fistula. Nevertheless, there is evidence that surveillance and early intervention for stenosis can extend the lives of AV grafts, so that secondary patency rates will match those of equivalent fistulas. Guidance from Europe, the United Kingdom and the United States would suggest that fistulas are to be preferred, requiring less maintenance interventions for low flow than AV grafts. The guidelines for avoiding trouble due to thrombosis are usually to intervene if the flow rates drop by 25% or more between consecutive ultrasound surveillance scans, and to consider intervention for tight stenosis (greater than 75% cross-sectional area reduction) with flows of less than 600ml per minute [4].

Interventions should be endovascular wherever possible and the outcome of the procedure should be checked with a further duplex scan within a few weeks, although flow monitoring during haemodialysis is an acceptable alternative. Surgery is reserved for patients in whom angioplasty has failed. The procedure should be planned to minimise interference with the segments of access used for dialysis. It is often possible to resect short stenoses and preserve a functioning fistula for dialysis.

Problems due to high flow

Flow changes in arterial access grafts are seen almost instantaneously after implantation and in arteriovenous fistulas the majority of increase in flow is seen within the first 48-72 hours. Occasionally, flow can increase significantly to a level that causes high output cardiac failure. This can usually be diagnosed clinically with the patient complaining of increasing breathlessness associated with a marked tachycardia. Occlusion of the fistula or graft will alleviate the tachycardia. Occasionally in more severe examples the patient can suffer other organ decompensation such as liver failure. The treatment of severe rapid onset high output cardiac failure is immediate ligation of the fistula or graft. One way to avoid this problem is to avoid using a large diameter graft. The ideal size of an access graft is 6mm and larger diameter grafts should only be used with significant caution in patients with a cardiac history.

In milder examples of high output cardiac failure, where it can be demonstrated that fistula occlusion is associated with a slowing of the pulse rate (due to reduced venous return), a flow reduction procedure can be undertaken. A short segment smaller diameter interposition graft will reduce flow if placed into an established AV graft or large fistula. Alternatives include extending the graft distally by disconnecting it and placing it onto a forearm artery using a smaller anastomosis. Banding procedures, where the fistula is surrounded by a band of synthetic material tightened using sutures, can be successful, but it can be difficult to set the band tension correctly, with over-tightening causing thrombosis, or under-tightening leaving the patient with the original problem. For this reason we have largely abandoned banding procedures and now place a small interposition graft or perform a distal extension.

Vascular steal

Another problem related to flow is vascular steal. This occurs when, following access placement, the blood supply to the hand, or foot in lower limb access, is inadequate resulting in ischaemia, loss of function and in severe cases distal necrosis, ulceration and gangrene. If left untreated, this condition can cause permanent neurological damage or result in the loss of the hand. There is a rare aggressive variant called ischaemic monomelic neuropathy which is thought to be due to nerve ischaemia at the time of surgery. This usually presents as severe pain and paralysis in the affected arm within a few hours of surgery. Treatment involves immediate ligation of the fistula otherwise function in the hand will be lost.

For milder cases that come on after some days to weeks, steal syndrome can develop due to an inadequacy of the collateral circulation at the elbow to provide forward flow into the hand. The discovery of reverse flow in the artery immediately distal to the fistula is not diagnostic of steal syndrome, as this is a common ultrasound finding in patients who do not have the syndrome. Clinical diagnosis can be difficult. In the most straightforward cases arm elevation will produce whiteness of the hand with a positive Buerger's test on placing the hand dependent (see case vignette). Elevating the arm until it blanches and then occluding the fistula may be helpful, as if there is an immediate return of pinkness to the hand, that clinches the diagnosis. Some patients complain of milder symptoms, such as tingling in the fingers or pain only after a period on dialysis. In this situation, the diagnosis may be more difficult and other tests may be helpful such as measuring the digital pressures (a level of less than 0.6 is thought to be diagnostic) or looking at the variation in digital waveforms and pressures with the fistula patent and occluded.

The treatment of vascular steal syndrome is either to ligate the fistula/graft, or to try and improve the flow towards the hand without compromising the access site. Ligation carries the risk of shifting the problem to the contralateral limb when new access is formed. For this reason, the author believes that attempts to relieve the problem in the affected limb are preferable. The technique is to reduce the load on the collateral circulation, or to improve flow into the forearm without compromise to the established access. The commonest procedure for this is the distal revascularisation interval ligation (DRIL) procedure [5], where a bypass graft is taken from the artery above the fistula (at least 8-10cm to avoid stealing from the bypass graft) and anastomosed to either the brachial or one of the forearm arteries distal to the fistula anastomosis. As the fistula may steal from the distal end of the graft as well, the surgeon must ligate the artery between the fistula anastomosis and the distal anastomosis of the brachial artery bypass graft. This procedure is fairly reliable and will usually benefit the majority of patients. If there have been prolonged neurological symptoms, these may not, or only partially, resolve with time.

Alternative procedures involve refashioning of the fistula anastomosis more distally onto one of the individual forearm arteries [6]. Occasionally it may be possible to take the fistula up in a loop and perform the arterial anastomosis in the axilla moving it more proximal than the collateral circuit to the elbow. All patients undergoing such bypass procedures should be entered into a surveillance programme to ensure that the graft bypassing the fistula does not become stenosed causing further problems.

Infective problems

Infection around vascular access sites can be a disaster and, when associated with significant haemorrhage, may be immediately life-threatening. For this reason, patients presenting with large scabs over needling points, inflammation of their fistula/graft or sudden painful aneurysmal dilatation of their fistula should be admitted urgently to hospital. These changes are an indication for rapid intervention to prevent secondary haemorrhage and its consequences. There is a limited amount of information in the literature to describe what to do and most approaches need to be individualised.

Localised fistula inflammation can often be managed with antibiotics alone. Occasionally abscess formation may dictate ligation or drainage with skip grafting of the infected segment. Grafts can only be used if they can be safely tunnelled through uninvolved tissues away from the infected area. They are not recommended where there is widespread inflammation.

The rapidly expanding infected aneurysmal fistula should be excised and an interposition graft used to maintain the patency of the rest of the fistula. Failing this, a new fistula will need to be created and the patient will probably need an interim central venous catheter.

Localised sepsis of a graft is not always an indication for removing the whole graft, especially if this is an access procedure performed urgently in a patient with limited alternative access sites. High-dose intravenous antibiotics after blood cultures are indicated, particularly if the patient has evidence of sepsis. If the sepsis is not controlled rapidly, then fistula ligation is probably a sensible option. If the inflammation around the graft subsides quickly, it may be possible to excise a small area of graft and place a skip graft around the infected area. Decision making can be difficult and it is important that the patient is fully informed of the risks and benefits of proposed procedures, to allow an informed choice about the best strategy to pursue.

If on surgical exploration, the graft is found to be loose in the subcutaneous tissues, with or without the presence of pus, infection throughout the graft is likely, and this graft should be removed. If, however, the graft is well incorporated and there is a localised abscess around the needling area of the fistula, it may be legitimate to excise this area and leave the wound open. The graft is then cut back using two separate clean incisions and a new interposition graft tunnelled in a circuitous route away from the infected field to maintain graft function. The infected area is packed with an antiseptic dressing for a few days and allowed to heal by secondary intention. Using this technique we have salvaged a number of grafts including some associated with MRSA abscesses. There is, however, an ever present risk of further sepsis and it is the author's view that the patient should be kept in hospital for a period of observation until satisfactory wound healing can be confirmed.

If the remaining non-infected segments of the graft are sufficiently close to the skin, they can be used for dialysis without the need to place a central line. The new portion of graft should be given about 10-14 days to bed in and become incorporated into the tissues before being used. Newer graft materials that allow immediate needling can be implanted if required and these can be used for dialysis as soon as the procedure is completed.

Other problems encountered in vascular access

The aneurysmal fistula

A non-infected, progressively aneurysmal AV fistula may be caused by idiopathic aneurysmal dilatation or by central venous stenosis. All such fistulas should be examined with duplex ultrasound and if there is no clear diagnosis of central stenosis, a venogram should be obtained. Angioplasty may allow the aneurysm dilatation to stabilise, but regression is rarely seen. If the aneurysm continues to dilate despite central venous angioplasty, or in the absence of central venous obstruction, the fistula should be excised or an aneurysmorrhaphy performed (Figures 2 and 3). The procedure is to expose, mobilise and excise part of

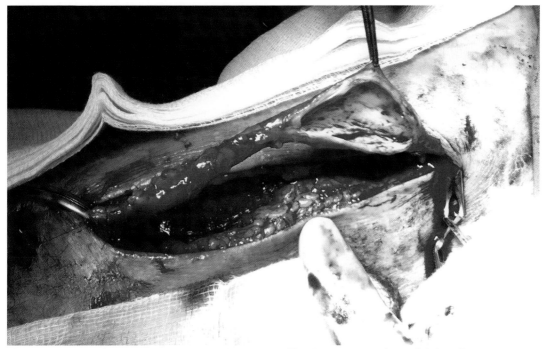

Figure 2. Operative photograph showing a mobilised segment of AV fistula after aneurysm excision. The distal half has been closed with direct suture.

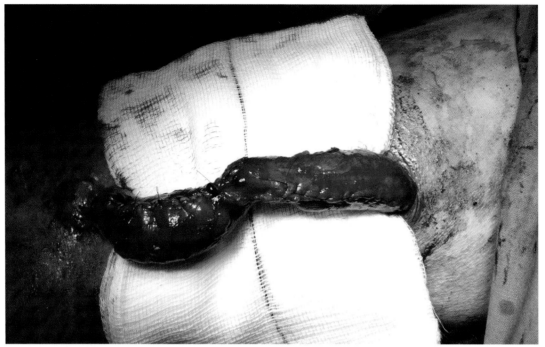

Figure 3. Operative photograph showing completed aneurysmorrhaphy. The fistula may be replaced and the wound closed, or reinforced with a mesh wrap.

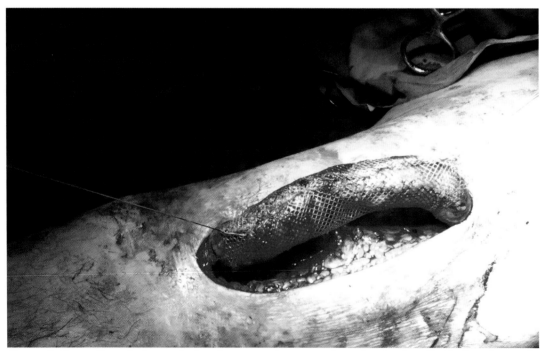

Figure 4. Operative photograph showing a mesh wrap, using standard synthetic hernia mesh. The wound is closed directly over the fistula which may be used for dialysis after 14 days.

the fistula followed by a reconstruction of a normal fistula by direct suture; this can also be supported with a loose wrap Prolene mesh (Figure 4) [7]. Aneurysmorrhaphy without mesh wrap has also been described with equally good results.

The deep lying fistula

In current practice, surgeons are seeing increasing numbers of obese patients presenting for haemodialysis. The formation of an AV fistula may be successful, but it is often difficult to dialyse the patient due to the deep lying position of their veins. In such situations, either a secondary transposition procedure or the use of suction lipectomy is required [8]. Surgical fistula transposition is more commonly required in the arm and occasionally in the forearm in some very obese patients. There is a choice of procedural techniques. The first is to make an incision adjacent to the fistula, bring it up to the skin, (reforming the anastomosis if necessary) and then mobilise the fat at a superficial level and suturing it under the fistula to hold it up against the skin; the wound is then closed. An alternative technique is to incise over a fistula that has not been used, mobilise it and disconnect the anastomosis. The fistula is then tunnelled superficially, as for a basilic vein or great saphenous vein transposition fistula. A new anastomosis is then fashioned at the appropriate position. These techniques can allow for successful fistula dialysis for the very obese, whereas otherwise they would require a graft or a central venous catheter.

Desperate access

Occasionally patients seem to run out of veins and places for grafts to be placed easily for access. In these situations, ingenuity of surgical and radiological colleagues can be invaluable in helping the patient obtain satisfactory access. A variety of procedures may be required, some of which can be quite challenging. The author has placed access grafts between the aorta and IVC tunnelled on the abdominal wall and between the brachial artery and the innominate vein/right atrium intrathoracically to provide access in extreme circumstances.

Axillofemoral access grafts are described, as are necklace grafts across the upper chest wall. Occasionally attempts to construct access in the upper limb can lead to central vein obstruction manifesting as gross head and neck swelling. For these patients, an interventional radiologist or cardiologist can be invaluable to dilate stenoses or recanalise occlusions of the great veins within the chest. This can result in both the relief of discomfort for the patient and provides an outflow tract for either an access graft fistula or a central venous catheter. These techniques have been successfully employed to recanalise the innominate vein, superior vena cava and even to deal with caval occlusions at the cava atrial junction.

Vascular complications of renal transplantation

It is unusual for vascular surgeons without a transplant practice, to be involved in the acute care of transplant patients. The increasing age of the recipient population and the liberalisation of criteria for acceptable donors (so called marginal donors), is likely to increase demand for expert vascular surgical input.

Problems with the donated kidney

It is more common to be offered kidneys with severe atheroma, which may cause marked stenosis of the renal artery. The options are to either perform a local endarterectomy or to excise the proximal renal artery beyond the plaque (it rarely extends far into the renal artery). The author's preference is to keep both the renal artery and vein at similar length for ease of transplantation.

Occasionally the vascular surgeon may be asked to help with vascular injury inflicted at organ retrieval. The principles are to repair primarily, or to use adjacent vascular tissue to reconstruct (e.g. the gonadal vein can be used to extend a transected polar artery) damaged vessels.

Vascular problems during transplantation

This is probably the commonest situation in which a vascular surgical opinion will be sought. Technical difficulties due to arterial or venous disease are seen increasingly in older and diabetic patients. The principles are to provide adequate inflow and outflow without undue risk to the life of the recipient. The most commonly performed procedure is local arterial endarterectomy, and occasionally reconstruction, if need be with synthetic graft material, onto which the donor artery is grafted. Unidentified disease in the recipient should be rare, but venous occlusion from silent DVT is occasionally seen. If this extends to the IVC, then the transplant should be performed in the contralateral iliac fossa. If confined to the external iliac vein, then the transplant can be performed at the common iliac level. This can make for a technically challenging procedure. The author has used both the aorta and internal iliac artery as arterial donor sites in times of difficulty; both sites are more commonly used in paediatric renal transplantation.

Vascular problems post-transplantation

In the acute phase, arterial or venous thrombosis can occur. Surgical re-exploration nearly always ends with nephrectomy as the kidney will have infarcted.

In the longer term, renal artery stenosis is a recognised cause of hypertension and sudden deterioration in renal function. This can be confirmed by CT angiography or direct catheter angiography. The treatment of choice is angioplasty and stenting, not a direct surgical approach which can be very challenging.

The other problem seen in vascular clinics is arterial stenosis or occlusion causing intermittent claudication in transplant recipients (Figure 5), or aortic aneurysms above renal transplants. In this situation, the patient should be assessed initially with ultrasound, and contrast studies minimised to reduce acute kidney injury. An endovascular approach is preferable, minimising renal ischaemia. If there is likely to be prolonged ischaemia, it is sensible to provide alternative perfusion using an extra-anatomic graft for part of the procedure (e.g. a temporary axillofemoral graft during aortic cross-clamping). If undertaking endovascular aneurysm grafting, then attention should focus on re-establishing renal perfusion quickly, which may dictate the side through which the main body of the graft is inserted.

Conclusions

There are a number of situations in which patients can get into difficulty attempting haemodialysis access. The best way to manage this is by having clear protocols and agreements within the team providing care for the patient. This requires a multidisciplinary approach, usually with the help of an access co-ordinator who can ensure that all parties remain informed about the process of care. They can

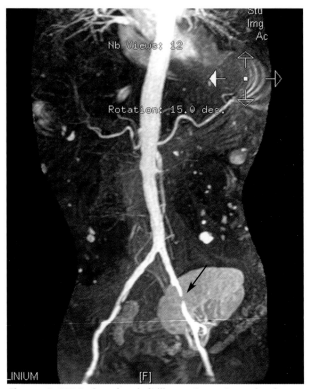

Figure 5. MRA showing left iliac artery stenosis above a kidney transplant.

provide an invaluable communication link to the patients and their families. The team should consist, as a minimum, of an access co-ordinator, nephrologist, vascular access surgeon and an interventional radiologist. Most problems can be addressed within the team and most problems confronting surgeons undertaking access surgery can be managed successfully using the techniques at their disposal.

In renal transplantation, there are a number of specific situations where vascular surgical input may be helpful. Surgeons should work from first principles using standard vascular surgical techniques. It is rare that a transplant cannot be completed, but very occasionally it may be safer to abandon a transplant rather than take undue risks with the patient's immediate wellbeing.

Key points

- The key to providing a well-organised service is to have a clear pathway and co-ordinator to ensure the smooth running of the pathway
- A regular MDT meeting is useful to resolve management issues in complex cases.
- Most vascular access problems can be diagnosed through careful history and clinical examination.
- Duplex ultrasound remains the key investigation in the majority of cases.
- Timely intervention for identified problems in vascular access reduces the need for emergency interventions.
- Most vascular problems in renal transplant recipients can be managed using standard vascular and endovascular techniques. Units undertaking these interventions should have both surgical and renal medical support available on site.
- Surgical exploration of arteries adjacent to a renal transplant can be technically challenging. Where possible an endovascular approach is to be preferred.

References

1. The organisation and delivery of the vascular access service for maintenance haemodialysis patients, 2006. http://www.vascularsociety.org.uk/library/vascular-society-publications.html.
2. NKF KDOQI Clinical Practice Guidelines and Clinical Practice Recommendations: Vascular Access, 2006. http://www.kidney.org/professionals/KDOQI/guideline_upHD_PD_VA/index.htm.
3. Fistula first project 2011. http://fistulafirst.org/AboutAVFistulaFirst/History.aspx.
4. Neyra NR, Ikixler TA, May RE, *et al.* Changes in access blood flow over time predicts vascular access thrombosis. *Kidney Int* 1998; 54: 1714-9.
5. Schnazer H, Schwartz M, Harrington E, *et al.* Treatment of ischemia due to 'steal' by arteriovenous fistula with distal artery ligation and revascularisation. *J Vasc Surg* 1988; 7: 770-3.
6. Minion DJ, Moore E, Endean E. Revision using distal inflow: a novel approach to dialysis associated steal syndrome. *Ann Vasc Surg* 2005; 19: 625-8.
7. Berard X, Brizzi V, Mayeux S, *et al.* Salvage treatment for venous aneurysm complicating vascular access arteriovenous fistula: use of an exoprosthesis to reinforce the vein after aneurysmorrhaphy. *Eur J Vasc Endovasc Surg* 2010; 40: 100-6.
8. Barnard KJ, Taubman KE, Jennings WC. Accessible autogenous vascular access for hemodialysis in obese individuals using lipectomy. *Am J Surg* 2010; 200: 798-802.

Case vignette Vascular steal

David C. Mitchell MA MS FRCS, Consultant Vascular and Transplant Surgeon
Southmead Hospital, Bristol, UK

A 40-year-old diabetic woman presented with a necrotic index finger-tip 8 months after the formation of a right-sided brachiocephalic AV fistula. She complained of pain in the hand and coldness with recent onset of necrosis at the site of finger prick testing for blood sugar levels. She was otherwise stable on thrice-weekly haemodialysis.

Examination showed a cool right hand with a necrotic tip to the index finger. The AV fistula was easily palpable at the elbow. The radial pulse was not palpable, but could be felt with manual occlusion of the fistula. Elevation of the hand produced blanching (Figure 1a) with dependent rubor. The elevated hand returned to a normal colour and warmth with AV fistula occlusion (Figure 1b).

Digital pressures were measured at 42mmHg without fistula occlusion and 103mmHg after occlusion (Figure 2). A diagnosis of vascular steal syndrome was made.

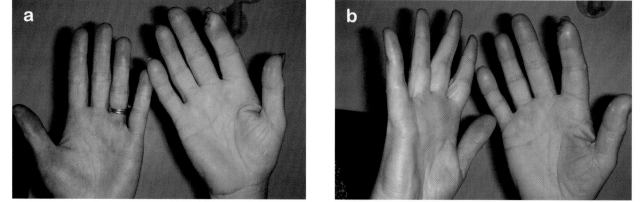

Figure 1. Elevated ischaemic right hand with necrosis of the index finger due to steal syndrome, before (a) and after (b) fistula compression (normal hand shown for comparison).

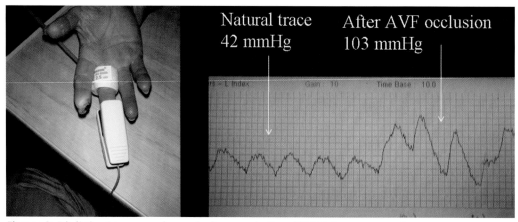

Figure 2. Digital artery waveforms before and after AV fistula compression.

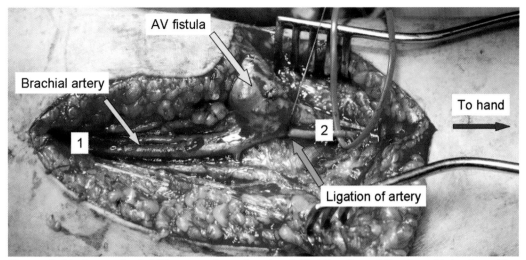

Figure 3. Photograph of DRIL procedure showing initial ligation of the brachial artery. The graft will run from 1 to 2.

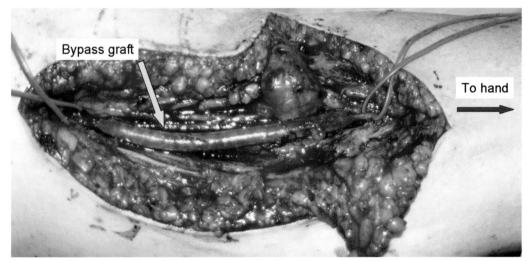

Figure 4. Photograph showing bypass graft *in situ*.

The patient agreed to a distal revascularisation interval ligation (DRIL) procedure which was performed under general anaesthesia, harvesting the basilic vein from the upper arm. The brachial artery was ligated distal to the AV fistula (Figure 3) and then a bypass graft performed from the brachial artery in the mid arm, 10cm above the fistula, to the artery distal to the point of ligation (Figure 4). At the end of the procedure, the patient had a palpable radial pulse.

The patient continued to dialyse satisfactorily using the AV fistula throughout the peri-operative phase and the index finger healed within 4 weeks.

Chapter 27 Amputation

Catherine Western BSc MBBS MRCS, Specialist Registrar in Vascular Surgery, Southwest Peninsula Deanery
Kenneth R. Woodburn MD FRCSG(Gen), Consultant Vascular and Endovascular Surgeon
Cornwall Vascular Unit, Honorary Clinical Lecturer, Peninsula Medical School, Royal Cornwall Hospitals Trust, Truro, Cornwall, UK

Introduction

Major limb amputation may be required in patients presenting with advanced tissue destruction, or as the ultimate outcome following a series of failed vascular interventions. In both categories, the patient is usually at the end of a long and painful journey, and major limb amputation can often be the first stage in the return to a relatively pain-free and meaningful existence.

It is, therefore, imperative that operative complications are minimised in this psychologically (and often physically) frail patient group, if optimum outcomes are to be obtained. The aim of this chapter is to highlight the potential complications encountered following amputation in patients with vascular disease, and offer strategies to minimise their occurrence.

Risks to life

Pre-operatively

Outcomes following major limb amputation have remained largely unchanged over the last 30 years and a recent epidemiological study from the United Kingdom found an overall mortality rate of 16.8% [1]. Consequently, suitability for amputation should be assessed on an individual basis and some extremely frail patients whose outcome will not be improved by such a procedure can be managed with palliative care and not subjected to destructive limb surgery.

As with other patients undergoing major vascular surgery, prospective amputees should undergo comprehensive assessment of renal, coronary and cerebrovascular status prior to surgery. In addition, attention to glycaemic control in the diabetic is vital as it influences wound healing and the risk of sepsis. Nutritional status is also often compromised and should be assessed. Similarly, DVT prophylaxis must not be overlooked and should be commenced on admission to mitigate the effects of prolonged immobility [2].

Intra-operatively

A planned, rather than emergency procedure with early anaesthetic assessment is advised, allowing time for further investigations which may otherwise delay surgery. Various local blocks can be employed during amputation and regional spinal/epidural anaesthesia utilised, alongside sedation if needed. If available, a dedicated vascular anaesthetist should be sought.

Postoperatively

Cardiovascular and respiratory complications are common and monitoring should therefore be continued until the patient is stable. Ideally this should occur in a dedicated high dependency facility in the early postoperative period. Cardiovascular risk factors need to be addressed, aspirin and statins restarted, and smoking cessation assistance provided.

Bleeding

Pre-operatively

Antiplatelet agents do not need to be stopped peri-operatively, as these rarely cause significant bleeding during amputation [3]. For patients on warfarin, or with a history of bleeding diatheses or hepatic disease, clotting should be checked pre-operatively and any derangement corrected. Clotting abnormalities will preclude the use of spinal or epidural anaesthesia, as well as increasing the risk of operative blood loss and the incidence of stump haematoma.

Intra-operatively

Bleeding is rarely a problem during amputation when performed for critical ischaemia and can usually be controlled by local pressure and subsequent vessel ligation. It is desirable to avoid the use of a tourniquet unless there is normal proximal vasculature, when limited tourniquet time may assist with vessel control. Once control is secured, the tourniquet should be removed to allow meticulous haemostasis. Vascular bundles and muscular bleeding points should be ligated individually or transfixed with absorbable sutures to avoid damage resulting from mass ligation or thermal injury from the use of electrocautery. Nerves should be excluded from vascular bundles before ligation and excised under tension to allow retraction, reducing the chance of neuroma formation. If absolute haemostasis cannot be achieved, consideration should be given to the placement of suction drains, which can generally be removed at 24-48 hours.

Postoperatively

If a significant haematoma develops, the wound may require re-exploration, haemostasis and possibly a blood transfusion. Haematoma formation can also increase the tension on the myocutaneous flaps and can precipitate flap failure, as well as providing a possible nidus for infection. If in doubt, a timely re-exploration should be undertaken.

Poor stump shape and function

Pre-operatively

Flexion deformity in the limb to be amputated should be addressed pre-operatively or a higher level of amputation selected. Fixed knee flexion of 15° precludes mobilisation on a below-knee prosthesis, while 45° or more predisposes to a non-healing stump secondary to pressure effects. The presence of a fixed flexion deformity at the hip will preclude mobilisation on a prosthesis following above-knee amputation.

Intra-operatively

Flexion deformity can sometimes be addressed through manipulation of the affected joint under anaesthetic, whilst hamstring tenotomy can reduce flexion deformity at the knee.

In the immobile patient, transfemoral amputation is preferable to transtibial due to the increased risk of failure of healing at the lower level [4], and the increased likelihood of flexion contracture formation postoperatively. Alternatively, a through-knee amputation, which offers greater stability when sitting, can be considered. This can be performed quickly with minimal blood loss, but does require a suction drain to manage synovial fluid collection in the early postoperative period.

The level of bone division should be selected with care. In transfemoral amputation the femur should be kept as long as possible to maximise stability, whilst ensuring healing. Bone division in transtibial amputation should be performed 10cm below the tibial tuberosity. If the stump is too long, there is a risk of stump failure. If it is too short, mobilisation is difficult given the short lever afforded by the more proximal division.

It is advisable to leave shaping of myocutaneous flaps until the end of the operation, so ensuring accurate division of tissues without risk of over-excision, subsequent undue suture line tension and stump breakdown. However, if excess tissue is not excised, 'dog-ear' formation may occur. This can be readily corrected by excision of redundant tissue under tension, enabling completion of a neat suture line (Figure 1).

Transfemoral amputation

An equal anterior-posterior flap (fish mouth) technique is usually performed alongside myodesis [5], whereby the four muscle compartments of the thigh are anchored to the distal femur through creation of transfemoral channels using a drill. This allows balanced muscle contraction, so minimising stump deformity and ensures good femoral coverage, decreasing the risk of pressure necrosis and bony erosion.

Transtibial amputation

The long posterior flap or skew flap method can be employed according to surgeon preference as there is no clear evidence demonstrating benefit of one

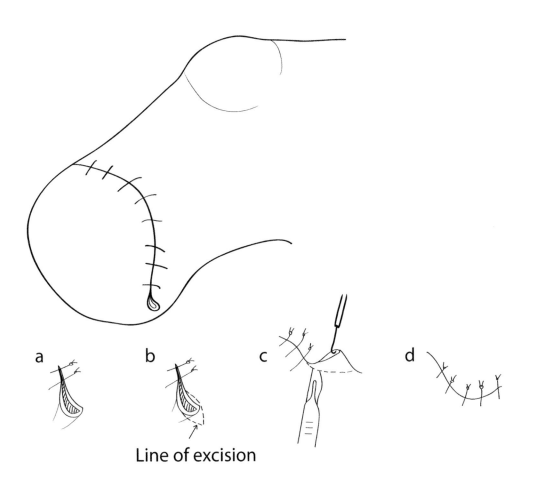

Line of excision

Figure 1. a) Dog-ear at the lateral aspect of a transtibial amputation suture line. b) Excision method 1 – excise an ellipse of skin centred on the suture line, taking more from the shorter edge and elongating the wound. c) Excision method 2 – using a hook, draw up the apex of the wound and excise the excess skin cutting parallel to the limb and elongating the wound. d) Completion of suture line following dog-ear excision.

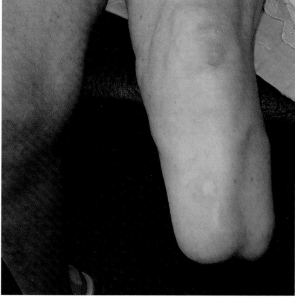

Figure 2. Healed transtibial amputation stump illustrating a misshapen stump due to failure of adequate fibula shortening. *Photo courtesy of Clayton Smith, © 2011.*

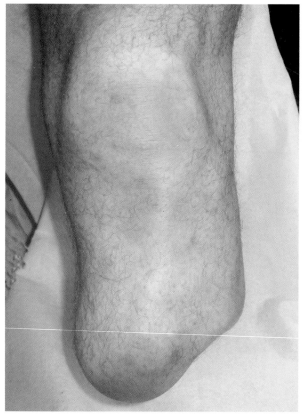

Figure 3. Healed transtibial amputation stump illustrating a misshapen stump due to transection of the fibula too proximally. *Photo courtesy of Clayton Smith, © 2011.*

technique over the other [6]. It is important that the level selected for fibular transection is about 2cm shorter than that selected for the tibia to avoid problematic stump deformities (Figures 2 and 3). If the long posterior flap technique is performed, the authors would recommend development of the plane between gastrocnemius and soleus and excision of soleus with the amputated limb, as this leaves a less bulky muscle pad, better suited for prosthesis fitting.

Following transtibial amputation, a rigid cast dressing may be applied with the knee held in 10° of flexion. This technique has been suggested to reduce oedema and prevent contractures, potentially reducing time to wound healing and limb-fitting [7, 8].

Transmetatarsal amputation

A variety of flaps can be utilised to close forefoot amputations, but in all cases the deep tissues must be healthy, adequately perfused and tension-free to minimise complications. As with transtibial amputation, a rigid plaster dressing can prove useful to protect the stump, reduce oedema and aid with heel weight-bearing after 7-10 days of elevation.

Ray and digital amputation

If performing ray or forefoot amputation, effort should be made to spare the metatarsal base(s) in order to preserve muscle insertion and assist with mobility. This is particularly pertinent with fifth ray amputation, where preservation of the peroneus brevis insertion maintains foot eversion.

Postoperatively

Early physiotherapy, ideally starting pre-operatively, is key to a good outcome, and exercises should resume as early as possible to rebuild muscle strength. Application of a stump stocking assists with stump moulding and the pneumatic post-amputation mobility aid (PPAM Aid) can also be used in the early stages of rehabilitation, allowing mobilisation. Early referral to the limb-fitting centre should be instigated and patients can often be seen and counselled by the rehabilitation staff prior to their amputation.

Pain

Pre-operatively

There is little evidence that pre-operative epidural placement reduces the incidence of phantom pain following amputation [9], although it may have a role in the control of pre-operative pain. This must be adequately controlled using the analgesic ladder and this often requires regular use of opiate-based preparations.

Intra-operatively

Operative technique can influence postoperative pain. Bone forceps should be avoided when dividing the fibula as they cause splintering and fractures, neuroma formation can be minimised by excising nerves under tension allowing retraction into the wound, while the application of a rigid plaster dressing following below-knee or transmetatarsal amputation may also reduce discomfort.

Postoperatively

The anaesthetic team are usually responsible for pain control in the initial postoperative period. Methods employed include patient-controlled analgesia (PCA), epidural or spinal anaesthesia. Phantom limb pain can usually be controlled with neuropathic modulators such as gabapentin or amitripyline.

Failure of healing

Pre-operatively

Failure of stump healing (Figure 4) often necessitates further surgical intervention with shortening of the residual limb, impacting on mobility. A number of measures can be undertaken to minimise risk of poor healing.

Nutritional status should be optimised prior to surgery (if there is time) and the nutrition team can advise on the use of protein and carbohydrate

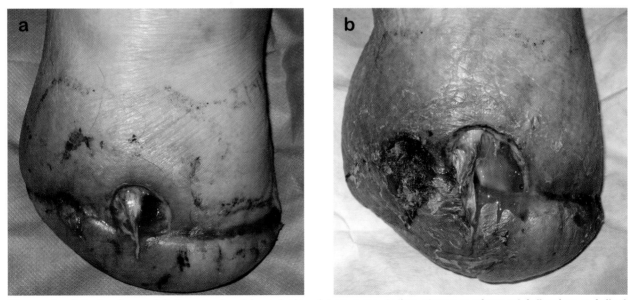

Figure 4. a) Early signs of failure to heal in a below-knee amputation stump performed following a failed revascularisation for acute limb ischaemia. b) The same stump 11 days later, before revision to an above-knee level.

supplements, nasogastric or even total parenteral nutrition if needed.

Proximal revascularisation should be considered to enable amputation at the most distal level compatible with healing. Rest pain, tissue loss and lack of femoral pulse are all indicators of poor healing in transtibial amputation [10]. Less than a quarter of transtibial amputations will heal in the absence of a femoral pulse but the presence of a popliteal pulse is a very good indicator for healing [11]. Other assessment tools are also available (e.g. $TcPO_2$ measurement, laser Doppler, xenon Xe 133 clearance), but selection of amputation level by an experienced clinician remains one of the most accurate predictors of stump healing.

Intra-operatively

A surgical technique that avoids the use of diathermy and minimises tissue handling should be utilised to preserve surrounding tissues. Muscle division should be performed cleanly with a blade to limit collateral damage and bone should be divided with an electric saw where possible; bone cutters can lead to splinter formation or proximal spiral fractures and hand saws may result in surrounding tissue trauma. Bone ends should be smoothed with a rasp to reduce muscle abrasion and saline irrigation performed after division to remove bone dust and fragments which can lead to heterotopic calcification.

In digital amputations, joint disarticulation should be avoided, as ongoing fluid production from residual synovial membrane impairs healing. Periosteum, bone fragments and cartilage within the wound impair healing and, therefore, if sesamoid bones are visible or palpable, they should be excised. Similarly, tendons are excised on the stretch to allow them to retract into surrounding tissues. Prosthetic material due to a previous failed bypass should be removed to reduce the risk of infection and to aid healing. If haemostasis cannot be secured, suction drains should be placed to reduce the chance of haematoma formation and subsequent flap tension.

On closure, skin tension should be avoided at all costs as it precipitates flap failure. The skin edges should be apposed using interrupted monofilament

sutures by preference or left open in the presence of infection. Adhesive paper tapes (steristrips) can be used as an adjunct to sutures to achieve a tension-free closure.

Postoperatively

Wound infections should be treated early to minimise their impact on healing and to reduce the risk of stump collection and osteomyelitis. The risk of subsequent trauma to the stump can be minimised by the application of a rigid plaster dressing (Figure 5). Direct weight bearing should be avoided until the wound has healed to minimise the effects of pressure on vulnerable stump tissues.

If revision for non-healing is required, tissues should be excised to a level where adequate tissue perfusion will ensure healing. This can be a local revision, but often necessitates division at a higher amputation level. Occasionally split-skin grafts can be employed to close a failing wound in the presence of an adequate blood supply.

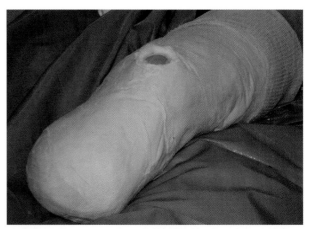

Figure 5. Postoperative rigid stump dressing applied to a below-knee amputation immediately postoperatively.

Infection

Pre-operatively

A short peri-operative course of antibiotic prophylaxis has been shown to reduce the stump infection rate [12]. The choice of antibiotic use for such prophylaxis and for the treatment of pre-existing infection should be based on local policy and culture results. If amputation becomes necessary for osteomyelitis, it is advisable to preserve all viable skin and leave the wound open to allow ongoing drainage of infection. Dry gangrene in the presence of chronic vascular insufficiency can be managed conservatively and may progress to auto-amputation. However, in the diabetic patient, or if wet gangrene or cellulitis intervene, urgent digital amputation and excision of all necrotic tissue must be undertaken, with the wounds left open to heal by secondary intention.

Intra-operatively

Life-threatening sepsis requiring major amputation may warrant a two-stage guillotine procedure. The limb is divided as distally as possible to excise all non-viable tissue and when the sepsis settles, a subsequent procedure can be undertaken to re-shape the stump to enable subsequent limb-fitting. Alternatively, definitive amputation can be performed, but the wound left open, or partially open, with delayed closure at 5-7 days. In the absence of infected tissues, stump wounds can be closed with clips, absorbable or non-absorbable sutures. Healing of open wounds can often be assisted with negative pressure dressings, which remove wound exudates, but also promote healing through stimulation of granulation [13].

Postoperatively

Selected sutures can be removed to allow drainage of pus collections or infected stump haematomas and antibiotics commenced on the basis of likely sensitivities.

If wound infection is suspected in the presence of a rigid stump dressing, the cast can be bivalved and then bandaged back in place following wound inspection. Rigid dressings can remain in place for up to 2 weeks postoperatively.

Psychological morbidity

Pre-operatively

Major amputation is seen by many as an end-of-life procedure. Emphasis should therefore be placed on it being a means of relieving longstanding pain and infection, and offering the opportunity to regain mobility and independence. It is of vital importance that amputation is approached in a multidisciplinary way and that patients are given the opportunity to voice concerns and fears, even in the emergency setting.

Many units employ a clinical psychologist to counsel potential amputees and there is usually a dedicated team of occupational therapists and physiotherapists who can help to allay fears regarding loss of function post-amputation. These health professionals play a key role in patient motivation and should be involved at an early stage for all amputations. Patients may benefit from the opportunity to meet previous amputees prior to surgery to discuss their experiences. Written information is also available, which can be read and reflected upon in the patients' own time.

Cancellations, whilst sometimes unavoidable, are very detrimental and pre-operative planning should ensure adequate theatre time to minimise risk.

Intra-operatively

If there is potential for conversion from transtibial to transfemoral amputation based on intra-operative findings, this must be communicated to the patient and the implications fully explained in order to ensure realistic postoperative expectations.

Postoperatively

Many hospitals have access to rehabilitation centres and, once medically fit, most patients will benefit from an inpatient referral to focus on both psychological and mobility issues before full discharge home. This time is also useful for families and carers to familiarise themselves with the equipment and mobilization techniques, whilst under the close supervision of the rehabilitation staff.

Conclusions

Most complications associated with amputation surgery can be prevented by thorough patient assessment and pre-operative planning, often involving multiple specialties. Application of basic surgical principles combined with meticulous and atraumatic surgical technique, using powered tools where appropriate, will reduce the development of complications, and enable their successful correction. Failure of stump healing leading to revision surgery can be minimised by careful assessment of the vascular status and tissue viability at the time of surgery, but remains the least predictable of complications.

Acknowledgement

The authors would like to thank Mr Clayton Smith, Senior Prosthetist, Disablement Services Centre, Brest Road, Plymouth, for his assistance in providing illustrations for this chapter.

Key points

- The mortality rate following major limb amputation has not fallen significantly over three decades. Therefore, appropriate selection of patients for operative intervention is vital.
- Thorough pre-operative assessment and planning by senior clinicians will minimise complications of amputation surgery.
- Once a decision has been made to amputate a limb, surgery should be carried out as soon as safely possible to minimise physiological and psychological deterioration.
- Surgical technique plays a major role in reducing complications following amputation surgery.
- Peri-operative antibiotic prophylaxis reduces stump infection rates.
- The use of rigid dressings can protect the amputation stump and minimise complications.
- Adequate pain control, using a variety of methods, is required to optimise outcome in the amputee.
- A multidisciplinary approach improves outcomes in this group of patients.

References

1. Moxey PW, Hofman D, Hinchcliffe RJ, *et al.* Epidemiological study of lower limb amputation in England between 2003 and 2008. *Br J Surg* 2010; 97: 1348-53.

2. Yeager RA, Moneta GL, Edwards *et al.* Deep vein thrombosis associated with lower extremity amputation. *J Vasc Surg* 1995; 22: 612-5.

3. Edmunds I, Avakian Z. Hand surgery on anticoagulated patients: a prospective study of 121 operations. *Hand Surg* 2010; 15: 109-13.

4. Nehler MR, Coll JR, Hiatt WR, *et al.* Functional outcome in a contemporary series of major lower extremity amputations. *J Vasc Surg* 2003; 38: 7-14.

5. Konduru S, Jain AS. Trans-femoral amputation in elderly dysvascular patients: reliable results with a technique of myodesis. *Prosthet Orthot Int* 2007; 31: 45-50.

6. Ruckley CV, Stonebridge PA, Prescott RJ. Skewflap versus long posterior flap in below-knee amputations: multicentre trial. *J Vasc Surg* 1991; 13: 423-7.

7. Nawijn SE, van der Linde H, Emmelot CH, *et al.* Stump management after trans-tibial amputation: a systematic review. *Prosthet Orthot Int* 2005; 29: 13-26.

8. Woodburn KR, Sockalingham S, Gilmore H, *et al.* A randomised trial of rigid stump dressing following transtibial amputation for peripheral arterial insufficiency. *Br J Surg* 2003; 90: 506.

9. Jahangiri H, Jayatunga AP, Bradley JW, *et al.* Prevention of phantom limb pain after major lower limb amputation by epidural infusion of diamorphine, clonidine and bupivacaine. *Ann R Coll Surg Engl* 1994; 76: 324-6.

10. Yip VS, Teo NB, Johnstone R, *et al.* An analysis of risk factors associated with failure of below knee amputations. *World J Surg* 2006; 30: 1081-7.

11. Dwars BJ, van den Broek TA, Rauwerda JA, *et al.* Criteria for reliable selection of the lowest level of amputation in peripheral vascular disease. *J Vasc Surg* 1992; 15: 536-42.

12. McIntosh J, Earnshaw JJ. Antibiotic prophylaxis for the prevention of infection after major limb amputation. *Eur J Vasc Endovasc Surg* 2009; 37: 696-703.

13. Argenta LC, Morykwas MJ. Vacuum-assisted closure: a new method for wound control and treatment: clinical experience. *Ann Plast Surg* 1997; 38: 563-76.

Case vignette Stump dehiscence

Catherine Western BSc MBBS MRCS, Specialist Registrar in Vascular Surgery, Southwest Peninsula Deanery
Kenneth R. Woodburn MD FRCSG(Gen), Consultant Vascular and Endovascular Surgeon
Cornwall Vascular Unit, Honorary Clinical Lecturer, Peninsula Medical School, Royal Cornwall Hospitals Trust, Truro, Cornwall, UK

A 62-year-old diabetic gentleman presented with extensive tissue necrosis on the right foot; this extended to include the heel, which was necrotic down to bone. A good femoral pulse was present, but colour duplex indicated a distal superficial femoral occlusion. As preservation of a functional foot was not possible he underwent a below-knee amputation with primary closure of the skin. His stump was well perfused and a rigid stump dressing was applied.

On the tenth postoperative day, the stump dressing was removed to reveal a clean, well-healing wound. The skin sutures were removed on the fourteenth postoperative day. The following evening, the patient fell sustaining minor trauma to his amputation stump; this resulted in complete dehiscence of his wound (Figure 1).

Minor stump trauma is common following surgery, as patients often take time to adjust to their amputation stump. Despite the appearance of a healed wound, dehiscence can occur with little provocation, and early removal of skin sutures may exacerbate this.

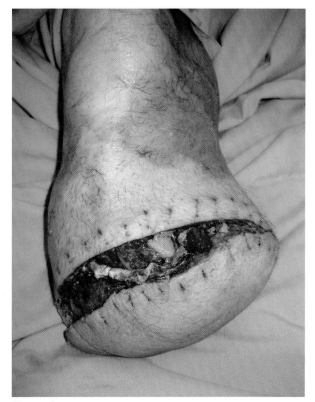

Figure 1.